Printed Name

MW00611293

Printed Name   Signature/Date

Printed Name   Signature/Date

Simplified Diet Manual

Twelfth Edition

Iowa Academy of Nutrition and Dietetics

Edited by
Paula Watkins, RD, LD, CDE

Editor: Paula Watkins, RD, LD, CDE is a dietitian and diabetes educator at Marengo Memorial Hospital in Marengo, Iowa.

This edition first published 2016 © 2016 by Iowa Academy of Nutrition and Dietetics

First edition, ©1958 Iowa State University Press
Second edition, ©1961 Iowa State University Press
Third edition, ©1969 Iowa State University Press
Fourth edition, ©1975 Iowa State University Press
Fifth edition, ©1984 Iowa State University Press
Sixth edition, ©1990 Iowa State University Press
Seventh edition, ©1995 Iowa State University Press
Eighth edition, ©1999 Iowa State University Press
Ninth edition, ©2002 Iowa State Press
Tenth edition, ©2007 Blackwell Publishing
Eleventh edition, ©2012 Iowa Dietetic Association

For information about how to apply for permission to reuse the copyright material in this book please see our website at http://eatrightiowa.org/conact/

For ordering information, see our website at http://eatrightiowa.org/store/

Designations used by companies to distinguish their products are often claimed as trademarks. All brand names and product names used in this book are trade names, service marks, trademarks or registered trademarks of their respective owners. The publisher is not associated with any product or vendor mentioned in this book. This publication is designed to provide accurate and authoritative information in regard to the subject matter covered. It is sold on the understanding that the publisher is not engaged in rendering professional services. If professional advice or other expert assistance is required, the services of a competent professional should be sought.

ISBN-13: 978-1- 4951-9134-3 (hard bound)

ISBN-13: 978-1- 4951-9135-0 (spiral bound)

Table of Contents

13 Dining Assistance/Special Needs   167

This book has a companion website providing patient education handouts only available online at http://eatrightiowa.org/simplifieddiet/

 When you see this icon in the diet manual, there is a corresponding patient education handout on the website.

Contributors

Study Guide Questions and Suggested Responses

Alicia Aguiar, MS, RD, LD
Kirkwood Community College Instructor
Cedar Rapids, Iowa

Guidelines for Diet Planning
General Diet
Nutrient Content of Selected Foods

Andrea K. Maher, RD LD
Consultant Dietitian
Huxley, IA

Guidelines for Pregnancy and Lactation
Guidelines for Peptic Ulcer, GERD, Hiatal Hernia

Martha McClurg, MPH, RD, LD
Registered Dietitian
Hy-Vee, Inc.
Cedar Rapids and Marion, Iowa

Recommendations for Feeding Normal Infants
Nutrition Guidelines for Children

Patricia J. Hildebrand, MS, RD, LD
Consultant
Des Moines, Iowa

Meeting Nutritional Needs of Older Adults
Finger Food Diet

Kathleen C. Niedert, PhD, MBA, RD, CSG, LD, FADA
Executive Director, Parkview Manor Campus
Western Home Communities
Reinbeck, Iowa

Liquid Diets and Modifications

Deborah D. Ashby, MS, RD, LD, CNSC
Clinical Dietitian
Central Iowa Healthcare
Marshalltown, Iowa

Modified Renal Diet
Weight Management Diet

Joyce A. Sankey, MBA, RDN, LD
Consultant Dietitian
HCR Manor Care Rehabilitation and Skilled Care
Cedar Rapids, Iowa

Bariatric Diet

Patricia "Pat" Peters, RD, LD
Clinical Dietitian
Sartori Memorial Hospital
Cedar Falls, Iowa

Diets for Diabetes

April Fuegen, RD, LD, CDE
Clinical Dietitian
Mercy Medical Center
Clinton, Iowa

Fat Restricted Diets

Char Kooima, RDN, LD, LN
CK Consulting, Inc.
Sioux Center, Iowa

Sodium Restricted Diets

Susan Boardsen, MPH, RD, LD
Consultant Dietitian
Clinton, Iowa

Guidelines for Liver Disease

Susan "Sue" B. Little, MS, RDN, LD, CNSC
Clinical Dietitian II
University of Iowa Hospital and Clinics
Iowa City, Iowa

Fiber Modified Diets

Jolene A. Wolf, MPH, RD, LD, CDE
Clinical Dietitian
Mary Greeley Medical Center
Ames, Iowa

Food Allergies and Intolerances
Lactose Restricted Diet

Renee Fields-Hu, RD, LD
Dietitian
St. Luke's Hospital
Cedar Rapids, IA

Gluten Restricted Diet

Judy Fitzgibbons, MS, RD, LD
Dietitian
Hy-Vee, Inc.
Cedar Rapids, Iowa

Fructose Malabsorption and Low FODMAP Diet

Tina Bauermeister, MS, RDN, LD
Registered Dietitian Nutritionist
Avera Holy Family Hospital
Estherville, IA

High Nutrient Diet
Guidelines for Individuals with Dementia

Mary Sand, MS, RD, LD
Consultant Dietitian
Ames, Iowa

Vegetarian Diets

Wendy Brewer, RDN, LD
Clinical Dietitian and Nutritionist
Grundy County Memorial Hospital
Grundy Center, Iowa

Halal Diet

Leigh Wright, RD, LD
Clinical Dietitian
Virginia Gay Hospital
Vinton, Iowa

Kosher Diet

Becky Idso, RD, LD
Consultant
Iowa Jewish Senior Life Center
Clive, Iowa

Phenylalanine Restricted Diet

Cheryl Stimson, MS, RD, LD
Metabolic Dietitian
University of Iowa Hospitals and Clinics
Iowa City, Iowa

Guidelines for Vitamin K and Prothrombin Time

Holly Romer, RD, LD, CDE
Diabetes Educator
Medical Associates
Clinton, IA

Guidelines for Gout

Lori Winborn, MPH, RDN, LD
Dietitian
University of Iowa Hospital and Clinics
Iowa City, Iowa

Nutrition for Individuals with Developmental Disabilities

Stephany Brimeyer, MPH, RD, LD
Early ACCESS Nutrition Consultant/
CHSC Nutrition Consultant
Child Health Specialty Clinics
Bettendorf, Iowa

About the Book

The twelfth edition of the *Simplified Diet Manual* marks 63 years of its publication by the Iowa Academy of Nutrition and Dietetics. In 1953 Nina Kagarice Bigsby, the dietary consultant to small hospitals and nursing homes for the Iowa State Department of Health, began a survey of diets that were being prescribed by physicians in Iowa. A trial manual was compiled, used for several months in ten Iowa hospitals, and evaluated by a special committee of the Iowa Academy of Nutrition and Dietetics; then a manuscript was prepared for publication.

Hospitals and long-term care facilities in every state and many foreign countries now use the *Simplified Diet Manual*. The Iowa Academy of Nutrition and Dietetics receives the royalties from its publication and uses them for the organization's mission: "Empower members to be Iowa's food and nutrition leaders."

Through the twelve editions, many thoughtful, practical, and insightful Iowa dietitians have contributed their expertise, ideas, and experience to keep the *Simplified Diet Manual* up to date while retaining its straightforward and uncomplicated style.

Educational handouts are available with the diet manual. Visit the website http://eatright iowa.org/simplifieddiet/ for patient education handouts that correspond with the therapeutic diets in the *Simplified Diet Manual*.

Study Guide Questions have been incorporated within the diet manual to give practice in applying the information. The material included has been carefully selected to cover basic information on the General Diet and its modifications for individually prescribed diets. Successful completion of this study will improve the skill of foodservice employees and other healthcare workers.

Instructions for Students:

1. Read and study each chapter of the *Simplified Diet Manual*.

2. Review the Study Guide Questions that follow each chapter, and answer as specified. Refer back to the chapter as needed. In some questions several answers are possible.

3. See Appendix 15 for the Suggested Responses; they may be removed from the manual. For incorrect answers, review with the instructor. If the answer section is left in the book, students should complete each section and then compare the answers with those in the answer section. The instructor should review answers with the students to provide additional clarification and explanation as needed.

The twelfth edition was edited by Paula Watkins, RD, LD, CDE. It reflects the comments and recommendations of Iowa Academy of Nutrition and Dietetics members and other users of this manual. These suggestions led to the revisions and additions that make this edition as comprehensive and useful as possible, consistent with current advances in Medical Nutrition Therapy.

The twelfth edition was endorsed by the Iowa Academy of Nutrition and Dietetics Publications Committee, Monica Lursen, RDN, LD, CLF, Chair; the Iowa Academy of Nutrition and Dietetics Board, Anne Cundiff, RD, LD, FAND, President; Iowa Dietetics in Health Care Communities, Renee Greiner, RD, LD, Chair; Barbara Thomsen CDM, CFPP,

State Spokesperson and Past-President, Iowa Association of Nutrition and Foodservice Professionals.

RD (registered dietitian) and RDN (registered dietitian nutritionist) are both approved credentials by The Commission on Dietetic Registration. Dietitians may choose to use either credential. To reduce confusion, the credential RDN is used in the text of the *Simplified Diet Manual* 12th edition.

The major changes in this edition are outlined in detail in the Preface.

Preface

In the early 1980s, the Iowa Dietetic Association adopted the policy of reviewing and revising its publications, including the *Simplified Diet Manual*, on a regular basis. The twelfth edition reflects the eighth time the manual has been revised under this policy. The diet manual is kept up to date and on the cutting edge by registered dietitians from the Iowa Academy of Nutrition and Dietetics that have expertise in the therapeutic diets in which they contribute.

The twelfth edition of the *Simplified Diet Manual* strives to keep up with the changes in the science of nutrition using evidence-based research. Its basic purpose is to provide consistency among diet terminology, in a simplified manner, for the prescription and interpretation of diets or nutrition plans.

Individuals' nutrition plans must meet their needs physiologically, psychosocially, and functionally. Nutritional adequacy must be emphasized, but the consideration of these needs will contribute to the greatest success. In all cases, we advocate the most liberal, least restrictive diets to meet nutritional needs, especially for residents in long-term care facilities.

Several changes were made to this edition:

- Addition of the Dysphagia Diet which replaced the National Dysphagia Diets.
- Addition of the Low Protein Modified Renal Diet.
- Addition of the Halal Diet.
- Addition of Vitamin K and Prothrombin Time Guidelines.
- Addition of Nutrition Guidelines for Gout.
- The Low Sodium Diet is 2300 mg sodium per day.
- Revision of the Fat Modified Diets.
- Expansion of Food Allergies and Intolerances into a chapter with the addition of Fructose Malabsorption and Low FODMAP Diet, and Wheat Allergy Guidelines.
- Expansion of the High Nutrient Diet to include nutritional recommendations for wound healing.
- Inclusion of *Choose Your Foods*, Food Lists for Diabetes (© 2014, Academy of Nutrition and Dietetics, American Diabetes Association).

The *Simplified Diet Manual* includes sample menus with most diets. As the use of the manual has spread, we realize that the names we use for meals do not always fit those used in other regions and countries. For meal planning purposes, we define meal names as follows:

Breakfast: *The first meal of the day, served shortly after rising.*

Lunch: *The meal served at midday.*

Supper: *The meal served in the evening, often a lighter meal than the midday meal.*

Snacks: *A small amount of food offered in addition to main meals.*

Guidelines for Diet Planning

Current dietary recommendations for Americans are based on two complementary resources: the Dietary Reference Intakes (DRIs) and the *2015-2020 Dietary Guidelines for Americans* (DGA).

The DRIs are published by the Food and Nutrition Board of the Institute of Medicine, National Academy of Sciences. They are intended to serve as a guide for good nutrition and provide the scientific basis for the development of food guidelines in both the United States and Canada. The DRIs, which vary by age and gender, provide reference values of recommended dietary allowances (RDA), adequate intakes (AI), and tolerable upper intake levels (UL) for nutrients and food components. (1) The DRI tables can be accessed at https://fnic.nal.usda.gov/dietary-guidance/dietary-reference-intakes. (2)

DIETARY GUIDELINES FOR AMERICANS

The *2015-2020 Dietary Guidelines for Americans* (DGA) provide evidence-based food and beverage recommendations for Americans ages 2 and older. These recommendations aim to promote health, prevent chronic disease, and help people reach and maintain a healthy weight. A Federal Advisory Committee, which is composed of nutrition and medical researchers, academics, and practitioners, develops a report that includes current scientific and medical evidence in nutrition. The U.S. Department of Health and Human Services (HHS) and the U.S. Department of Agriculture (USDA) uses information in the Advisory Report, along with public and federal agency comments, to jointly publish the DGA every 5 years. The DGA is developed for use by policymakers and health professionals, as well as communication with the general public, including businesses, schools, community groups, media, the food industry, and state and local governments.

The *2015-2020 Dietary Guidelines for Americans (8ᵗʰ edition)* was released in January 2016 and is available at www.health.gov/dietaryguidelines. (3) Healthy eating as a whole, versus singling out specific food and nutrients, is a focus of the DGA. This edition outlines how people can improve their overall eating patterns, the complete combination of foods and drinks in their diet, and physical activity patterns in five overarching guidelines:

1. **Follow a healthy eating pattern across the lifespan.** All food and beverage choices matter. Choose a healthy eating pattern at an appropriate calorie level to help achieve and maintain a healthy body weight, support nutrient adequacy, and reduce the risk of chronic disease.

2. **Focus on variety, nutrient density, and amount.** To meet nutrient needs within calorie limits, choose a variety of nutrient-dense foods across and within all food groups in recommended amounts.

3. **Limit calories from added sugars and saturated fats and reduce sodium intake.** Consume an eating pattern low in added sugars, saturated fats, and sodium. Cut back on foods and beverages higher in these components to amounts that fit within healthy eating patterns.

4. **Shift to healthier food and beverage choices.** Choose nutrient-dense foods and beverages across and within all food groups in place of less healthy choices. Consider cultural and personal preferences to make these shifts easier to accomplish and maintain.

Simplified Diet Manual, Twelfth Edition. Edited by Paula Watkins.
© 2016 Iowa Academy of Nutrition and Dietetics.

5. **Support healthy eating patterns for all.** Everyone has a role in helping to create and support healthy eating patterns in multiple settings nationwide, from home to school to work to communities.

> The *2015-2020 Dietary Guidelines for Americans* empower Americans to make **shifts** in their eating patterns to promote healthy eating. Small shifts in food choices can make a big difference over time.

Chronic diet-related diseases have risen in the U.S. population, due in part to changes in lifestyle behaviors. About half of all American adults have one or more preventable chronic diseases, including cardiovascular disease, high blood pressure, type 2 diabetes, some cancers, and poor bone health. (3) The typical American does not consume food groups in the amounts recommended by the DGA. This is illustrated in Figure 1.1.

USDA FOOD PATTERNS

The USDA Food Pattern from the previous *Dietary Guidelines* is now referred to as the Healthy U.S.-Style Eating Pattern. The *2015-2020 Dietary Guidelines for Americans* includes two variations of the Healthy U.S.-Style Eating Pattern that serve as examples of adaptations that can be made to accommodate personal preferences.

The *Dietary Guidelines* list Key Recommendations which describe the elements of what should be included in its entirety in any of the healthy eating patterns to promote a healthy, well-balanced diet.

1. Consume a healthy eating pattern that accounts for all foods and beverages within an appropriate calorie level.

2. A healthy eating pattern includes:

    *   A variety of vegetables from all the subgroups - dark green, red and orange, legumes (beans and peas), starchy, and other

    *   Fruits, especially whole fruits

    *   Grains, at least half of which are whole grains

    *   Fat-free or low-fat dairy, including milk, yogurt, cheese, and/or fortified soy beverages

    *   A variety of protein foods, including seafood, lean meats and poultry, eggs, legumes (beans and peas), and nuts, seeds, and soy products

    *   Oils

3. A healthy eating pattern limits:

    *   Saturated fats and *trans* fats, added sugars, and sodium

        *   Consume less than 10 percent of calories per day from added sugars

        *   Consume less than 10 percent of calories per day from saturated fats

        *   Consume less than 2,300 milligrams (mg) per day of sodium

    *   If alcohol is consumed, it should be consumed in moderation--up to one drink per day for women and up to two drinks per day for men--and only by adults of legal drinking age.

Healthy U.S.-Style Eating Pattern

The Healthy U.S.-Style Eating Pattern is consistent with the types of foods typically consumed by Americans, but in nutrient-dense forms--with little or no solid fats and added sugars, refined starches, and sodium--and in appropriate amounts. The typical American will need to shift their current intake patterns to those recommended by the Healthy U.S-Style Eating

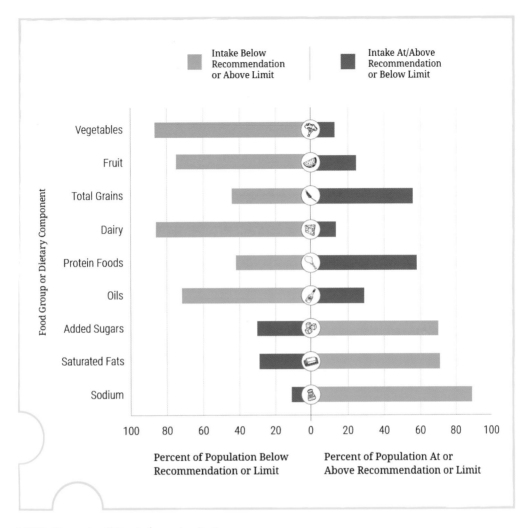

NOTE: The center (0) line is the goal or limit.

DATA SOURCES: What We Eat in American, NHANES 2007-2010 for average intakes by age-sex group. Healthy U.S.-Style Food Patterns which vary based on age, sex, and activity level, for recommended intakes and limits.

Accessed February 19, 2016 at http://health.gov/dietaryguidelines/2015/guidelines/chapter-2/current-eating-patterns-in-the-united-states/ (3)

Figure 1.1 Dietary Intakes Compared to Recommendations. Percent of the U.S. Population Ages 1 Year and Older Who are Below, At, or Above Each Dietary Goal or Limit

Pattern. Some shifts that are needed are minor and can be accomplished by making simple substitutions, while others will require greater effort to accomplish. (3)

The Healthy U.S.-Style Eating Pattern includes calorie levels ranging from 1,000-3,200 (see Table 1.1). It is designed to meet the Recommended Dietary Allowances (RDA) and Adequate Intakes (AI) for essential nutrients, as well as Acceptable Macronutrient Distribution Ranges (AMDR) set by the Food and Nutrition Board of the Institute of Medicine. (3)

Two Additional Healthy Eating Patterns

Two additional USDA Food Patterns are included that recognize cultural and personal preferences that are different than the typical American eating pattern. The Healthy Mediterranean-Style Eating Pattern and the Healthy Vegetarian Eating Pattern variations were modified from the Healthy U.S.-Style Eating Pattern. These patterns were designed to consider the types and proportions of foods Americans typically consume, but in nutrient-dense forms and appropriate amounts, which result in patterns that are relevant in the U.S. population. (3)

Mediterranean-style eating patterns were recognized for their beneficial health outcomes in the previous edition of the *Dietary Guidelines*. The *2015-2020 Dietary Guidelines for Americans* now include a Healthy Mediterranean-Style Eating Pattern. This eating pattern was designed based on a Mediterranean-style type of diet. A typical Mediterranean-style diet is abundant in nuts, berries, seeds, legumes, rice, seafood, and olive oil with small servings of meat and poultry. The Healthy Mediterranean-Style Eating Pattern contains more fruits and seafood and less dairy than does the Healthy U.S.-Style Eating Pattern. The amount of oil is the same as the Healthy U.S.-Style Eating Pattern but higher than what the typical American consumes. Levels of calcium and Vitamin D in the Healthy Mediterranean-Style Pattern are lower because less dairy is included. (3) The Healthy Mediterranean-Style Eating Pattern includes calorie levels ranging from 1,000-3,200. For specifics, refer to the Healthy Mediterranean-Style Eating Pattern in this chapter, Table 1.2.

The Healthy Vegetarian Eating Pattern replaces the Lacto-Ovo Vegetarian Adaption from the *2010 Dietary Guidelines*. The Healthy Vegetarian Eating Pattern includes dairy and eggs which are commonly consumed in the diets of many vegetarians; however, fortified soy beverages or plant-based dairy substitutes can be substituted for a vegan. The Healthy Vegetarian Eating Pattern includes more legumes (beans and peas), soy products, nuts and seeds, and whole grains than the Healthy U.S.-Style Eating Pattern and excludes meats, poultry, and seafood. A Healthy Vegetarian Eating Pattern is similar in nutrient content to the Healthy U.S.-Style Pattern, but somewhat higher in calcium and dietary fiber and lower in Vitamin D. (3) Refer to Chapter 12 for Vegetarian Diets. The Healthy Vegetarian Eating Pattern includes calorie levels ranging from 1,000-3,200. It can be accessed at http://health.gov/dietaryguidelines/2015/guidelines/appendix-5/ (3)

Table 1.1 Healthy U.S.-Style Eating Pattern (3)

Calorie level of pattern[a]	1,000	1,200	1,400	1,600	1,800	2,000	2,200	2,400	2,600	2,800	3,000	3,200
Food Group[b]	Daily Amount[c] of Food From Each Group (vegetable and protein foods subgroup amounts are per week)											
Vegetables	1 c-eq	1½ c-eq	1½ c-eq	2 c-eq	2½ c-eq	2½ c-eq	3 c-eq	3 c-eq	3½ c-eq	3½ c-eq	4 c-eq	4 c-eq
Dark-green vegetables (c-eq/wk)	½	1	1	1½	1½	1½	2	2	2½	2½	2½	2½
Red and orange vegetables (c-eq/wk)	2½	3	3	4	5½	5½	6	6	7	7	7½	7½
Legumes (beans and peas) (c-eq/wk)	½	½	½	1	1½	1½	2	2	2½	2½	3	3
Starchy vegetables (c-eq/wk)	2	3½	3½	4	5	5	6	6	7	7	8	8
Other vegetables (c-eq/wk)	1½	2½	2½	3½	4	4	5	5	5½	5½	7	7
Fruits	1 c-eq	1 c-eq	1½ c-eq	1½ c-eq	1½ c-eq	2 c-eq	2 c-eq	2 c-eq	2 c-eq	2½ c-eq	2½ c-eq	2½ c-eq
Grains	3 oz-eq	4 oz-eq	5 oz-eq	5 oz-eq	6 oz-eq	6 oz-eq	7 oz-eq	8 oz-eq	9 oz-eq	10 oz-eq	10 oz-eq	10 oz-eq
Whole grains[d] (oz-eq/day)	1½	2	2½	3	3	3	3½	4	4½	5	5	5
Refined grains (oz-eq/day)	1½	2	2½	2	3	3	3½	4	4½	5	5	5
Dairy	2 c-eq	2½ c-eq	2½ c-eq	3 c-eq	3 c-eq	3 c-eq	3 c-eq	3 c-eq	3 c-eq	3 c-eq	3 c-eq	3 c-eq
Protein Foods	2 oz-eq	3 oz-eq	4 oz-eq	5 oz-eq	5 oz-eq	5½ oz-eq	6 oz-eq	6½ oz-eq	6½ oz-eq	7 oz-eq	7 oz-eq	7 oz-eq
Seafood (oz-eq/wk)	3	4	6	8	8	8	9	10	10	10	10	10
Meat, poultry, eggs (oz-eq/wk)	10	14	19	23	23	26	28	31	31	33	33	33
Nuts, seeds, soy products (oz-eq/wk)	2	2	3	4	4	5	5	5	5	6	6	6
Oils	15 g	17 g	17 g	22 g	24 g	27 g	29 g	31 g	34 g	36 g	44 g	51 g
Limit on Calories for Other Uses, calories (% of calories)[e,f]	150 (15%)	100 (8%)	110 (8%)	130 (8%)	170 (9%)	270 (14%)	280 (13%)	350 (15%)	380 (15%)	400 (14%)	470 (16%)	610 (19%)

Continued on next page

a. Food intake patterns at 1,000, 1,200, and 1,400 calories are designed to meet the nutritional needs of 2- to 8-year old children. Patterns from 1,600 to 3,200 calories are designed to meet the nutritional needs of children 9 years and older and adults. If a child 4 to 8 years of age needs more calories and, therefore, is following a pattern at 1,600 calories or more, his/her recommended amount from the dairy group should be 2.5 cups per day. Children 9 years and older and adults should not use the 1,000-1,200, or 1,400-calorie patterns.

b. Foods in each group and subgroup will be discussed in the next section of this chapter.

c. Food group amounts shown in cup-(c) or ounce-equivalents (oz-eq). Oils are shown in grams (g). Quantity equivalents for each food group are:

- Grains, 1 ounce-equivalent is: ½ cup cooked rice, pasta, or cereal; 1 ounce dry pasta or rice; 1 medium (1 ounce) slice bread; 1 ounce of ready-to-eat cereal (about 1 cup of flaked cereal).

- Vegetables and fruits, 1 cup-equivalent is: 1 cup raw or cooked vegetable or fruit; 1 cup vegetable or fruit juice; 2 cups leafy salad greens, ½ cup dried fruit or vegetable.

- Protein Foods, 1 ounce-equivalent is: 1 ounce lean meat, poultry, or seafood; 1 egg; ¼ cup cooked beans or tofu; 1 Tbsp peanut butter; ½ ounce nuts or seeds.

- Dairy, 1 cup equivalent is: 1 cup milk, yogurt, or fortified soymilk; 1 ½ ounces natural cheese such as cheddar cheese or 2 ounces of processed cheese.

d. Amounts of whole grains in the Patterns for children are less than the minimum of 3 oz-eq in all Patterns recommended for adults.

e. All foods are assumed to be in nutrient-dense forms, lean or low-fat and prepared without added fats, sugars, refined starches, or salt. If all food choices to meet food group recommendations are in nutrient-dense forms, a small number of calories remain within the overall calorie limit of the Pattern (i.e., limit on calories for other uses). The number of these calories depends on the overall calorie limit in the Pattern and the amounts of food from each food group required to meet nutritional goals. Nutritional goals are higher for the 1,200- to 1,600-calorie Patterns than for the 1,000-calorie Pattern, so the limit on calories for other uses is lower in the 1,200-to 1,600-calorie Patterns. Calories up to the specified limit can be used for added sugars, added refined starches, solid fats, alcohol, or to eat more than the recommended amount of food in a food group. The overall eating pattern also should not exceed the limits of less than 10 percent of calories from added sugars and less than 10 percent of calories from saturated fats. At most calorie levels, amounts that can be accommodated are less than these limits. For adults of legal drinking age who choose to drink alcohol, a limit of up to 1 drink per day for women and up to 2 drinks for day for men within limits on calories for other uses applies; and calories from protein, carbohydrate, and total fats should be within the Acceptable Macronutrient Distribution Ranges (AMDRs).

f. Values are rounded.

U.S. Department of Health and Human Services and U.S. Department of Agriculture. *2015-2020 Dietary Guidelines for Americans*. 8th ed. Published December 2015. Accessed January 13, 2016 at http://health.gov/dietaryguidelines/2015/guidelines/appendix-3/ (3)

Table 1.2 Healthy Mediterranean-Style Eating Pattern (3)

Calorie level of pattern[a]	1,000	1,200	1,400	1,600	1,800	2,000	2,200	2,400	2,600	2,800	3,000	3,200
Food Group[b]	Daily Amount[c] of Food From Each Group (vegetable and protein foods subgroup amounts are per week)											
Vegetables	1 c-eq	1½ c-eq	1½ c-eq	2 c-eq	2½ c-eq	2½ c-eq	3 c-eq	3 c-eq	3½ c-eq	3½ c-eq	4 c-eq	4 c-eq
Dark-green vegetables (c-eq/wk)	½	1	1	1½	1½	1½	2	2	2 ½	2 ½	2 ½	2 ½
Red and orange vegetables (c-eq/wk)	2½	3	3	4	5 ½	5 ½	6	6	7	7	7½	7 ½
Legumes (beans and peas) (c-eq/wk)	½	½	½	1	1½	1½	2	2	2½	2½	3	3
Starchy vegetables (c-eq/wk)	2	3½	3½	4	5	5	6	6	7	7	8	8
Other vegetables (c-eq/wk)	1½	2½	2½	3½	4	4	5	5	5½	5½	7	7
Fruits	1 c-eq	1 c-eq	1½ c-eq	2 c-eq	2 c-eq	2½ c-eq	2½ c-eq	2½ c-eq	2½ c-eq	3 c-eq	3 c-eq	3 c-eq
Grains	3 oz-eq	4 oz-eq	5 oz-eq	5 oz-eq	6 oz-eq	6 oz-eq	7 oz-eq	8 oz-eq	9 oz-eq	10 oz-eq	10 oz-eq	10 oz-eq
Whole grains[d] (oz-eq/day)	1½	2	2½	3	3	3	3½	4	4½	5	5	5
Refined grains (oz-eq/day)	1½	2	2½	2	3	3	3½	4	4½	5	5	5
Dairy	2 c-eq	2½ c-eq	2½ c-eq	2 c-eq	2 c-eq	2 c-eq	2 c-eq	2½ c-eq	2½ c-eq	2½ c-eq	2½ c-eq	2½ c-eq
Protein Foods	2 oz-eq	3 oz-eq	4 oz-eq	5½ oz-eq	6 oz-eq	6½ oz-eq	7 oz-eq	7½ oz-eq	7½ oz-eq	8 oz-eq	8 oz-eq	8 oz-eq
Seafood (oz-eq/wk)*	3	4	6	11	15	15	16	16	17	17	17	17
Meat, poultry, eggs (oz-eq/wk)	10	14	19	23	23	26	28	31	31	33	33	33
Nuts, seeds, soy products (oz-eq/wk)	2	2	3	4	4	5	5	5	5	6	6	6
Oils	15 g	17 g	17 g	22 g	24 g	27 g	29 g	31 g	34 g	36 g	44 g	51 g
Limit on Calories for Other	150	100	110	140	160	260	270	300	330	350	430	570
Uses, calories (% of calories)[e,f]	(15%)	(8%)	(8%)	(9%)	(9%)	(13%)	(12%)	(13%)	(13%)	(13%)	(14%)	(18%)

Continued on next page

Continued from previous page

a,b,c,d,e,f See Table 1.1. Healthy U.S.-Style Eating Pattern, notes a through f.   *The U.S. Food and Drug Administration (FDA) and the U.S. Environmental Protection Agency (EPA) provide joint guidance regarding seafood consumption for women who are pregnant or breastfeeding and young children. For more information, see the FDA or EPA websites www.FDA.gov/fishadvice; www.EPA.gov/fishadvice.

Food Groups Defined

Each of the three recommended USDA Food Patterns include foods from five food groups: vegetables, fruit, grains, dairy, and protein foods. A variety of foods should be selected within each food group. This helps ensure that the foods and beverages selected by individuals over time meet nutrient requirements to promote health.

Vegetables

The Vegetable Group includes fresh, frozen, and canned vegetables and 100% vegetable juice. Most vegetables are naturally low in fat and calories and provide rich sources of many nutrients including potassium, dietary fiber, folate, vitamin A, vitamin K, vitamin B_6, vitamin E, and vitamin C. The eating patterns recommend weekly intake amounts for the five vegetable subgroups to provide a wide range of nutrients. For example, Vitamin A content is highest in the dark-green and red and orange vegetable subgroups. Shifting to more vegetables instead of some other higher-calorie foods may be useful in helping to lower calorie intake.

Table 1.3 Vegetable Subgroups

Dark-green	Red and Orange	Legumes (beans and peas)	Starchy	Other
Arugula	Acorn squash	Black beans	Cassava	Alfalfa sprouts
Bok choy	Butternut squash	Black-eyed peas	Corn	Artichokes
Broccoli	Carrots	Edamame	Green Bananas	Asparagus
Collard greens	Chili Peppers	Garbanzo beans	Green lima beans	Avocado
Dark green leafy lettuce	Pumpkin	Kidney beans	Green peas	Beets
Endive	Red peppers	Lentils	Jicama	Brussels sprouts
Escarole	Sweet Potatoes	Lima beans (mature)	Plantains	Cabbage
Kale	Tomato Juice	Navy beans	Potatoes (white)	Cauliflower
Mesclun	Tomatoes	Pinto beans	Taro	Celery
Mixed greens	100% vegetable juice	Soy beans	Water chestnuts	Cucumbers
Mustard greens	Yams	Split peas		Eggplant
Radicchio		Tofu		Green beans
Romaine lettuce		White beans		Green peppers
Spinach				Iceberg lettuce
Swiss Chard				Mushrooms
Turnip greens				Okra
Watercress				Onions

Continued on next page

Table 1.3 Vegetable Subgroups Continued from previous page

Dark-green	Red and Orange	Legumes (beans and peas)	Starchy	Other
				Radishes
				Red cabbage
				Scallions
				Snow peas
				Wax beans
				Yellow squash
				Zucchini

US Department of Agriculture. Choose My Plate website. Vegetables Gallery. www.choosemyplate.gov/foodgallery-vegetables Accessed February 5, 2016. (5)

Fruit

The Fruit Group includes fresh, frozen, canned, and dried fruits and 100% fruit juices. Fruits are rich in many nutrients, including potassium, dietary fiber, vitamin C, and folate. Selecting more fruit rather than juice is recommended. Only 100% fruit juices count as fruit servings. Most fruit drinks, punches, cocktails, and "ades" contain very little juice and a great deal of sugar. Beverages made from powdered fruit-flavored mixes or fruit-flavored carbonated beverages also do not count as fruit servings. Shift to consume more fruits, mostly whole fruits, and those lowest in added sugars.

Grains

The Grain Group includes any food made from wheat, rice, oats, cornmeal, barley, or another cereal grain (e.g., bread, pasta, breakfast cereals, tortillas, and grits). Grains are divided into two subgroups: whole grains and refined grains. Shift to make half of all grains consumed be whole grains.

Whole grains contain the entire grain kernel. Some examples of whole grains include whole-wheat bread, oatmeal, whole-grain cereal and crackers, brown rice, popcorn, and quinoa. Whole grains are a source of dietary fiber, iron, zinc, folate, niacin, vitamin B_6, riboflavin, and vitamin A.

Refined grains have been milled, a process that removes the bran and germ from the kernel, and reduces its nutritive value. Some examples of refined grains include white flour, white rice, refined grain cereals and crackers, pasta and degermed cornmeal.

Most refined grains are *enriched*. This means certain B-vitamins (thiamin, riboflavin, niacin, and folic acid) and iron are added back after processing. Fiber is not usually added back to most enriched grains.

Dairy

The Dairy Group includes all fluid milk, including lactose-free and lactose-reduced products and fortified soy beverages; yogurt; dairy desserts; and cheeses. Most choices should be fat-free or low-fat (1%) vitamin D-fortified milk or yogurt instead of cheese. Milk-based foods that are low in calcium content (such as cream cheese, cream, and butter) are not included. Foods in the dairy group provide calcium, potassium, vitamin D, vitamin A, phosphorus, riboflavin, and protein. Shift to consume more dairy in fat-free or low-fat forms.

Protein Foods

The Protein Group includes a variety of protein foods for improved nutrient intake and health benefits and includes several subgroups: meat, poultry, and eggs; seafood; and nuts, seeds, and soy products. Legumes (beans and peas) are part of this group as well as the Vegetable Group, but should be counted in one group or the other when planning meals. Most meat and poultry choices should be lean or low-fat. Foods in the protein group provide B vitamins (niacin, riboflavin, Vitamin B_{12} and B_6), vitamin E, iron, zinc, and magnesium.

Shift to increase variety in protein food choices. Selecting 8 or more ounces per week of seafood (including fresh water fish) is recommended for the 2,000-calorie level Healthy U.S.-Style Eating Pattern. Seafood provides omega-3 fatty acids (EPA and DHA) which are associated with reduced risk of cardiovascular disease.

Vitamins and Minerals

Nutrient needs should be met primarily through consuming foods in nutrient-dense forms. In certain cases, fortified foods and dietary supplements may be useful in providing one or more nutrients that otherwise might be consumed in less than recommended amounts (e.g., vitamin D and folic acid for women capable of becoming pregnant, iron for pregnant women, and B_{12} for individuals older than age 50 years).

Oils

Oils are liquid at room temperature. Although not a food group, oils are part of healthy eating patterns as they provide essential fatty acids and vitamin E. Naturally occurring food sources of oils include nuts, seeds, avocados, and seafood. Oils are also extracted from plants, such as olive, peanuts, corn, safflower, canola, soybean, sesame, and sunflower. Most oils provide a high percentage of monounsaturated and polyunsaturated fats. Exceptions to this rule are coconut oil, palm kernel oil, and palm oil which have a high percentage of saturated fat. Americans should shift from solid fats to oils in food preparation where possible.

Definition of Solid Fat

Solid fats are fats that are usually not liquid at room temperature. Solid fats are found in most animal foods but also can be made from vegetable oils through hydrogenation. Some common solid fats include: butter, lard, stick margarine, coconut oil, palm oil, palm kernel oil, and shortening. Solid fats are the major source of saturated fats.

Saturated Fats, *Trans* Fats and Added Sugars are of Particular Concern

Over-consumption of saturated fats and added sugars can contribute to excessive weight gain. As the amount of solid fats or added sugars increases in the diet, eating foods with sufficient dietary fiber and essential nutrients, without exceeding calorie needs, becomes difficult.

Saturated fats account on average for 11 percent of calories in the U.S. population. (3) The major sources of saturated fats for Americans are snacks and desserts made with butter, margarine, and shortening; mixed dishes containing fatty meat and regular cheeses such as casseroles, pizza and burgers; processed meats (e.g., sausages, hot dogs, bacon); and ice cream. Saturated fats can raise blood cholesterol levels. Americans should *shift* to reduce saturated fats to less than 10 percent of calories per day. Choose lean meats and include more vegetables in mixed dishes.

Trans fats are made in a process that changes vegetable oils to semisolid fats. *Trans* fats can raise blood cholesterol levels. There is no established safe intake of *trans* fat. Limit foods as much as possible that contain partially hydrogenated oils (a major source of *trans* fat) such as some margarines, snack foods, and prepared desserts. Check the Nutrition Facts label to choose foods with little or no saturated fat and *trans* fat.

Added sugars account on average for almost 270 calories, or more than 13 percent of calories per day in the U.S. population. (3) Added sugars are abundant in grain-based desserts, dairy desserts, and sugar-sweetened beverages such as soft drinks, coffee and tea with added sugar, sport and energy drinks, and alcoholic beverages. Americans should shift to reduce sugar consumption to less than 10 percent of calories per day. Choose beverages with no added sugars, limit dairy desserts and sweet snacks, and select fruits and fruit juices without added sugars.

Physical Activity

Nutrition is the primary focus of the *Dietary Guidelines*, however physical activity receives strong emphasis because of its critical and complementary role in promoting good health and preventing disease, including many diet-related chronic diseases. Most individuals would benefit from making shifts to increase the amount of physical activity they engage in each week. The Physical Activity Guidelines for Americans define regular physical activity as at least 150 minutes (2.5 hours) per week of moderate-intensity physical activity (e.g., brisk walking). (4) Reduce time spent in sedentary behaviors (e.g., watching television or using video games).

Food Safety

Food safety is discussed in the *Dietary Guidelines for Americans* because the prevention of foodborne illness depends on proper food handling. Some individuals, including women who are pregnant, young children, older adults, and individuals with compromised immune systems, are at increased risk for foodborne illness. The following four basic food safety principles are the cornerstones of *Fight* BAC!®: (3)

- **Clean** hands, food contact surfaces, and vegetables and fruits.
- **Separate** raw, cooked, and ready-to-eat foods while shopping, storing, and preparing foods.
- **Cook** foods to a safe temperature.
- **Chill** (refrigerate) perishable foods promptly.

Federal food safety information including safe minimum cooking temperatures can be found at http://www.foodsafety.gov website.

MYPLATE

MyPlate is a federal symbol that serves as a reminder to Americans to make shifts in their daily food and beverage choices to align with the *Dietary Guidelines*.

MyPlate illustrates the five food groups using a familiar mealtime visual, a place setting. The plate is divided into four sections, representing vegetables, fruit, grains, and protein foods. The protein group includes a variety of foods such as meat, seafood, legumes, and processed soy products. A circle shape next to the plate represents dairy products. Consumer messages such as, "Make half your plate fruits and vegetables," and "Switch to fat-free or low-fat (1%) milk," help consumers translate the *Dietary Guidelines* and MyPlate icon into healthy behaviors. Viewing MyPlate online allows consumers and professionals to obtain the most current information on the *Dietary Guidelines*.

Interactive tools on the website, http://www.choosemyplate.gov allow an individual to create a customized food plan with the amount of each food group they need daily. MyPlate includes plans for special populations such as preschoolers, kids, and women who are pregnant or breastfeeding.

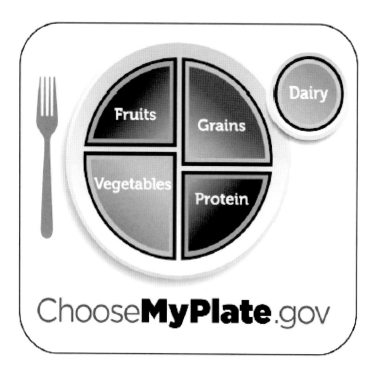

Figure 1.2 MyPlate serves as a reminder to help consumers make healthier food choices. To see this graphic in color, go to www.choosemyplate.gov website. (5)

REFERENCES

1. Nutrient Recommendations: Dietary Reference Intakes. National Institutes of Health, Office of Dietary Supplements website. https://ods.od.nih.gov/Health_Information/Dietary_Reference_Intakes.aspx/ Accessed February 18, 2016.

2. Dietary Reference Intakes. U.S. Department of Agriculture, National Agriculture Library website. https://fnic.nal.usda.gov/dietary-guidance/dietary-reference-intakes Updated January 29, 2016. Accessed February 18, 2016.

3. U. S. Department of Health and Human Services and U. S. Department of Agriculture. *2015 – 2020 Dietary Guidelines for Americans*, 8th ed. http://health.gov/dietaryguidelines/2015/guidelines/appendix-14/ Published December 2015. Accessed January 13, 2016.

4. Office of Disease Prevention and Health Promotion (ODPHP), Physical Activity Guidelines for Americans. Available at http://health.gov/paguidelines/. Accessed 2/13/2016.

5. U.S. Department of Agriculture Choose My Plate.gov website. http://www.choosemyplate.gov/ Published June 2, 2011. Accessed February 5, 2016.

ADDITIONAL WEBSITES:

Dietary Guidelines for Americans: http://www.cnpp.usda.gov/dietaryguidelines.htm

Super Tracker: http://www.choosemyplate.gov/supertracker-other-tools

USDA Center for Nutrition Policy and Promotion (DNPP): http://www.cnpp.usda.gov

Fight BAC!®: http://www.fightbac.org

USDA Nutrition Evidence Library: http://www.nel.gov

Academy of Nutrition and Dietetics: www.eatright.org

USDA Food Safety: http://www.foodsafety.gov

Study Guide Questions

A. Which website do you access to find personalized meal plans, based on *the 2015-2020 Dietary Guidelines for Americans*?

B. What are the names of the five food groups?

C. Using the Healthy U.S.-Style Eating Pattern table in this chapter, indicate the recommended amount (cups per week) for each vegetable subgroup in a 2000-calorie diet. Note that when you combine the amount from each subgroup in a week, it equals 2 ½ cup-equivalents daily.

- Dark-green vegetables: __ cups per week

- Red and Orange vegetables: __ cups per week

- Legumes (beans and peas): __ cups per week

- Starchy vegetables: __ cups per week

- Other vegetables: __ cups per week

D. How much seafood is recommended for a 2,000-calorie diet on the Healthy U.S.-Style Eating Pattern compared to the Healthy Mediterranean-Style Eating Pattern?

E. Vitamin A is highest in which two vegetable subgroups? List four vegetables high in Vitamin A.

Study Guide Suggested Responses can be found in Appendix 15.

Nutrition for the Life Span

2

GENERAL DIET

Use

The General Diet is designed for people who require no dietary modifications and to reduce the risk of the development of chronic, nutrition-related diseases. This diet may also be referred to as a Regular Diet in some facilities.

Adequacy

The suggested food plan includes food in amounts that will provide the Dietary Reference Intakes (DRIs) recommended by the National Academy of Sciences for ages 2 years and older.

Diet Principles

1. The diet should incorporate the principles of the *2015-2020 Dietary Guidelines for Americans*, focusing on nutrient-dense foods and beverages and maintaining calorie balance to achieve and sustain a healthy weight. Refer to Chapter 1.

2. The quantity of food selected from each food group depends on the energy needs. Individuals should follow a food pattern that meets their estimated calorie needs.

3. Select a variety of foods within each food group and subgroup over time in recommended amounts. This allows for personal choice and helps to ensure that the foods and beverages selected by individuals provide a mix of nutrients that will meet their needs. Healthy U.S.-Style Eating Pattern and Healthy Mediterranean-Style Eating Pattern tables are included in Chapter 1.

4. The diet should provide color and be pleasing in texture and flavor. Choose an eating style low in saturated fat, sodium, and added sugars.

Table 2.1 General Diet

Food for the Day	Recommended - Select a Variety of Nutrient-Dense Foods	Choose Less Often
Vegetables *1–4 cups* *Include a variety of vegetables from all of the five subgroups*	**Dark-green vegetables:** arugula, bok choy, broccoli, collard greens, dark-green leafy lettuce, endive, escarole, kale, leeks, mesclun, mixed greens, mustard greens, radicchio, romaine lettuce, spinach, Swiss chard, turnip greens, watercress. **Red and orange vegetables:** acorn squash, butternut squash, carrot juice, carrots, chili peppers, pattypan squash,	Canned vegetables—rinse to decrease sodium content or choose those labeled "reduced sodium," "low sodium," or "no salt added." Vegetables served with added creamy sauces, salt-based seasonings, condiments or dressings high in saturated or *trans* fat.

Continued on next page

Table 2.1 General Diet Continued from previous page

Food for the Day	Recommended - Select a Variety of Nutrient-Dense Foods	Choose Less Often
	pumpkin, red peppers (sweet, bell), sweet potato, tomato juice, tomatoes, 100% vegetable juice, yams.	
	Legumes** (beans and peas): black beans, black-eyed peas (mature, dry), chickpeas (garbanzo beans), kidney beans, lentils, navy beans, pinto beans, soy beans, split peas, white beans.	
	Starchy vegetables: cassava, corn, green bananas, green lima beans, green peas, jicama, plantains, potatoes (white), taro, water chestnuts.	
	Other vegetables: alfalfa sprouts, artichokes, asparagus, avocado, bamboo shoots, bean sprouts, beets, Brussels sprouts, cabbage, cauliflower, celery, cucumbers, eggplant, garlic, green beans, green peppers, iceberg lettuce, mungbean sprouts, mushrooms, okra, onions, radishes, red cabbage, scallions, snow peas, tomatillos, turnips, wax beans, yellow squash, zucchini.	
Fruits *1–2.5 cups* *At least half of all fruit intake should come from whole fruits*	All fresh, frozen, canned (in own juices or light syrup), dried (with no sugar added) or 100% fruit juice. Apple, apricot, banana, blackberries, blueberries, cantaloupe, cherries, cranberries, currants, date, fig, goji berries, grapes, grapefruit, guava, honeydew, kiwi fruit, lemon, lime, mandarin orange, mango, nectarine, orange, papaya, peach, pear, persimmons, pineapple, plum, pomegranate, raspberries, starfruit (carambola), strawberries, tangerine, watermelon; Dried fruit (e.g., raisins, prunes, apricots); 100% fruit juice (e.g., apple, grape, cranberry, grapefruit, orange, pineapple, pomegranate).	Fruit canned in heavy syrup or dried fruits with added sugar.
Grains *3–10 ounce-equivalents* *At least half of all grains eaten should be whole grains*	**Whole grains:** amaranth, brown rice, buckwheat, bulgur (cracked wheat), kamut, millet, muesli, oatmeal, popcorn, quinoa, rolled oats, spelt, teff, whole grain barley, whole grain cornmeal, whole rye, whole wheat bread, whole wheat cereal flakes, whole wheat	Processed/packaged baked goods and snack foods. Limit refined grains to servings suggested in Healthy U.S.-Style Eating Patterns. Average intake of refined grains are well above recommended limits for most age-sex groups.

Continued on next page

Table 2.1 General Diet Continued from previous page

Food for the Day	Recommended - Select a Variety of Nutrient-Dense Foods	Choose Less Often
Some foods are made with a mixture of whole and refined grains **These products are usually made from refined grains, but may be made with whole grains*	crackers, whole wheat pasta, whole wheat rolls, whole wheat tortillas, wild rice. **Enriched refined grains:** bagels*, biscuits*, breadcrumbs*, cakes, challah, cookies, corn flakes, corn tortillas*, cornbread*, couscous*, crackers*, English muffin, flour tortillas*, grits, hominy*, matzo, naan, noodles*, pancakes, pastas* (e.g., noodles, spaghetti, macaroni), pitas*, pizza crust*, pretzels, rice paper (spring roll wrappers), rice vermicelli, white bread, white rice, white sandwich buns and rolls.	
Dairy*** *2–3 cups*	Fluid milk: fat-free (skim) and low-fat (1%), (except for those 1 year of age), lactose-reduced and lactose-free milks. Soymilk. Yogurt: fat-free, low-fat, kefir, soy, Greek. Low-fat or part-skim cheeses.	Fluid milk: reduced fat (2%) or whole milk (unless 1 year of age), flavored milks. Reduced fat and whole milk yogurts. Full fat cheese, processed cheese (American and cheese spreads). Milk-based desserts: puddings, frozen yogurt, ice cream, lassi, sherbet.
Protein Foods *2–7 ounce-equivalents* *Select a variety of protein foods to improve nutrient intake and health benefits* *Choose seafood at least twice per week*	**Nuts, Seeds, Soy Products:** almond butter, almonds, cashews, chia seeds, hazelnuts, peanut butter, peanuts, pecans, pistachios, pumpkin seeds, sesame seeds, sunflower seeds, walnuts, tempeh, texturized vegetable protein (TVP), tofu, veggie burgers. **Seafood:** Fish: anchovies, catfish, cod, flounder, haddock, halibut, herring, mackerel, pollock, porgy, salmon, sardines, sea bass, snapper, swordfish, tilapia, trout, tuna. Shellfish: clams, crayfish, lobster, mussels, octopus, oysters, scallops, shrimp, squid (calamari). **Meats, Poultry, Eggs:** lean or low-fat meat (e.g., round and loin cuts of beef and pork) and poultry (skinless). Eggs. **Legumes** (beans and peas):** bean burgers, black beans, black-eyed peas, chickpeas (garbanzo beans), edamame, falafel, hummus (chickpea spread), kidney beans, lentils, lima beans	Higher fat meat (e.g., regular ground beef that is 75-80% lean), ribs, poultry with skin. Processed meats (e.g., ham, sausage, luncheon meat, hot dogs, bacon) higher in fat and/or sodium or meats enhanced with a salt-containing solution. Frying protein foods in solid fat. Salted nuts and seeds.

Continued on next page

Table 2.1 General Diet Continued from previous page

Food for the Day	Recommended - Select a Variety of Nutrient-Dense Foods	Choose Less Often
	(mature), navy beans, pinto beans, soy beans, split peas, white beans.	
Oils/Solid Fats *Limit saturated fats to less than 10% of calories per day. Limit intake of trans fat as low as possible.*	Vegetable oils: canola, corn, cottonseed, olive, safflower, soybean and sunflower. Flavoring oils: walnut and sesame. Soft margarine (tub or squeeze) with no *trans* fat, mayonnaise, salad dressing.	Beef fat (suet), butter, chicken fat, coconut oil, cream, cream cheese, margarine with *trans* fat, palm kernel oil, palm oil, partially hydrogenated oil, pork fat (lard), shortening, sour cream.
Added Sugars *This does not include natural sugars found in milk and fruit.*	Added sugars add calories without adding essential nutrients. Limit added sugars to less than 10% of calories per day.	Brown sugar, corn sweetener, corn syrup, dextrose, fructose, glucose, high fructose corn syrup, honey, invert sugar, malt syrup, maltose, molasses, pancake syrup, powdered sugar, raw sugar, sucrose and foods made with these sugars. Fruit drinks, energy drinks, sports drinks, and soft drinks with added sugars.

US Department of Agriculture. Choose My Plate.gov website. Food Galleries. www.choosemyplate.gov/food-gallery Updated June 3, 2016. Accessed February 5, 2016. (1)

Note: Limit sodium to 2,300 mg/day.

** Legumes (beans and peas) can be considered a part of the vegetable group or the protein group, but should be counted in one group only.

*** Other products sold as "milks" but made from plants (e.g., almond, rice, coconut, and hemp "milks") may contain calcium and be consumed as a source of calcium, but they are not included as part of the dairy group because their overall nutritional content is not similar to dairy milk and fortified soy beverages (soymilk).

Table 2.2 Sample Menu for General Diet*

Breakfast	Supper
½ c. orange juice	2 oz. tuna on 2 slices whole wheat bread,
1 egg	2 tsp mayonnaise
½ c. oatmeal	2 tomato slices
1 slice whole wheat toast	1 c. leafy greens salad
1 tsp. soft margarine	1 Tbsp. oil and vinegar dressing
2 tsp. jelly	½ c. fruit cocktail
1 c. low-fat milk	1 c. low-fat milk
Sugar, pepper (optional)	Water
Hot beverage	

Continued on next page

Table 2.2 Sample Menu for General Diet*

Lunch	Snack Ideas
2 oz. roasted chicken breast	½ c. cantaloupe
½ c. mashed potatoes with 2 oz. fat-free gravy	½ c. carrot sticks
½ c. mixed vegetables	3 c. popcorn, no *trans*-fat
1 oz. wheat roll	
1 tsp. soft margarine	
1 c. low-fat milk	
Water	

*Based on 1,800 calorie diet

REFERENCES

1. US Department of Agriculture. Choose My Plate.gov website. Food Galleries. www.choosemyplate.gov/food-gallery Updated June 3, 2015. Accessed February 5, 2016.

NUTRITION GUIDELINES FOR PREGNANCY AND LACTATION

The nutrition recommendations for pregnant and lactating women are based on the *2015-2020 Dietary Guidelines for Americans* (DGAs) in Chapter 1 and include increased amounts of protein, vitamins, and minerals. The suggested food plan includes foods in amounts that will provide the DRIs recommended by the National Academy of Sciences for women who are pregnant or lactating, depending on food choices. Special attention should be given to intakes of iron, folate, choline, calcium, vitamin D, and iodine to ensure adequacy. (1) Women with multiple gestation pregnancies have greater nutrition needs and should be assessed to insure adequate nutritional intake. Most doctors recommend women who are pregnant take a daily prenatal vitamin and mineral supplement in addition to eating a healthy diet. Women who are pregnant should consume 600 mcg dietary folate equivalents (DFEs) daily. (1) This may be achieved by consuming 400 mcg daily of synthetic folic acid (from fortified foods and/or supplements) in addition to food forms of folate from a varied diet. See Appendix 5 "Folate Content of Selected Foods." Women who are pregnant and breastfeeding may also need an additional iron supplement, if recommended by their physician.

Diet Principles

1. Weight gain during pregnancy should be individualized according to a woman's prepregnancy body mass index (BMI). The recommended weight gain during pregnancy for normal-weight (BMI 18.5-24.9) women is 25–35 pounds; women who are underweight (BMI <18.5) are advised to gain 28–40 pounds; women who are overweight (BMI 25-29.9) are advised to gain 15–25 pounds; and women who are obese (BMI ≥30) are advised to gain 11-20 pounds. (2)

    Women who are pregnant with twins and are in the normal BMI category should gain 37-54 pounds; women who are overweight should gain 31-50 pounds; and women who are obese should gain 25-42 pounds. (2) If weight gain exceeds recommended ranges, a detailed diet history/recall may be needed to evaluate excessive calorie intake.

2. High caffeine consumption is associated with delayed conception, spontaneous miscarriage, and low birth weight. Women who are pregnant and lactating are advised to limit caffeine consumption to less than 200 mg per day. This would translate into less than 16 ounces of coffee per day. (3)

3. It is advisable to avoid alcohol consumption during pregnancy and limit alcohol intake while breastfeeding. Alcohol has harmful effects on the developing fetus and excessive intake may cause Fetal Alcohol Syndrome or other neurological damage.

4. Pregnant women should be advised to limit herbal supplements until they are proven safe during pregnancy.

5. Refer to Chapter 6 for the management of gestational diabetes which includes a sample meal plan.

6. Pregnant and breastfeeding women should also limit white (albacore) tuna to 6 ounces per week and avoid tilefish, shark, swordfish, and king mackerel due to their high mercury content. Fish caught from local waters should be consumed in quantities of 6 ounces or less per week if no safety information is available. (4) EPA and FDA issued updated draft advice on fish consumption in June 2014. The 2014 draft advice recommends that pregnant women eat at least 8 ounces and up to 12 ounces (2 to 3 servings) per week of a variety of fish/seafood that are lower in mercury to support fetal growth and development. (5) This is consistent with the recommendations in the DGAs.

7. Food safety is of optimal importance for pregnant and breastfeeding women. Clean hands and cooking surfaces, avoidance of cross-contamination, cooking foods to proper temperatures, and quick cooling and proper storage of foods should be encouraged. Some foods should be avoided during pregnancy. This includes raw milk, cheese made from unpasteurized milk (e.g., feta, brie, camembert, blue-veined varieties, queso fresco, queso blanco, panela), raw or rare meat, raw or undercooked eggs, raw sprouts (e.g., bean, alfalfa), raw fish (e.g., sushi), and raw shellfish (e.g., oysters). Some ready-to-eat foods require reheating to 165°F before eating (e.g., hot dogs, bologna, deli meats, dry sausages). More information on foods to avoid is available from the U.S. Food and Drug Administration. (6)

8. The daily food plan for pregnancy and lactation is individualized based on the mother's height, weight, age, activity level, and stage of pregnancy or breastfeeding status. For help in determining individual needs, go to ChooseMyPlate.gov for Daily Food Plans for Pregnancy and Breastfeeding. (7) Most women will need food plans that provide 2200 to 2900 calories per day. The equation to estimate calorie needs during pregnancy may be found in the practice paper Nutrition and Lifestyle for a Healthy Pregnancy Outcome. (8) Lactating women should insure that they are well-hydrated, due to the volume of fluid required for milk production. See Chapter 1 for more information on USDA Food Patterns.

REFERENCES

1. Procter SB, Campbell CG. Position of the Academy of Nutrition and Dietetics: Nutrition and Lifestyle for a Healthy Pregnancy Outcome. *J Acad Nutr Diet*. 2014; 114(7):1099-1103.

2. Institute of Medicine. *Weight gain during pregnancy: reexamining the guidelines*. Washington, DC. National Academies Press; 2009. http://iom.nationalacademies.org/Reports/2009/Weight-Gain-During-Pregnancy-Reexamining-the-Guidelines.aspx

3. American College of Obstetricians and Gynecologists. ACOG Committee Opinion No. 462: Moderate caffeine consumption during pregnancy. *Obstet Gynecol* 2010; 116(2 Pt 1):467-468. doi: 10.1097/AOG.0b013e3181eeb2a1

4. What You Need to Know about Mercury in Fish and Shellfish 2004 EPA and FDA Advice. United States Environmental Protection Agency website. http://water.epa.gov/scitech/swguidance/fishshellfish/outreach/advice_index.cfm Updated November 20, 2013. Accessed August 28, 2015.

5. EPA-FDA Advisory on Mercury in Fish and Shellfish. U.S. Environmental Protection Agency website. http://www.epa.gov/fish-tech/epa-fda-advisory-mercury-fish-and-shellfish Updated October 6, 2015. Accessed December 14, 2015.

6. Food Safety for Moms-To-Be: While You're Pregnant. U.S. Food and Drug Administration website. http://www.fda.gov/Food/FoodborneIllnessContaminants/PeopleAtRisk/ucm083308.htm Updated June 11 2014. Accessed August 28, 2015.

7. U.S. Department of Agriculture. Choose My Plate.gov website. http://www.choosemyplate.gov/moms-pregnancy-breastfeeding Updated July 17, 2015. Accessed December 15, 2015.

8. Academy of Nutrition and Dietetics. Practice Paper of the Academy of Nutrition and Dietetics: Nutrition and lifestyle for a healthy pregnancy outcome. http://www.eatrightpro.org/resource/practice/position-and-practice-papers/practice-papers/practice-paper-nutrition-and-lifestyle-for-a-healthy-pregnancy-outcome Published July 1, 2014. Accessed December 12, 2015

Websites

Nutrition.gov: http://www.nutrition.gov/life-stages/women/women-pregnancy

Office of Dietary Supplements: http://ods.od.nih.gov

WIC Works Resource System: https://wicworks.fns.usda.gov/about-wic-works

RECOMMENDATIONS FOR FEEDING NORMAL INFANTS

Nutrition intake during infancy is more important for health, growth, and development than at any other time in the lifecycle. Ideal feeding experiences are those that meet nutrient demands while focusing on the individual developmental readiness of the infant. (1) These recommendations will provide the quantities of nutrients recommended by the American Academy of Pediatrics (AAP) for infants.

Diet Principles

The AAP, the American College of Obstetricians and Gynecologists (ACOG), and the Academy of Nutrition and Dietetics (AND) strongly recommend breastfeeding as the preferred feeding for all infants over formula feeding. (2) The AAP further recommends that after the first 6 months, mothers continue to breastfeed after the addition of complementary foods for at least a year or until mutually desired by mother and child. Successful breastfeeding requires education, support, and an environment that values and understands breastfeeding. (3) There are unavoidable instances when breastfeeding is not possible due to medical conditions or adoption. If families decide not to breastfeed their infant, iron-fortified formula is recommended. It is recommended the registered dietitian nutritionist (RDN) be consulted to determine the most suitable commercial formula for the infant.

Breast-Fed Infant: Birth to 12 Months

1. Human milk has a changing nutrient composition that may vary through lactation, over the course of a day, within a feeding, and from woman to woman. The variable composition of human milk provides nutrients specifically adapted to the changing needs of the infant, and also provides an array of flavors and tastes to stimulate the baby's senses. Colostrum, which is produced in the first few days of lactation, provides high amounts of protein and antibodies to protect the infant from infection. The transition to mature milk begins around days 3 to 5 postpartum, and mature milk appears about 10 days after birth. (3) Milk and its changing concentrations of protein, fat, carbohydrates, minerals, and other properties continue to change over time. (4)

2. Breastfeeding should begin within the first hour after birth, unless the medical condition of the mother or infant indicates otherwise. Infants who are placed on their mother's abdomen and who attach to the breast within 1 hour of birth have better breastfeeding outcomes than infants who do not. Encourage nursing in the delivery room, and avoid the separation of the mother and infant in the first few hours following birth. Skin-to-skin contact in the delivery room also maintains the baby's body temperature in a normal range. (3)

3. Typically, newborns will nurse 8 to 12 times or more in 24 hours, for at least 10 to 15 minutes per breast. The time between feedings is calculated from the beginning of one nursing to the beginning of the next. Frequent breastfeeding in the first few days reduces the baby's weight loss, decreases bilirubin levels, and helps establish a good milk supply. Although the average feeding is every 2 to 3 hours, the time will vary with each infant. (3) Following the ten steps to successful breastfeeding provides a structure for healthcare facilities to support mothers choosing to breastfeed. (Table 2.3) Provide the mother contact information for the lactation consultant or other breastfeeding resources available in your community.

4. Breastmilk empties from the stomach faster than infant formula. It is common for mothers to compare feeding schedules to bottle-fed infants. They may believe that because their child eats frequently they do not have a sufficient milk supply. As the infant becomes older, the frequency and duration of feedings decreases as the infant becomes more efficient at breastfeeding. (3)

5. The recommendation for feeding infants with human milk is made because human milk has been proven to be beneficial to infant nutrition, gastrointestinal function, the immune system, and has the potential beneficial influence on the development of the brain and spinal cord. Additionally, human milk has the potential benefit to prevent chronic diseases of childhood. (2)

6. An iron-fortified commercial formula is recommended for those who chose not to breastfeed. The introduction of formula should be considered if it is a substitute for human milk in infants with medical conditions which contraindicate breastfeeding. Infant formulas may also be helpful as a supplement to breastfed infants who are unable to obtain adequate calories to promote weight gain.

Table 2.3 Ten Steps to Successful Breastfeeding in Healthcare Facilities

Step 1	Have a written breastfeeding policy that is routinely communicated to all healthcare staff.
Step 2	Train all healthcare professionals in skills necessary to implement this policy.
Step 3	Inform all pregnant women about the benefits and management of breastfeeding.
Step 4	Help mothers initiate breastfeeding within ½ hour of birth, preferably in the delivery room.
Step 5	Show mothers how to breastfeed and how to maintain lactation even if they are separated from their infants.
Step 6	Give newborn infants no food or drink other than human milk, unless medically indicated.
Step 7	Practice rooming-in—allow mothers and infants to remain together 24 hours a day.
Step 8	Encourage breastfeeding on demand.
Step 9	Give no artificial teats or pacifiers to breastfeeding infants.
Step 10	Foster the establishment of breastfeeding support groups and refer mothers to them on discharge from the hospital or birth center.

Reprinted from *Protecting, Promoting and Supporting Breastfeeding: The Special Role of Maternity Services*, World Health Organization and UNICEF, Ten Steps to Successful Breastfeeding, page iv, 1989. http://apps.who. int/iris/bitstream/10665/39679/1/9241561300.pdf?ua=1&ua=1 (5) Used with permission.

Breastfeeding in a Disaster

A disaster, whether natural or human-made, makes access to food, clean water, heat, shelter, clothing, medicine, and other things necessary to survive more difficult to obtain. (3) Infants are especially at risk. For additional information on breastfeeding in a disaster, consult *Infant Feeding in Disasters and Emergencies*. (6)

Bottle-Fed Infant: Birth to 12 Months

1. The composition of human breast milk provides the basis for commercial infant formulas. There are several differences between the two that cannot be replicated. They include:

   a. First, human milk contains a number of components (such as hormones, growth factors, antibodies, enzymes, and live cells) that are difficult, if not impossible, to add to infant formula.

   b. Second, infant formulas are made from cow milk or are soy-based which do not have the same chemical properties and composition to the corresponding nutrients in human milk.

   c. Third, human milk is usually consumed within hours of being produced, whereas infant formulas are heat-treated and must have long shelf lives, generally at least 1 year.

   d. Fourth, the bioavailability of some nutrients in infant formula may be lower than that of the nutrients in human milk. (7)

2. The most common human milk substitute is standard cow's milk formula. In these formulas the cow's milk is altered by removing the butterfat, adding vegetable oils and carbohydrate, and decreasing the protein. Standard formulas vary in their ratio of casein to whey. The current requirements for protein in infant formulas range from 1.7 to 3.4 grams per 100 calories. Taurine, a free amino acid present in human milk, is often added to standard formulas. It is recommended to choose an iron-fortified formula prepared with fluoridated water.

3. Infant milk-based formulas are available in three forms. They are: concentrated liquid, ready-to-feed, and powder. Ready-to-feed formulas provide 20 calories per fluid ounce. Concentrate and powder formulas also provide 20 calories per fluid ounce when reconstituted as directed. Each manufacturer must ensure by analysis that all 29 essential nutrients are present in each batch of formula as referenced in the Infant Formula Act, and make a quantitative declaration for each nutrient on the label. In the United States, this "label claim" must be accurate until the end of the shelf life of the formula. Some vitamins degrade very little over the shelf life such as vitamin K, but others such as riboflavin, vitamin B_{12}, and vitamin C experience considerable loss. (6) *Note: In 2013 Abbott Nutrition changed the calories in some of their formulas to 19 calories per fluid ounce.*

4. Soy formulas also provide 20 calories per ounce, and are available in the same forms as milk based formulas. Carnitine, which plays a role in lipid metabolism, is added due to its low content in soy-based formulas. (7)

5. Heating formula in a microwave oven is not recommended because the formula heats unevenly which may cause mouth burns. The bottle may feel cool on the outside, yet the formula may be very hot.

6. As the infant grows, the recommended number of feedings and volume change. (Table 2.4a and Table 2.4b)

Table 2.4a Guide for formula feeding (0 to 5 months)

Age	Number of feedings per day	Volume in ounces per feeding
Birth–1 month	6 to 8 times	2 to 4 ounces
2 months	5 to 6 times	5 to 6 ounces
3 to 5 months	5 to 6 times	6 to 7 ounces

Table 2.4b Guide for formula feeding (4 to 12 months)

Age	Number of feedings per day	Volume in ounces per day
4 to 6 months	4 to 6 times	28 to 32 ounces per day
7 to 9 months	3 to 5 times	30 to 32 ounces per day
10 to 12 months	3 to 4 times	24 to 30 ounces per day

Tables 2.4a and 2.4b Modified from Recommended feeding guide for the first year. Johns Hopkins Medicine website. http://m.hopkinsmedicine.org/healthlibrary/conditions/pediatrics/feeding_guide_for_the_first_year_90,P02209/ (8) Used with permission.

Supplements for All Infants

Some supplements are suggested for both breastfed and formula fed infants. (Table 2.5)

Table 2.5 Suggested Vitamin and Mineral Supplementation for Full-Term Infants (0–12 Months) (9,10,11,12,13,14,15,16)

Vitamin or Mineral	Started at	Breastfed Infants	Infants Fed Infant Formula
Vitamin K	Birth	Dose given to prevent the possibility of bleeding.	Dose given to prevent the possibility of bleeding.
Vitamin D	Birth	400 IU/day unless consuming 1 qt. per day of vitamin D-fortified formula.	400 IU/day when consuming less than 1 qt. per day of vitamin D-fortified formula.
Iron	4 to 6 months	1 mg/kg/day	Total of at least 11 mg/day as iron-fortified formula (12 mg/qt).
Iron	6 to 12 months	1 mg/kg/day or consuming infant cereal totaling 11 mg/day.	Total of at least 11 mg/day as iron-fortified formula (12 mg/qt) or infant cereal.
Fluoride	6 months	If local water has < 0.3 ppm fluoride; 0.25 mg/day.	Fluoride throughout life helps control and prevent tooth decay. Infants can get fluoride through drinking infant formulas. Consult your family physician for fluoride recommendations related to type of formula used and level of fluoride in the water used in mixing.

All Infants

1. Feed infants when they provide hunger cues rather than on a specific schedule. These cues include rooting, mouth opening, lip licking, placing hands to mouth, and motor activity.

2. Making the correct food choices for infants during the first year of her/his life is important because more growth occurs during the first year than any other time of a child's life.

After Age 4 to 6 Months

1. Breast milk or iron-fortified formula is recommended for infants to age 1 year. Cow's milk in any form (whole, reduced-fat [2%], low-fat [1%], or fat-free [skim]) and goat's milk should not be given to infants during their first 12 months.

2. Introduce solid foods, using a spoon, when infants are developmentally ready. This is usually between 4 and 6 months of age or when birth weight has doubled. Signs of developmental readiness include moving food from the front to the back of the mouth and swallowing it, sitting alone or with minimal support, reaching to grasp the spoon, and turning the head away to refuse food. Generally, when an infant begins solids, the amount of formula will not exceed 32 ounces per day.

3. A commercially prepared, single-grain infant cereal (usually rice) fortified with iron should be the first solid food introduced. The order of introduction of other solid foods is not important.

4. Introduce no more than one single-ingredient food at a time. Offer new foods at weekly intervals to identify food intolerances. The new food can be offered several days in a row.

5. Begin teaching infants to drink from a cup at about 6 months.

6. Small, frequent feedings are preferable for infants. Let infants decide when they have had enough. "Full" cues include refusing to open mouth, turning head away, and spitting food out.

7. When infant foods are prepared at home, no salt or sugar should be added. Start with fresh or frozen foods as much as possible. Fruits canned in fruit juice and vegetables canned without salt can be used. Fruit canned in heavy syrup and vegetables canned with salt are not appropriate for infants.

8. In the last several months of their first year, infants can progress from smooth foods to foods with more texture. Provide mashed foods first, followed by "chunky" foods. Offer cut-up soft table foods after infants have mastered eating chunky textures.

9. After the age of 12 months, foods should be the primary source of nourishment, even if a child continues to be breast- or bottle-fed.

10. By age 12 months, children make the transition from demand feeding to the family schedule of meals and snacks. By this time weaning from the bottle often occurs automatically as children become interested in eating table foods. Nursing from bottle or breast, if continued, should be in place of a scheduled snack and no longer given on demand.

11. To protect children's teeth, frequent nursing from breast or bottle should not be permitted, and bottles should not be allowed in bed. (17)

Safety Concerns

1. Honey should not be given to children under the age of 2 years. It may contain spores of the bacteria *Clostridium botulism*, which can produce a dangerous toxin in the gastrointestinal tracts of infants.

2. Water that has been in household pipes for more than 6 hours can contain lead. To ensure low levels of lead in formula and foods, prepare them with cold water that has run until

it reaches its maximal coldness. Well water should be tested for nitrate and bacteria levels. Boiling well water for formula is not recommended because nitrates and other substances can become concentrated.

3. Do not give infants round, slippery, or hard foods such as carrot slices, olives, hot dogs, peanuts, and hard candies. These foods can become lodged in the throat and block the air passage.

NUTRITION GUIDELINES FOR CHILDREN

These nutrition guidelines are designed for children aged 1 to 8 years who require no special dietary modifications. The servings suggested for various age groups include foods in amounts that will provide the nutrients recommended by the AAP for the average child. Individual children from ages 2 years to puberty gain an average of 4.5–6.5 pounds and grow 2.5–3.5 inches per year on the average. This is a time when physical growth is a much slower than in infancy and appetites decrease often making feeding challenging and unpredictable. (7) Daily estimates for calories without considering exercise can be found below (Table 2.6). Calorie estimates increase with the addition of exercise. Information concerning weight and calories, physical activity, healthy eating tips, and tracking tools for child nutrition can be accessed at ChooseMyPlate.gov website. (18)

Table 2.6 Daily Estimated Calories for Children Based on Sedentary Lifestyle

Age	Daily Estimated Calories
1 Year Old	900
2-3 Years Old	1000
4-5 Years Old	1200
6-7 Years Old	1200 (Female) 1400 (Male)
8 Years Old	1400

Sources: U. S. Department of Health and Human Services and U. S. Department of Agriculture. *2015 – 2020 Dietary Guidelines for Americans,* 8th ed. http://health.gov/dietaryguidelines/2015/guidelines/ Published December 2015 and Gidding SS, Dennison BA, Birch LL, et al. Dietary recommendations for children and adolescents: a guide for practitioners. *Pediatrics.* 2006; 117(2):544–559. (19)

Diet Principles

1. The diet should provide adequate nourishment, variety, color, and be pleasing in texture and flavor.

2. Make mealtime enjoyable by creating a pleasant setting. Children's appetites vary from day to day and go through phases of likes and dislikes. Serve small portions and allow children to ask for more food as they are ready. Avoid nagging, forcing, and bribing children to eat. Focusing attention on a child's poor appetite or eating problem will likely make the problem last longer.

3. Successful eating patterns are set by a division of eating responsibilities. The caregiver has the responsibility of providing a variety of nutritious foods and creating the mealtime environment. Children make food choices from what is offered and determine how much is consumed. (20)

4. Include snacks with high nutrient value in menu plans. The nutrient requirements of children cannot be met by meals alone because their small stomach capacity limits the amount of food they can eat at any one time.

5. Fat and cholesterol should not be limited in the diets of children under the age of 2 years; however, high fat foods with limited amounts of nutrients (pastries, gravies, fried foods, sweets) should be offered only in limited amounts.

6. The *2015-2020 Dietary Guidelines for Americans* (Chapter 1) recommend keeping total fat intake between 30 and 40% of total calories for children 2 to 3 years of age, and between 25 and 35% of total calories for children and adolescents 4 to 18 years of age, with most fats coming from sources of unsaturated fatty acids, such as fish, nuts, and vegetable oils.

7. A sick child may regress in his or her level of eating performance, and this regression may progress throughout a long illness. For instance, a 6-year-old child may regress to the level of a 4- or 5-year-old so far as eating is concerned.

8. When a child begins cow's milk at 1 year, it should be whole cow's milk and not 2% or skim to provide essential fat and calories. (21)

9. For younger children it is important that meat be tender, moist, and cut into strips or bite-sized pieces to facilitate chewing and prevent choking.

10. Young children like crisp finger foods; serve them often.

11. Highly seasoned foods may not be well accepted; use seasonings in moderate amounts.

12. Dieting at a young age can be dangerous to children's development, both physically and psychologically. If a child is overweight, maintaining weight during growth in height is recommended rather than encouraging weight loss, unless a child is severely overweight. Any weight management efforts in children should occur under the monitoring of the family physician or a pediatric weight management program.

13. Vitamin and mineral supplements may be prescribed by a physician.

14. Fluoride supplements may be needed for children whose tap water contains ≤ 0.6 ppm fluoride. (16) You can find the amount of fluoride in your water at My Water's Fluoride. (22)

15. The recommended average daily intake from food groups at various calorie levels can be found in the USDA Food Patterns in Chapter 1.

Child Safety, Feeding Recommendations and Resources

1. Parents may encounter common feeding concerns in young children such as refusing meat, drinking too little or too much milk, and refusing vegetables and fruits. Possible solutions for these concerns are listed in Table 2.7.

2. Toddlers and preschoolers can choke on medium to large pieces of food. Cut foods into small pieces and remove seeds, skin, and small bones. Cut round foods like hot dogs, carrots, and string cheese into short strips; chop whole grapes and berries into small pieces. Wait until closer to age 4 to serve risky foods like popcorn, pretzels, nuts, seeds, dried fruit, and round or hard candy.

3. Peanut butter can stick in the mouth and be hard to swallow. Wait until children are closer to 2 years to offer peanut butter. Spread it thinly on crackers, bread, or toast.

4. Require children to sit down when they eat to avoid choking and supervise them while eating.

5. Counseling tips when working with parents dealing with feeding concerns are available from the U.S. Department of Agriculture Food and Nutrition Service on the "Core Nutrition Messages" web site. Messages and tips are grouped by the following topics: Child Feeding, Fruits and Vegetables, Milk, and Whole Grain. (23)

Table 2.7 Common Feeding Concerns in Young Children

Common concerns	Possible Solutions
Refuses meats	• Offer small, bite-size pieces of moist, tender meat, or poultry. • Incorporate into meatloaf, spaghetti sauce, stews, casseroles, burritos, or pizza. • Include legumes, eggs, and cheese. • Offer boneless fish (including canned tuna and salmon).
Drinks too little milk	• Offer cheeses and yogurt, including cheese in cooking (e.g., macaroni and cheese, cheese sauce, pizza). Use milk to cook hot cereals. Offer cream soups and milk-based puddings and custards. • Allow child to pour milk from a pitcher and use a straw. • Include powdered milk in cooking and baking (e.g., biscuits, muffins, pancakes, meatloaf, casseroles).
Drinks too much milk	• Offer water if thirsty between meals. • Limit milk to one serving with meals or offer at end of meal; offer water for seconds. • If bottle is still used, wean to cup.
Refuses vegetables and fruits	• If child refuses vegetables, offer more fruits, and vice versa. • Prepare vegetables that are tender but not overcooked. • Steam vegetable strips (or offer raw if appropriate) and allow child to eat with fingers. • Offer sauces and dips (e.g., cheese sauce for cooked vegetables, dip for raw vegetables, yogurt to dip fruit). • Include vegetables in soups and casseroles. • Add fresh or dried fruit to cereals. • Prepare fruits in a variety of ways (e.g., fresh, cooked, juice, in gelatin, as a salad). • Continue to offer a variety of fruits and vegetables.
Eats too many sweets	• Limit purchase and preparation of sweet foods in the home. • Avoid using as a bribe or reward. • Incorporate into meals instead of snacks for better dental health. • Reduce sugar by half in recipes for cookies, muffins, quick breads, and the like. • Limit excessive juice consumption. • Work with staff of day care, preschools, and others to reduce use of sweets.

Modified from Samour PQ and King K, *Pediatric Nutrition*, 4th Edition, 2012, Jones and Bartlett Publishers, Burlington, MA. www.jblearning.com. Reprinted with permission. p. 108, Table 6-4. (21)

REFERENCES

1. Akers S, Groh-Wargo S. Normal nutrition during infancy. In: Samour PQ, King KK, ed. *Pediatric Nutrition*, 4th ed. Sudbury, MA: Jones and Bartlett Publishers, Inc.; 2012:71-101.

2. American Academy of Pediatrics. Policy statement: breastfeeding and the use of human milk: section on breastfeeding. *Pediatrics*. 2012;129(3): e827-e841.doi: 10.1542/peds.2011-3552

3. American Academy of Pediatrics, American College of Obstetricians and Gynecologists. *Breastfeeding Handbook for Physicians*, 2nd Edition. Elk Grove Village, IL: American Academy of Pediatrics; 2014.

4. Lawrence RA, Lawrence RM. *Breastfeeding: A Guide for the Medical Profession*, 7th ed. St. Louis, MO: Mosby; 2010.

5. World Health Organization and UNICEF. *Protecting, Promoting and Supporting Breastfeeding: The Special Role of Maternity Services,* Geneva, Switzerland: World Health Organization; 1989.

6. Infant Feeding in Disasters and Emergencies. http://www.aap.org/breastfeeding/files/pdf/InfantNutritionDisaster.pdf Published 2015. Accessed August 5, 2015.

7. Kleinman RE, *Pediatric Nutrition Handbook*, 6th ed. Elk Grove Village, IL: American Academy of Pediatrics; 2009.

8. Recommended feeding guide for the first year. Johns Hopkins Medicine website. http://m.hopkinsmedicine.org/healthlibrary/conditions/pediatrics/feeding_guide_for_the_first_year_90,P02209/ Accessed August 31, 2015.

9. Medical Care and Your Newborn. Nemours Foundation, Kids Health website. http://kidshealth.org/parent/growth/medical/mednewborn.html Published January 2015. Accessed September 21, 2015.

10. Prophylactic vitamin K for vitamin K deficiency bleeding in neonates. Cochran website. http://www.cochrane.org/CD002776/NEONATAL_prophylactic-vitamin-k-for-vitamin-k-deficiency-bleeding-in-neonates Accessed September 20, 2015.

11. Vitamin D: Fact Sheet for Health Professionals. National Institute of Health Office of Dietary Supplements website. https://ods.od.nih.gov/factsheets/VitaminD-HealthProfessional/ Published November 10, 2014. Accessed September 20, 2015.

12. Wagner CL, Greer FR, and the Section on Breastfeeding and Committee on Nutrition. From the American Academy of Pediatrics: Prevention of rickets and vitamin D deficiency in infants, children, and adolescents. *Pediatrics.* 2008; 122(5):1142-1152. doi: 10.1542/peds.2008-1862

13. Iron: Dietary Supplement Fact Sheet. National Institutes of Health, Office of Dietary Supplements website. https://ods.od.nih.gov/pdf/factsheets/Iron-HealthProfessional.pdf Reviewed February 19, 2015. Accessed September 21, 2015.

14. Baker RD, Greer FR, and the Committee on Nutrition. From the American Academy of Pediatrics: Clinical Report—Diagnosis and prevention of iron deficiency and iron-deficiency anemia in infants and young children (0–3 Years of Age). *Pediatrics.* 2010; 126(5):1040-1050. doi: 10.1542/peds.2010-2576

15. Overview: Infant Formula and Fluorosis. Centers for Disease Control and Prevention, Community Water Fluoridation. http://www.cdc.gov/fluoridation/safety/infant_formula.htm Updated July 31, 2015. Accessed September 20, 2015.

16. Clark MB, Slayton RL, and Section on Oral Health. From the American Academy of Pediatrics: Clinical Report: Fluoride Use in Caries Prevention in the Primary Care Setting. *Pediatrics.* 2014; 134 (3):626-633. doi:10.1542/peds.2014-1699

17. Keep Your Baby Smiling—Prevent Early Childhood Tooth Decay. Iowa Department of Public Health Web site. http://www.idph.state.ia.us/IDPHChannelsService/file.ashx?file=7CABD60B-CDC2-457B-9F04-567E85B9CF47 Published June 2000. Accessed August 8, 2015.

18. U.S. Department of Agriculture Choose My Plate.gov website. http://www.choosemyplate.gov/ Published June 2, 2011. Accessed August 5, 2015.

19. Gidding SS, Dennison BA, Birch LL, et al. Dietary recommendations for children and adolescents: a guide for practitioners. *Pediatrics.* 2006; 117(2):544–559.

20. Carruth BR, Skinner JD. Feeding behaviors and other motor development in healthy children (2–24 months). *J Am Coll Nutr*. 2002; 21:88–96.

21. Samour PQ, King KK, *Pediatric Nutrition*, 4th ed. Sudbury, MA: Jones and Bartlett Publishers; 2012.

22. My Water's Fluoride. Centers for Disease Control and Prevention website. https://nccd.cdc.gov/DOH_MWF/Default/Default.aspx Accessed September 21, 2015.

23. U.S. Department of Agriculture Food and Nutrition Service Core Nutrition Messages. http://www.fns.usda.gov/core-nutrition/core-nutrition-messages Published May 14, 2014. Accessed August 5, 2015.

ADDITIONAL RESOURCES

Children's Feeding Guide Age 1 to 5, Iowa Department of Public Health-Iowa WIC Program. http://www.idph.state.ia.us/IDPHChannelsService/file.ashx?file=40CC6EC0-96CE-4512-9C05-122961A52BC9. Published 2008.

American Dietetic Association. Benchmarks for nutrition programs in child care settings. *J Am Diet Assoc*. 2005; 105(6):979–986.

Yan J, Liu L, Zhu Y, Huang G, Wang PP. The association between breastfeeding and childhood obesity: a meta-analysis. *BMC Public Health*. 2014; 14:1267-1277.

Pan L, Blanck HM, Sherry B, Dalenius K, Grummer-Strawn LM. Trends in the prevalence of extreme obesity among US preschool children living in low-income families, 1998-2010. *JAMA* 2012; 308(24); 2563-2565.

Position of the American Dietetic Association: Nutrition and lifestyle for a healthy pregnancy outcome. *J Am Diet Assoc*. 2008; 108(3):553–561.

Position of the American Dietetic Association: Promoting and supporting breastfeeding. *J Am Diet Assoc*. 2009; 109(11):1926–1942.

Quick Tips for Feeding a Picky Eater. WebMD website. http://www.webmd.com/parenting/ss/slideshow-picky-eaters Updated April 7, 2014.

Websites

Baby-Friendly USA: http://www.babyfriendlyusa.org/

Choose My Plate.gov: http://www.choosemyplate.gov/

MEETING NUTRITIONAL NEEDS OF OLDER ADULTS

Food and dining requirements are core components of quality of life and quality of care in nursing facilities. Both are integral parts of individualized care and self-directed living. In 2011, the New Dining Practice Standards established nationally agreed upon standards of practice supporting individualized care and self-directed living versus traditional diagnosis-focused treatment for older adults. (1) This corresponds to Tag F242 Self-Determination and Participation. The resident also has the right to choose health care consistent with his/her interests, including making choices about diet and diet restrictions. (2)

As people age, their nutritional needs change. The aging process can affect the older adult in numerous ways: economic, functional, physiological, and psychosocial. (3, 4, 5, 6) These changes often influence not only nutritional status but also the risk for malnutrition. Since total and resting energy requirements decrease progressively with age, it can be challenging to maintain nutritional status since vitamin and mineral needs often remain constant, or may even increase for many nutrients. (7) Even when older adults follow standard nutritional recommendations, they may still develop a nutritional disorder. (6)

Studies show that food and fluid intake decreases even in the healthy older adult. (7) Dehydration, a form of malnutrition, is a major problem in older adults, especially persons greater than 85 years old, as well as institutionalized older adults. (7) In older adults, a diet consistent with current guidelines including high amounts of vegetables, fruits, whole grains, poultry, fish, and low-fat dairy products may be associated with improved nutritional status, quality of life, and survival. (8)

Body composition also changes as people age. Older adults who are either underweight or obese are at risk for sarcopenia, a decrease in lean body mass (primarily loss of skeletal muscle). Loss of lean body mass affects muscle strength and ability to complete daily activities. To prevent a loss in lean body mass, adequate energy and protein intake is essential. Routine nutrition screening and assessment should be completed to ensure appropriate intake of food. (6)

Involuntary weight loss among older adults has been demonstrated to increase mortality risk. (9) When a resident is losing weight, dietary restrictions may be lifted and the diet liberalized to improve the resident's food intake in an effort to stabilize weight. The theory of "real food first" should be the first intervention when weight loss is occurring. When this doesn't work, research suggests that whole protein and energy nutritional products may be used to supplement intake in this group of residents. Further research has supported this intervention in improving body weight and increasing both protein and energy intake in older adults with illness-related malnutrition. This increase in weight gain is at times small, but it has significant effect on mortality in this age group. (10)

The caloric needs for weight maintenance of healthy older adults range from 25 to 35 calories per kg per day in females and 30 to 40 calories per kg per day in males with physical activity levels ranging from sedentary to very active. (11, 12) The caloric needs for weight maintenance of underweight older adults range from 25 to 30 calories per kg per day, or higher calorie levels for weight gain, with physical activity levels ranging from sedentary to very active. (11, 12)

MyPlate for Older Adults (13, 14)

In late 2011, nutrition scientists at the Jean Mayer USDA Human Nutrition Research Center on Aging (USDA HNRCA) at Tufts University introduced the MyPlate for Older Adults which corresponds with MyPlate. The MyPlate for Older Adults icon illustrates the recommendations of the federal government's 2010 Dietary Guidelines for Americans and MyPlate specifically tailored to adults older than 70 years emphasizing topics such as adequate fluid and convenient, affordable, and readily available foods. It calls attention to the decline in caloric needs due to a slow-down in metabolism and physical activity while emphasizing that nutritional requirements remain the same or in some cases increase. (13)

MyPlate for Older Adults provides examples of foods that contain high levels of vitamins and minerals per serving; recommends limiting foods high in *trans* and saturated fats, salt and added sugars, and emphasizes whole grains. MyPlate for Older Adults is intended to be a guide for healthy, older adults who are living independently and looking for examples of good food choices and physical activities.

MyPlate for Older Adults

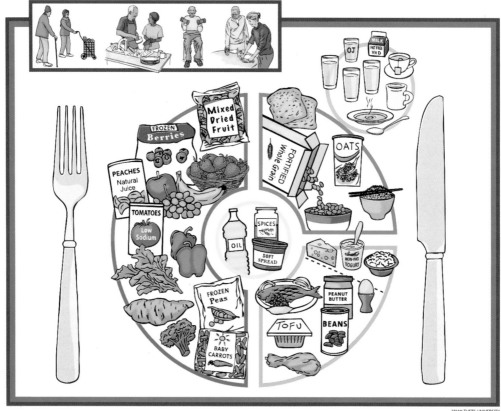

Copyright 2011 Tufts University. For details about the MyPlate for Older Adults, please see http://nutrition. tufts.edu/research/myplate-older-adults. Used with permission.

Figure 2.1 MyPlate for Older Adults.

The following foods, fluids, and physical activities are represented by icons on MyPlate for Older Adults:

- Bright-colored vegetables such as carrots and broccoli.
- Deep-colored fruit such as berries and peaches.
- Whole, enriched and fortified grains and cereals such as brown rice and 100% whole wheat bread.
- Low- and non-fat dairy products such as yogurt and low-lactose milk.
- Dry beans and nuts, fish, poultry, lean meat, and eggs.
- Liquid vegetable oils, soft spreads low in saturated and *trans* fat, and spices to replace salt.
- Fluids such as water, tea, coffee fat-free milk, and soup.
- Physical activity such as walking, resistance training and light cleaning as well as other daily errands and household chores.

Another version of MyPlate for Older Adults was developed by the Elder Nutrition and Food Safety (ENAFS) faculty and staff at the University of Florida. This includes the original drawings of foods that often are chosen by older adults for ease of purchasing, chewing/swallowing and/or preparing. (14) This edition of MyPlate for Older Adults includes a meal plan for 1800 calories.

Nutritional status is also affected when low income and food insecurity results in the older adult not having adequate means to obtain food. When a person's income is insufficient to meet basic needs, it is the responsibility of the nutrition professional to be proactive in helping individuals seek economic assistance. Good nutritional choices should be at the forefront of maintaining healthy aging. Awareness of the full range of options available (i.e., supplemental nutrition assistance program [SNAP], formerly known as food stamps, home-delivered meals, congregate meals, and food pantries) and the patterns of use within the community may ensure nutritional needs will be met. (15)

Many diseases or conditions that would be considered abnormal or alarming in younger adult populations are often seen as a part of the "normal aging process" in the older adult. (15) Use of nutrition care protocols can help with the identification of inadequate intake patterns and unintentional weight loss. (16) The nutrition professional must determine the underlying causes of weight changes (i.e., bowel elimination, uncontrolled disease processes, economic, oral, cognition, anorexia of aging, etc.).

Medications can affect intake, nutrient absorption, metabolism, and excretion which can alter the nutritional status of an older adult. An assessment of all medications (prescribed, over the counter, and nontraditional) is important because food and drug interactions in the older adult remain largely under recognized. (17, 18)

Given that most nursing home residents are at risk for malnutrition, and may in fact have different therapeutic targets for blood pressure, blood sugar, and cholesterol, a regular diet which allows for resident choice is most often the preferred option. (1) With this in mind, intensive treatment of diabetes, hypertension, heart failure, and hypercholesterolemia may not be appropriate for older adults in long term care facilities. It is important to consider the resident's cognitive and functional status, severity of disease, expressed preferences, and life expectancy. (6, 19)

Prior to prescribing a therapeutic diet, consider the person's quality of life, risk versus benefits, and the impact the diet will have on the overall nutritional status of the older adult. Prevention strategies should be based on individual functional status and the life goals of the older adults rather than on chronological age. For those in assisted living or nursing facilities, these groups should be offered as liberal a diet as possible. (6)

Consider the following guidelines when implementing food plans for older adults:

1. Use the General Diet as much as possible, especially for people older than 70 years of age living in long-term care facilities on a permanent basis. A diet that stresses higher amounts of fruits, vegetables, bread, cereals, potatoes, beans, nuts, and seeds should be considered (Mediterranean-style eating pattern – see Chapter 1). Olive oil, dairy products, fish, and poultry are consumed in moderate amounts. This also coincides with the Tufts MyPlate for Older Adults. (20) People living in long-term care facilities on a permanent basis desire a homelike atmosphere where they feel loved and important. Unless truly contraindicated, physicians should be encouraged to place these residents on the General Diet with only texture modifications, individualized to that resident. Serving popular, nutritious foods to some residents and not to others may cause anxiety, decreased food intake, and unhappiness. (6) Menus should be planned to include food in amounts that will provide the Dietary Reference Intakes (DRIs) recommended by the National Academy of Sciences for adults. If a nutrient analysis program is not available for menu planning, the USDA Food Pattern in Chapter 1 for a 1,800-calorie diet may be a useful tool for the older adult.

2. If modifications are needed for the older adult (especially the residents of long-term care facilities), the least restrictive diet is encouraged. Severely restricted diets and

combination diets are not well accepted on a long-term basis and are often the cause of malnutrition in the older adult. (6)

3. Minor changes to a well-planned General Diet may meet the needs of people with high blood cholesterol, diabetes, or for whom weight management is appropriate. (6, 20, 21)

4. Hypertension is often seen in older adults. According to the *2015-2020 Dietary Guidelines for Americans* adults with prehypertension and hypertension are recommended to reduce sodium in their diets to 1,500 mg daily, but this may need to be tempered in the institutionalized older adults. Dietary restriction may benefit some individuals, but more lenient blood pressure goals in the frail older adult may be desirable. The use of a 2000 mg sodium diet has been shown to reduce systolic blood pressures, on average, by only 5 mmHg and diastolic blood pressures by only 2.5 mmHg; this diet's effect on blood pressure is modest at best and has not actually been shown to improve cardiovascular outcomes in the nursing home resident. (1) These significantly restricted diets may be poorly tolerated in this population leading to loss of appetite, hyponatremia (low blood sodium level), or confusion. (1, 22)

5. A study by Zajacova and Ailshire concluded that weight loss is associated with particularly high mortality risk even when the typical body mass index (BMI) change is from obesity to overweight suggesting that a higher BMI may be protective among long-stay residents. (23, 24) Serving fat-free or low-fat dairy products, limiting gravies and margarine, reducing portion size of desserts, and offering reduced sugar sweeteners and condiments may be adequate for medical nutrition therapy.

6. Individualization is the key to dietary alterations for any person. The menu plan should be personalized with a focus on physical, mental, and social well-being. Choices from all the food groups provide variety in the diet.

7. Food habits influenced by ethnic, religious, and socioeconomic factors, are important because older adults place much emphasis on preserving their cultural traditions. Consider these factors when planning meals or dietary modifications to maximize quality of life.

8. Energy needs for the older adults are difficult to assess. In some cases, energy needs decrease as a result of decreased activity and lean body mass. In other cases, needs may increase because of infection and stress. (25) Meeting the needs of older adults is extremely challenging as requirements for many nutrients remain the same or increase. (7) For this reason, a balanced variety of foods should be consumed to ensure adequate nutrition.

9. As part of the DRIs, the Recommended Dietary Allowance (RDA) for protein needs of the older adult is 0.8 grams per kilogram (kg) of body weight per day. (26) Some experts suggest that protein intake of 1.0 to 1.6 grams per kg daily is safe and adequate to meet the needs of healthy adults. (7) Evidence suggests that the upper limit on how much protein can be synthesized at a single meal is approximately 30 grams. Some experts recommend that older adults consume 25-30 grams of high quality protein at each meal. (27) Good sources of protein include meat, poultry, fish, eggs, dairy, soybeans, nuts, seeds, and dry beans. See Appendix 13 "Protein Content of Selected Foods."

10. Dietary fat intake for older adults should be 20 to 35% of total daily caloric intake. Relevant research trends suggest the effects of traditional low cholesterol and low fat diets used to treat elevated cholesterol vary greatly and often decrease lipid levels only 10-15%. Aggressive reduction, if needed, can be more effectively achieved through the use of medication that has been shown to reduce lipid levels between 30-40% while still allowing the older adult to enjoy food preferences. (1) If there is decreased tolerance to fats, avoid fried foods and decrease amounts of fats added to or present in foods.

11. Intake of carbohydrates should compose 45 to 65% of total calories for the older adult to protect protein from being used as an energy source. Complex carbohydrates (e.g., whole grains, legumes, fresh fruits) should be a part of the older adult's daily intake. (3, 13)

12. The choice of a target level for glycemic control in the older adult should be individualized. Most research suggests a AlC of <7.5% is desired for those healthy older adults with few coexisting chronic diseases; <8% for complex/intermediate conditions who have multiple coexisting chronic illnesses; and <8.5% for the very complex/older adults in poor health who are in long term care facilities and/or have end stage chronic illnesses. Considerations must be given to the life expectancy of the older adult. (21)

13. Intake of calcium and vitamin D should be emphasized in the older adult. Older adults need to maintain serum 25(OH)D levels >30 ng/mL for optimal benefits. (28) Research is emerging regarding vitamin D deficiency and its effect on neuromuscular function, cardiovascular disease, inflammatory illnesses, and bone mineralization. Older adults with vitamin D deficiency are at risk for osteoporosis, increased falls, and periodontal disease. For adults aged 51–70 years, the DRI for vitamin D is 15 mcg and increases to 20 mcg for older adults. The recommended calcium intake for males aged 51–70 is 1000 mg and 1200 mg for older adults; calcium intake for females aged 51 and older is 1200 mg/day (29) which can be met with the General diet with three cups of dairy products daily. If an individual is unable to do this, supplementation is sometimes needed. (3, 28) See Appendix 3 "Calcium Content of Selected Foods" and Appendix 11 "Vitamin D Content of Selected Foods."

14. Older adults may be less tolerant of milk and milk products, although small servings of milk (up to 8 fluid oz. per serving) may be tolerated. Milk products that have been fermented (i.e., buttermilk, cheese, or yogurt) or cooked (i.e., pudding, custard, cream soup, and sauces) are often tolerated. Other options include the use of lactose-free milk or adding lactase enzyme tablets to fresh milk to aid digestion. The older adult should be encouraged to consume other calcium-rich food and beverage sources (dark green leafy vegetables, calcium-fortified foods/beverages) to help reduce the risk of osteoporosis. Restricting milk products may not be the answer if the older adult continues with such symptoms as diarrhea, abdominal cramping, etc. Consider medical causes such as gastroenteritis, *Clostridium difficile*, colitis, and other conditions that may result in abnormal elimination patterns. Also consider possible effects of medications such as antibiotics, antacids, antidepressants, diuretics, laxatives, tranquilizers, and those with large amounts of mannitol or sorbitol.

15. Folate (20) and vitamin B_{12} (30, 31) intake and utilization may be affected in the older adult. Vitamin B_{12} deficiency is frequent among older adults with a prevalence approaching 20%. (31) Intake of these vitamins should be ensured either through fortified foods or supplements. See Appendix 5 "Folate Content of Selected Foods" and Appendix 9 "Vitamin B_{12} Content of Selected Foods."

16. For persons with iron deficiency anemia, encourage intake of iron-rich foods. Include vitamin C-rich foods at meals as these increase iron absorption. Do not take iron inhibitors (e.g., tea and coffee), whether food or medication, with meals. Avoid excessive or inappropriate iron supplementation due to potential side effects, such as gastrointestinal distress, iron overload, etc. See Appendix 4 "Iron Content of Selected Foods" and Appendix 10 "Vitamin C Content of Selected Foods."

17. A daily fluid intake of 30 mL/kg of body weight or a minimum of 1500 mL/day is often recommended for the older adult. However, due to the lack of research, the use of physical signs and symptoms may actually assist the clinician in determining needs. A variety of beverages or foods may be used to meet fluid needs including broth, gelatin, ice cream, water, coffee, tea, carbonated beverages, and juices. Liberal fluid intake promotes gastrointestinal function and prevents dehydration. The nutrition professional

must be aware that no evidence has been found to establish or validate the three usual methods of estimating fluid needs for adults (Weight Method, RDA Method or Fluid Balance Method); however, these three equations have been cited extensively in many well-respected documents and widely used in clinical practice. Well-designed studies are needed to determine and validate predictive equations to estimate fluid requirements in the older adult. (5, 12, 33)

18. Encourage fiber rich fruits, vegetables, and whole grains for improved gastric motility if appropriate. Monitor and evaluate the intakes of the frail older adults and those with poor appetite so that high-fiber diet options do not lead to excess satiety, decreased overall food consumption, and limited nutrient intake. See Appendix 2 "Fiber Content of Selected Foods."

19. People who have difficulty chewing or swallowing may need adjustments in the consistency of the foods served to maintain adequate calories. (34) Meats may need to be chopped, ground, or pureed. Meats should be moist and well-seasoned. Texture modifications should be individualized and used only when needed. For modifications, refer to Consistency Altered Diets in Chapter 3.

20. Diet and nutrition intervention for older adults with compromised oral integrity must target individual needs based on all health problems and disabilities as well as oral signs and symptoms. (34, 35) Vegetables should be steamed, sautéed, or stir-fried to enhance their flavors. For those with dry mouth, offering very sweet or tart foods and beverages (lemonade or cranberry juice) may stimulate saliva production. Ice chips, sugar-free hard candy, gum, or popsicles may also provide relief. Adding cream, gravy, sauces, soups, and such to increase moisture of foods provided may help in the swallowing process. Numerous other artificial saliva preparations are available to help resolve/improve this problem.

21. Finger foods may be necessary for people with decreased dexterity. These foods are more easily consumed and increase independence. For more information, refer to the Finger Food Diet in Chapter 13.

22. Food intake is improved when served at regular meal times, including a bedtime snack. Intake may be enhanced by serving the larger meal at midday; or by serving smaller, more frequent meals. No more than 14 hours should elapse between a substantial evening meal and breakfast. Portion sizes at meals may vary based on an individual's nutritional needs. (36)

23. Social contact in a pleasant environment may stimulate the appetite. This is important for people who live in long-term care facilities as well as people who live independently.

24. Evaluation for depression and alcohol use and their effects on the intake of the older adult must be assessed. Regular alcohol use may be associated with changes in absorption/utilization of vitamins B_6, B_{12}, and C; thiamin deficiency, decreased zinc absorption, and increased iron absorption. (37)

REFERENCES

1. Pioneer Network Food and Dining Clinical Standards Task Force. *New Dining Practice Standards.* Pioneer Network and The Hulda B & Maurice L. Rothschild Foundation. August 2011. www.pioneernetwork.net/Data/Documents/NewDiningPracticeStandards.pdf Accessed June 27, 2015.

2. Centers for Medicare & Medicaid. *State Operations Manual*, Appendix PP, Tag 242 Self-Determination. www.cms.gov/Regulations-and-Guidance/Guidance/Manuals/downloads/som107ap_pp_guidelines_ltcf.pdf Page 88. Accessed June 27, 2015.

3. Wellman NS, Kamp BJ. Nutrition in aging. In Mahon K, Escott-Stump S, Raymond J, ed. *Krause's Food, Nutrition and Diet Therapy*, 13th ed., St Louis, MO, Elsevier; 2012: 442-459.

4. Chippendale T. Factors associated with depressive symptoms among elders in senior residences: the importance of feeling valued by others, *Clin Ger 2013; 36(2): 162-169 DOI:* 10.1080/07317115.2012.749321.

5. Chernoff R. Demographics of Aging. In: Chernoff R, ed. *Geriatric Nutrition,* 4th ed. Burlington, MA: Jones & Bartlett Learning; 2014:1-13.

6. Dorner, B. Position of the American Dietetic Association: Individualized nutrition approaches for older adults in health care communities. *J Am Diet Assoc.* 2010; 110: 1549-1553.

7. Bernstein M, Munoz, N. Position of the Academy of Nutrition and Dietetics: Food and nutrition for older adults: promoting health and wellness. *J Acad Nutr Diet.* 2012; 112:1255-1277.

8. Anderson AL, Harris TB, Tylavsky FA, et al. Dietary patterns and survival of older adults. *J Am Diet Assoc.* 2011; 111(1): 84-91. doi: 10.1016/j.jada.2010.10.012.

9. CMS State Operations Manual Appendix PP, Tag 325 Nutrition. www.cms.gov/ Regulations-and-Guidance/Guidance/Manuals/downloads/som107ap_pp_ guidelines_ltcf.pdf Page 357. Accessed July 5, 2015.

10. Silver HJ. Oral strategies to supplement older adults' dietary intakes: Comparing the evidence. *Nutr Rev.* 2009 Jan; 67(1):21–31.

11. Academy of Nutrition and Dietetics. Evidence Analysis Library. What are the caloric needs of healthy older adults (over age 65)? Conclusion Statement. http://www.andeal. org/template.cfm?template=guide_summary&key=2066 Published 2009. Accessed January 24, 2016.

12. Eckstein L, Adams K. *Pocket Resource for Nutrition Assessment*, 2013 Edition. Dietetics in Health Care Communities. Chicago, IL. 2013.

13. Tufts University nutrition scientists unveil MyPlate for older adults. Tufts Now website. http://now.tufts.edu/news-releases/tufts-university-nutrition-scientists-unveil- Accessed June 27, 2015.

14. MyPlate for Older Adults adapted by Department of Family, Youth and Community Services, Institute of Food and Agricultural Sciences, University of Florida 2011. http:// edis.ifas.ufl.edu/pdffiles/FY/FY126000.pdf Accessed June 27, 2015.

15. Kamp B. Position of the American Dietetic Association, American Society for Nutrition, and Society for Nutrition Education: Food and nutrition programs for community-residing older adults. *J Am Diet Assoc.* 2010; 110(3):463-472.

16. White JV, Guenter P, Jensen G, Malone A, Schofield M; Academy of Nutrition and Dietetics Malnutrition Work Group; A.S.P.E.N. Malnutrition Task Force; A.S.P.E.N. Board of Directors. Consensus statement of the Academy of Nutrition and Dietetics/ American Society for Parenteral and Enteral Nutrition: characteristics recommended for the identification and documentation of adult malnutrition (undernutrition). *J Acad Nutr Diet.* 2012; 112(5):730-738. doi.org/10.1016/j.jand.2012.03.012

17. McCabe-Sellers, B. Position of the American Dietetic Association: Integration of medical nutrition therapy and pharmacotherapy. *J Am Diet Assoc.* 2010 June; 110(6):950-956.

18. Couris R, Gura K, Blumberg J, Chernoff R. Pharmacology, nutrition and the elderly adult: Interactions and implications. In: Chernoff R, ed. *Geriatric Nutrition,* 4th ed. Burlington, MA: Jones & Bartlett Learning; 2014: 365–405.

19. American Medical Directors Association. *AMDA Clinical Practice Guidelines: Diabetes Management in the Long Term Care Setting.* Columbia, MD 2015.

20. Macpherson H, Lee J, Villalon L, Pase M, Pipingas, A, Schoola, A. The Influence of the Mediterranean Diet. In Preedy V, Watson R, ed. *Cognitive Health in the Mediterranean Diet: An Evidence-Based Approach.* Elsevier; New York, NY 2015:81-87.

21. American Diabetes Association. Older adults. Sec. 10. *In* Standards of Medical Care in Diabetes – 2015. *Diabetes Care.* 2015; 38(Suppl 1): S67-S69. DOI: 10.2337/dc15-S013.

22. Kalogeropoulos AP, Georgiopoulou VV, Murphy RA, et al. Dietary sodium content, mortality, and risk for cardiovascular events in older adults: the health, aging, and body composition (Health ABC) study. *JAMA Intern Med* 2015; 175(3): 410-419 doi: 10.1001/jamainternmed.2014.6278.

23. Zajacova A, Ailshire J. Body mass trajectories and mortality among older adults: a joint growth mixture-discrete-time survival analysis. *Gerontologist.* 2014; 54(2):221-231. doi: 10.1093/geront/gns164.

24. Flicker L, McCaul KA, Hankey GJ, et al. Body Mass Index and survival in men and women aged 70 to 75. *J Am Geriatric Soc.* 2010; 58(2):234–241.

25. Chernoff R. Carbohydrate, Fat, and Fluid Requirements in Older Adults. In: Chernoff R, ed. *Geriatric Nutrition,* 4th ed. Burlington, MA: Jones & Bartlett Learning; 2014:27-34.

26. U. S. Department of Health and Human Services and U. S. Department of Agriculture. *2015 – 2020 Dietary Guidelines for Americans,* 8th ed. http://health.gov/dietaryguidelines/2015/guidelines/ Published December 2015. Accessed January 13, 2016.

27. Padden-Jones D, Rasmussen B. Dietary protein recommendations and the prevention of sarcopenia. *Curr Opin Clin Nutr Metab Care.* 2009; 12(1): 86-90.

28. Houston DK, Tooze JA, Davis CC, et al. Serum 25-hydroxyvitamin D and physical function in older adults: the cardiovascular health study all stars. *J Am Geriatr* Soc 2011; 59(10): 1793-1801 doi: 10.1111/j.1532-5415.2011.03601.x

29. Institute of Medicine of the National Academies. http://www.iom.edu/Activities/Nutrition/SummaryDRIs/DRI-Tables.aspx Revised 2011. Accessed July 5, 2015.

30. Michelakos T, Kousoulis AA, Katsiardanis K, et al. Serum folate and B12 levels in association with cognitive impairments among seniors: results from the VELESTINKO study in Greece and meta-analysis. *J Aging Health.* 2013; 25(4)589-616. doi: 10.1177/0898264313482488

31. Allen L. How common is vitamin B12 deficiency: *Am J Clin* Nutri 2009; 89(2):693s-696s.

32. Vogel T, Dali-Youcef N, Kaltenbach G, Andrès E. Homocysteine, vitamin B12, folate and cognitive functions: a systematic and critical review of the literature. *Int J Clin Pract.* 2009; 63(7):1061–1067.

33. Academy of Nutrition and Dietetics Evidence Analysis Library. What is the best equation to estimate fluid requirements in adults 19 years and older? http://www.andeal.org/topic.cfm?cat=3217&conclusion_statement_id=250894&highlight=conclusion%20statement%20fluid&home=1 Accessed July 5, 2015.

34. Touger-Decker R, Mobley, C. Position of the Academy of Nutrition and Dietetics: Oral health and nutrition. *J Acad Nutr Diet.* 2013; 113(5):693-701.

35. Razak P, Richard K, Thankachan R, Hafiz K, Kumar K, Sameer K. Geriatric oral health: a review article. *J Int Oral Health* 2014; 6(6): 110-116.

36. Centers for Medicare & Medicaid. *State Operations Manual*, Appendix PP. Tag 368 Frequency of Meals. www.cms.gov/Manuals/Downloads/som107ap_pp_guidelines_ltcf.pdf Page 522 Accessed July 5, 2015.

37. Wagnerberger S, Kanuri G, Bergheim I. Alcohol drinking patterns and nutrition in alcoholic liver disease, trends. In: Shimizu I, ed. *Trends in Alcoholic Liver Disease Research-Clinical and Scientific Aspects.* InTech 2012.

ADDITIONAL RESOURCES

Centers for Medicare & Medicaid Services website. MDS 3.0 RAI Manual. https://www.cms.gov/Medicare/Quality-Initiatives-Patient-Assessment-Instruments/NursingHomeQualityInits/MDS30RAIManual.html

Study Guide Questions

A. During pregnancy, special attention should be paid to intakes of what micronutrients (vitamins and minerals) to ensure adequacy?

B. List 3 foods naturally high in folate.

C. What are three nutritional advantages for infants who are breastfed?

D. What safety precautions should be taken when feeding a child younger than 1 year of age?

E. Describe in detail at least three diet principles to consider when developing menus for school-aged children.

F. What are 3 common concerns associated with feeding young children and a possible solution for each?

G. List at least three key factors that contribute to increased nutritional risk for the older adult.

H. Describe in detail at least three guidelines for implementing food plans for the older adult.

I. Using the icons from MyPlate for Older Adults as a guide, plan an entire day's menu for an 1800-calorie diet. Include specific foods and portion sizes to meet the minimum recommended serving for each food category.

J. Discussion question: Why is it is so difficult to meet the nutrient needs of the elderly with diet alone and what can be done to promote nutrient density in foods?

Study Guide Suggested Responses can be found in Appendix 15.

Consistency Altered Diets

Altering the consistency of foods can greatly relieve problems related to chewing, managing food in the mouth, and swallowing. These problems may be due to stroke, head or neck injury, cancer, cerebral palsy, dementia, and other illness, or simply the result of aging. Aspiration (inhaling) of food or fluids into the lungs as a result of inadequate chewing and swallowing is now recognized as a major contribution to respiratory infections and pneumonia among institutionalized children and adults.

Difficulties in chewing and swallowing are often diagnosed as dysphagia, which occurs among all age groups but is seen more often among the elderly. It should be emphasized that the evaluation and treatment of dysphagia requires a team approach, which includes a physician, a swallowing therapist (speech language pathologist or occupational therapist), a registered dietitian nutritionist (RDN), and a nurse.

Treatment plans are designed to promote the safest texture level to prevent further aspiration events. Goals include returning to previously tolerated food and fluid consistency, or maintaining the best tolerated consistency of food and fluids without additional aspiration events. Treatment may include oral motor exercises, changes in eating techniques, and altering the consistency of food and fluids. The RDN and swallowing therapist will work closely together in assessing, recommending, and implementing the necessary texture changes on an individual client basis.

Before making major changes in food and/or fluid consistency, all possible factors contributing to the chewing and swallowing problems should be evaluated. Proper positioning during eating and drinking is essential to prevent aspiration. Food served must be well prepared, flavorful, and appealing. Appropriate assistive devices such as modified spoons, forks, and cups can make self-feeding easier.

PRINCIPLES OF CONSISTENCY ALTERATION

1. The goals of consistency alteration are to allow individuals to consume adequate nutrients and fluids to maintain nutritional status, reduce the risk of choking and aspiration, and provide food and fluids at the least restrictive level. The chewing and swallowing ability should be evaluated before prescribing a consistency altered diet. The consistency of foods included in any modified diet can be altered.

2. Extensive individualization to meet energy, nutrient, and consistency of food and fluid needs is essential. Modifications in either solid foods and/or liquids may be necessary to achieve optimal nutritional status. Based on complete assessment of chewing and swallowing ability, diets can include combinations of unaltered solid foods, mechanically soft foods, and pureed foods. Individuals vary greatly in chewing and swallowing ability.

3. Monitor food and fluid intake closely as intakes are often decreased due to reduced ability to tolerate or accept the altered consistency. Foods of high nutrient density should be included when inadequate oral intake is observed; refer to the High Nutrient Diet in Chapter 12.

4. Adequate fluid intake is essential. Close monitoring of those individuals on thickened liquids for signs and symptoms of dehydration is necessary. A free water protocol may be ordered in some instances (see page page 49).

5. Nutritional supplementation may be necessary to ensure adequate hydration and nutritional status. Oral intake of foods and fluids should be evaluated prior to implementing nutrition supplements. Additionally, some individuals may require a multivitamin supplement.

6. Some individuals may require additional nutrition support such as a tube feeding when swallowing problems are too severe to maintain adequate nutrition and/or hydration.

7. An individual's ability to chew and swallow safely may or may not improve. Reevaluation of chewing and swallowing capabilities should be conducted regularly with adjustments made in texture modification to meet the current skill level.

MECHANICAL SOFT DIET

Use

The use of this diet is for individuals who have difficulty chewing but are able to tolerate a wide variety of foods. Modifications in the diet need to be individualized according to the person's needs. The Mechanical Soft Diet may be used for individuals with missing teeth, ill-fitting dentures, and other chewing problems; it may be useful for individuals with esophageal stricture (narrowing of the esophagus).

Adequacy

The suggested food plan includes foods in amounts that will provide the Dietary Reference Intakes (DRIs) by the National Academy of Sciences for the adult if the individual consumes the proper amount and variety of foods.

Diet Principles

The Mechanical Soft Diet is designed to permit easy chewing. The General Diet is modified in consistency and texture by cooking, grinding, chopping, mincing, or mashing. The diet includes foods soft in texture such as cooked fruits and vegetables, moist ground meat, and soft bread and cereal products. Foods that "dissolve" readily when held in the mouth such as graham crackers and some ready-to-eat cereals are also appropriate. It is most important to individualize or adjust it to the tolerance of the individual.

Table 3.1 Mechanical Soft Diet

Food for the Day	Recommended	Avoid
Vegetables *1–4 cups*	Soft, cooked, tender, chopped, shredded vegetables. Creamed corn. Vegetable juice. Shredded lettuce.*	Most raw or undercooked vegetables and those with tough skins. Whole kernel corn and peas. Fried vegetables.
Fruits *1–2.5 cups*	Fruit juice and nectars. Cooked, tender, canned fruits. Chopped seedless ripe melon, ripe banana or other soft, raw fruits. Crushed pineapple.	Dried fruits. Coconut. Chunk pineapple. Fruit with tough skin such as whole grapes.
Grains *3–10 ounce-equivalents* *At least half of which are whole grains.*	Plain, soft breads, rolls, muffins, lightly toasted bread. Plain crackers. Cooked cereal and well-soaked dry cereals. Pastas, rice.	Breads, rolls, muffins with dry, hard crusts. Any containing seeds, nuts, dried fruits, coconut. Popcorn. Most granola-type cereals. Wild rice.

*avoid lettuce with esophageal stricture

Continued on next page

Table 3.1 Mechanical Soft Diet Continued from previous page

Food for the Day	Recommended	Avoid
Dairy Products *2–3 cups*	Milk, nondairy milks (soy, almond, rice), yogurt and cottage cheese, cheese.	Any containing nuts, seeds, pieces of fruit.
Protein Foods *2–7 ounce-equivalents*	Very tender, shredded or ground meats and poultry, moistened with gravy or sauce. Well-moistened fish. Eggs. Soft or mashed beans. Meat, fish, or egg salads without celery/onion chunks.	Whole meats and poultry. Hot dogs, bacon. Meats with thick hard breading. Dry or tough meats. Dry fish or fish with bones. Crunchy peanut butter. Tough legumes.
Oils, Solid Fats, Added Sugars	Butter, margarine, oils, mayonnaise. Plain, soft cookies, donuts, cakes. Soft pies, puddings, cheese cake, plain ice cream, sherbet, gelatin. Cheese puffs.	Any containing nuts, coconut, dried fruit. Bacon, olives. Dry, hard, crunchy, chunky or sticky products such as chips and pretzels.
Fluids/Soups	All.	No restrictions. Must evaluate any with lumps, chunks, or seeds.

PUREED DIET

Use

The Pureed Diet is designed for individuals with moderate to severe dysphagia, and for individuals with poor dentition, minimal or no ability to chew.

Adequacy

The suggested food plan includes foods in amounts that will provide the DRIs recommended by the National Academy of Sciences for the adult, if the individual consumes the proper amount and variety.

Diet Principles

1. The Pureed Diet is designed to permit easy swallowing and requires minimal or no chewing.

2. The General Diet or other appropriate diet is modified in consistency by pureeing or modifying foods to a smooth consistency. Some foods may need to be thickened after they are pureed (e.g., melon or tossed salad) to achieve desired consistency.

3. To improve appearance and appetite appeal, foods may be slurried (moistening foods and retaining their shape).

4. Individuals vary in their abilities to handle different puree consistencies. Thickeners or thinning liquids are useful in adapting pureed foods to individual needs.

5. It is most important to customize or adjust it to the tolerance of the individual.

Table 3.2 Pureed Diet

Food for the Day	Recommended	Avoid
Vegetables *1–4 cups*	Pureed vegetables without lumps. Mashed potatoes without lumps. Vegetable juices.	All vegetables that are not pureed.
Fruits *1–2.5 cups*	Pureed fruits without lumps. Fruit juice and nectars. Raw, ripe banana—mashed.	Dried fruits. Coconut. All non-pureed fruit except bananas.
Grains *3–10 ounce-equivalents*	Pureed or slurried breads, rolls, muffins. Plain crackers, if crushed and moistened. Moistened cracker or bread crumbs. Smooth, lump-free cooked cereals. Pureed oatmeal. Milk toast. Pureed pastas and rice.	Any containing seeds, nuts, dried fruits, coconut. Popcorn. Wild rice. Dry cereal.
Dairy Products *2–3 cups*	Milk, nondairy milks (soy, almond, rice), smooth yogurt. Smooth cheese paste such as smooth ricotta. Pureed cottage cheese. Cheese sauce.	Any containing nuts, seeds, pieces of fruit. All solid cheese.
Protein Foods *2–7 ounce-equivalents*	Pureed meats, pureed scrambled eggs. Smooth hummus or pureed lentils/legumes. Moistened soft tofu.	Meat, fish, poultry, legumes or lentils that are not pureed.
Oils, Solid Fats, Added Sugars	Most fats present no problem, for example butter, margarine, oils, mayonnaise. Plain puddings, custards, cheese cake, plain ice cream, sherbet, yogurt, gelatin, jelly. Plain cakes and cookies soaked in milk or juice.	Any containing nuts, olives, coconut, chocolate chips, bacon or other coarse or chunky pieces. Pastries, pies; any containing nuts, coconut, raisins. Jams with seeds or lumps. Fruit leather rolls.
Fluids/Soups	Soups that have been pureed or strained to remove lumps.	Any containing lumps, chunks, or seeds.

Note: **The National Dysphagia Diet** is no longer in print, therefore, it could not be printed in this edition of the Simplified Diet Manual. The Dysphagia Diet below may be used as a transition from pureed textures to mechanical soft textures.

DYSPHAGIA DIET

Use

This diet is a transition from the pureed textures to mechanical soft textures. Chewing ability is required; biting is not required. The textures on this level are appropriate for individuals with mild to moderate oral or pharyngeal dysphagia. Individuals should be assessed for tolerance to mixed textures. It is expected that some mixed textures are tolerated on this diet.

Adequacy

The suggested food plan includes foods in amounts that will provide the DRIs recommended by the National Academy of Sciences for the adult, if the individual consumes the proper amount and variety.

Diet Principles

This diet consists of foods that are moist, soft-textured, and easily formed into a bolus. No hard, tough, dry, crunchy, or chewy textures are allowed. Meats are ground or are minced no larger than ¼-inch pieces; they should be moist or served with a gravy or sauce to increase moisture. It is important to individualize or adjust it to the tolerance of the individual.

The diet was developed using the following resources: National Dysphagia Diets (1), International Dysphagia Diet Standardization Initiative (2) and Australian Standardised Terminology and Definitions for Texture Modified Foods and Fluids (3). All foods from the pureed diet are acceptable.

Food Textures for Dysphagia Diet

Table 3.3 Dysphagia Diet (1, 2, 3)

Food for the Day	Recommended	Avoid
Vegetables *1–4 cups*	All tender, well-cooked vegetables. Vegetables should be <½ inch. Should be easily mashed with a fork. Vegetable juices*. Well-cooked, moistened, boiled, baked, or mashed potatoes.	All raw vegetables. Corn, peas, broccoli, cabbage, Brussels sprouts, asparagus, or other fibrous, nontender or rubbery vegetables. Potato skins and chips. Fried or French-fried potatoes.
Fruits *1–2.5 cups*	Soft, drained, diced canned, or cooked fruits without seeds or skin. Fresh soft/ripe banana, seedless melon, or mango. Should be easily mashed with a fork. Fruit juices* and nectar*.	Fruit pieces larger than ½ inch. Fresh fruits except soft/ripe banana, seedless melon, and mango. Cooked fruit with skin or seeds. Frozen or dried fruits. Fresh, canned, or cooked pineapple. Whole round fruits such as grapes and cherries.
Grains *3–10 ounce-equivalents*	Moistened cracker or bread crumbs. Soft pancakes, well moistened with syrup or sauce. Pureed bread mixes, *pregelled* or *slurried* breads that are gelled through entire thickness. Cooked cereals with no hard lumps, including oatmeal (soft tender lumps less than ½ inch acceptable).	Bread, crackers. Whole-grain dry or coarse cereals. Cereals with nuts, seeds, dried fruit and/or coconut. Rice. Hard pieces or crusts formed during baking or cooking such as bread dressing.

Continued on next page

Table 3.3 Dysphagia Diet (1, 2, 3) Continued from previous page

Food for the Day	Recommended	Avoid
Grains *(Continued)*	Slightly moistened dry cereals with little texture such as corn flakes, crispy rice. Note: if thin liquids are restricted, it is important that all of the liquid is absorbed into the cereal. Milk/liquid should not separate off. Soft, moist pieces of pasta in a sauce such as moist macaroni and cheese.	
Dairy Products *2–3 cups*	Milk*, smooth yogurt, soft cheese with small lumps such as small-curd cottage cheese.	Any containing nuts, seeds, cereal, or pieces of hard fruit. Cheese slices and cubes.
Protein Foods *2–7 ounce-equivalents* *Meat pieces should not exceed ¼ inch cube and should be moist and tender.*	Moistened ground or cooked meat, poultry, or fish. Moist ground or tender meat may be served with gravy or sauce. Fish soft enough to break into small pieces with a fork. Casseroles without rice. Moist macaroni and cheese, well-cooked pasta with meat sauce, tuna-noodle casserole, soft, moist lasagna. Moist meatballs, meat loaf, or fish loaf. Protein salads such as tuna or egg without large chunks, celery, or onion. Smooth quiche or soufflé without large chunks. Poached, scrambled, or soft-cooked eggs (egg yolks should be moist and mashable with margarine, or other moisture added to them). (Cook eggs to 155°F or use pasteurized eggs for safety). Hummus and soft tofu. Well-cooked, slightly mashed, moist legumes such as baked beans.	Dry meats, tough meats (such as bacon, sausage, hot dogs, bratwurst). Dry casseroles or casseroles with rice or large chunks. Peanut butter and nuts. Hard-cooked or crisp fried eggs. Sandwiches. Pizza.
Oils, Solid Fats	Butter, margarine, cream*, gravy, cream sauces, mayonnaise, salad dressings, cream cheese, cream cheese spreads with soft additives, sour cream, sour cream dips with soft additives, whipped toppings.	All fats with coarse or chunky additives.

Continued on next page

Table 3.3 Dysphagia Diet (1, 2, 3) Continued from previous page

Food for the Day	Recommended	Avoid
Added Sugars/ Desserts	Pudding, custard.	Dry, coarse cakes and cookies.
	Soft fruit based desserts **without** hard bases, crumbly or flaky pastry.	Anything containing nuts, seeds, coconut, chocolate chips, rhubarb, pineapple, large hard fruit pieces, or dried fruit.
	Soft, moist cakes with icing or "slurried" cakes.	
	Pregelled cookies or soft, moist cookies that have been "dunked" in milk, coffee, or other liquid.	Rice pudding.
		Hard pieces or crusts formed during baking or cooking such as bread pudding.
	If thin liquids allowed, also may have: Ice cream, sherbet, shakes, nutritional supplements, frozen yogurt, and other ices.	
	Plain gelatin or gelatin with canned fruit, excluding pineapple.	
Fluids/Soup*	Soups* with easy-to-chew or easy-to-swallow meats or vegetables: meat in soups should be <¼ inch and vegetables should be <½ inch.	Soups with large chunks of meat and vegetables.
		Soups containing rice, corn, peas, or legumes.
	All beverages* with minimal amounts of texture, pulp, etc. (Any texture should be suspended in the liquid and should not precipitate out.)	
Miscellaneous	Jams and preserves without seeds or dried fruit, jelly.	Seeds, nuts, coconut, sticky foods.
	Sauces, salsas, etc., that may have small tender chunks <½ inch.	Chewy candies such as caramel and licorice.
	Soft, smooth chocolate bars that are easily chewed.	Popcorn.

*Liquids may need to be thickened to recommended consistency.

** Thickener may be added to achieve desired consistency.

Table 3.4 Sample Menus for Consistency Altered Diets Compared to General Diet

Meal	General	Mechanical Soft	Dysphagia	Pureed
Breakfast	½ c. orange juice	½ c. orange juice*	½ c. orange juice*	½ c. orange juice*
	1 scrambled egg	1 scrambled egg	1 moist scrambled egg pureed with 3 Tbsp. bread crumbs	1 moist scrambled egg pureed with 3 Tbsp. bread crumbs
	½ c. oatmeal	½ c. oatmeal	½ c. oatmeal (no hard lumps)	½ c. oatmeal, pureed
	1 slice whole wheat toast	1 slice whole wheat toast	1 tsp. soft margarine	1 tsp. soft margarine
	2 tsp. jelly	2 tsp. jelly	1 c. milk*	1 c. milk*
	1 tsp. soft margarine	1 tsp. soft margarine	Hot beverage*	Hot beverage*
	1 c. milk	1 c. milk*	Sugar, pepper (optional)	Sugar, pepper (optional)
	Hot beverage	Hot beverage*		
	Sugar, pepper (optional)	Sugar, pepper (optional)		
Lunch	2 oz. roasted chicken	2 oz. roasted chicken, ground	2 oz. roasted chicken, ground	2 oz. roasted chicken, pureed with 3 Tbsp. bread crumbs
	½ c. mashed potatoes with 2 oz. gravy	½ c. mashed potatoes with 2 oz. gravy	½ c. mashed potatoes with 2 oz. gravy	½ c. mashed potatoes with 2 oz. gravy
	½ c. mixed vegetables	½ c. mixed vegetables, no corn or peas, tender	½ c. cooked carrots, tender, diced	½ c. mixed vegetables, pureed
	1 oz. wheat roll	1 oz. wheat roll	1 oz. wheat roll, slurried	1 tsp. soft margarine
	1 tsp. soft margarine	1 tsp. soft margarine	1 tsp. soft margarine	1 c. milk*
	1 c. milk	1 c. milk*	1 c. milk*	Water*
	Water	Water*	Water*	
Supper	2 oz. tuna on 2 slices whole wheat bread, 2 tsp. mayonnaise	2 oz. tuna on 2 slices whole wheat bread, 2 tsp. mayonnaise	2 oz. tuna, ½ cup cooked tender pasta, mayonnaise to moisten	2 oz. tuna, 2 slices wheat bread and 2 tsp. mayonnaise, pureed
	2 tomato slices	½ c. tomatoes, chopped	6 oz. tomato soup*	2 slices tomato, 1 cup leafy green salad and 1 Tbsp. salad dressing, pureed**
	1 c. leafy greens salad	1 c. leafy greens, shredded	½ c. cooked green beans, tender, <½ inch long	
	1 Tbsp. salad dressing	1 Tbsp. salad dressing	½ c. peaches, canned, drained, diced	½ c. fruit cocktail, pureed
	½ c. fruit cocktail	½ c. fruit cocktail (without grapes)	1 c. milk*	1 c. milk*
	1 c. milk	1 c. milk*	Water*	Water*
	Water	Water*		

Continued on next page

Table 3.4 Sample Menus for Consistency Altered Diets Compared to General Diet
Continued from previous page

Meal	General	Mechanical Soft	Dysphagia	Pureed
Snacks	½ c. cantaloupe ½ c. carrots 3 c. popcorn	½ c. cantaloupe, soft, bite size pieces ½ c. vegetable juice* 1 sugar cookie, soft	½ c. soft ripe cantaloupe, diced ½ c. vegetable juice* 1 sugar cookie, soaked	½ c. cantaloupe, pureed** ½ c. vegetable juice* 1 sugar cookie, soaked

*Liquids may need to be thickened to recommended consistency.

** Thickener may be added to achieve desired consistency.

LIQUID CONSISTENCY LEVELS

Individuals with swallowing difficulty can often handle thickened beverages better than normal thin fluids such as water, milk, soup, or coffee. However, not everyone needs thickened liquids. The following terms and definitions are used to prescribe the appropriate consistency for liquids based on individual needs.

Definitions of Terms Used for Thickened Liquids

Table 3.7 Definitions and Terms Used for Thickened Liquids (1, 2, 3)

Thin or unmodified	Unmodified fluids do not have thickeners added to them. May drink by cup or straw.
Nectar-like or mildly thick	Fluids at this thickness run fast through the prongs of a fork and flow off a spoon. May be drank from a cup. Effort is required to drink from a straw.
Honey-like or moderately thick	Fluids at this thickness slowly drip through the prongs of a fork. Possible to drink from a cup but is difficult to drink from a straw.
Spoon-thick or pudding-like or extremely thick	There is no flow and it does not pour or go through the prongs of a fork. These fluids keep their shape on a spoon but will fall off the spoon when it is tilted. It is not possible to drink from a cup or straw. Spooning into the mouth is the best way to take this liquid. The spoon should NOT be able to stand upright in fluids at this thickness.

Liquids that change thickness at room temperature or body temperature may not be appropriate for persons on thickened liquids. Examples include milkshakes, ice cream, sherbet, frozen yogurt, and gelatin. A variety of commercial thickeners are available to modify liquids' consistencies. Follow the manufacturer's directions to achieve the preferred thickness.

FREE WATER PROTOCOLS

Thin water may be offered to individuals with thin liquid aspiration if a Free Water Protocol (FWP) is ordered. Aspiration of water does not necessarily lead to pneumonia. (4) Small amounts of water taken into the lungs are quickly absorbed in the body. (5) There is evidence that aspiration of thickened liquids (compared to thin liquids), and poor oral health/hygiene are more likely to lead to pneumonia. (6) Research has shown that persons on thickened liquids are more likely to become dehydrated. Persons with low mobility and severe neurological dysfunction are at higher risk of aspiration and are not good candidates for a FWP. (7)

A swallowing therapist is involved in assessing if a person is appropriate for a FWP. It needs to be determined if the person can follow the protocol independently or will require supervision. The FWP is initiated after receiving a physician order. Education to the individual, family, and staff is essential for success. Two commonly used FWP are the Frazier Water Protocol (5) and the GF Strong Water Protocol (6)

General guidelines for FWPs:

- Oral care is done first thing in the morning, before oral intake, after meals and snacks, and at bedtime. The mouth must be free of food particles before drinking water.

- Water from a cup is allowed between meals and after oral care.

- Water intake is **not** allowed during meals or snacks, or within 30 minutes following a meal or snack.

- The prescribed thickened liquid is provided with meals, snacks, and pills.

FOOD AND BEVERAGE PREPARATION TIPS

Thickeners for Consistency Altered Foods

A variety of methods and special products are available to prepare a wide range of food consistencies. Thickeners for pureed foods and liquids include:

For pureed foods:

- Commercial food thickeners, bread and cracker crumbs, instant potato flakes, instant infant cereal, and instant pudding mixes are good nutritious thickeners.

For liquids:

- Commercial thickeners, instant pudding mix, and instant potato flakes are acceptable thickeners. Yogurt, applesauce, and puddings are also acceptable, however they increase the volume of the products considerably; these may not be good choices for persons with poor appetite. Prethickened beverages are available.

- Addition of thickening agents, irrespective of type, to orally ingested fluids does not significantly alter the absorption rate of water from the gut. Client acceptance is always a concern. Introducing a new thickened beverage such as lemon-flavored thickened water or thickened fruit juice may be more acceptable than offering thickened coffee or milk, which would have a different mouth feel than is usually expected with those flavors.

Preparation of Texture Altered Foods

Because diminished appetite is often present in individuals requiring texture modification, it is of utmost importance that the food be prepared to enhance its natural flavor. Every attempt should be made to make the food as palatable as possible. Every effort should be made to minimize the total volume necessary to provide nutritional adequacy. Foods should be served as separate entities, on attractive dishes, garnished appropriately, and served at correct temperatures.

To achieve the desired consistency, use a food processor or immersion blender. Foods with a variety of consistencies can be prepared with the addition of very little liquid. The traditional blender usually requires more liquids, which dilutes nutrient density and increases the volume of foods.

Soaking or moistening recognizable foods in liquids, gravies, and slurries helps maintain their appeal. A slurry is a combination of a commercial thickener, common thickener, or gelatin, with liquids such as milk, juice, or broth. Slurries can be obtained by using 1 to 4 tablespoons of thickener or gelatin to 2 cups of liquid.

Cookies and cakes without nuts and chips can be soaked in milk. Bread or biscuits soaked in gravy, or pancakes soaked in syrup or slurry are often well tolerated. A slurry can also be used to moisten and soften such foods as bread, cakes, cookies, or crackers. In addition, it is used to gel pureed foods. This allows an individual to consume food items that are not routinely part of the puree texture modification. Before serving a dry, crumbly food with added slurry, be sure the slurry soaks through the entire thickness of the food.

Method for Determining the Portion Sizes of Consistency Altered Foods

Foods often change in volume when they have been modified in consistency and texture. To ensure that nutritional adequacy is maintained, the following guidelines may be used when several portions of a consistency altered food are needed. Puree is used in this example.

1. Measure out desired number of servings into container for pureeing. Puree the food. Add any necessary thickener or liquid to obtain desired consistency. In most cases, it is desirable to maintain or increase the caloric value of consistency altered foods. When thinning foods use liquids that add to the nutritional value as well as the flavor of foods. Appropriate liquids include milk, fruit or vegetable juice, broth, gravy, cream sauce, and liquid nutrient supplements. Plain water is not recommended for thinning.

2. Measure the volume of the food after it has been pureed.

3. Divide the total volume of the pureed food by the original number of portions. This is the new portion size. Note: Some foods may have a smaller, rather than larger, portion after pureeing.

4. After dividing portions, foods must be reheated or chilled to serving temperature per Hazard Analysis and Critical Control Points (HACCP) guidelines.

REFERENCES

1. American Dietetic Association. National Dysphagia Diet Task Force. *National Dysphagia Diet: standardization for optimal care.* Chicago, IL: American Dietetic Association; 2002.

2. IDDSI detailed descriptions. International Dysphagia Diet Initiative website. http://iddsi.org/wp-content/uploads/2015/06/IDDSI_Detailed_Descriptions.pdf Published June 2015. Accessed September 7, 2015.

3. Dietitians Association of Australia and The Speech Pathology Association of Australia Limited. Texture-modified foods and thickened fluids as used for individuals with dysphagia: Australian standardized labels and definitions. *Nutrition and Dietetics.* 2007; 64:S53-S76. doi: 10.1111/j.1747-0080.2007.00153.x

4. Frey KL, Ramsberger G. Comparison of outcomes before and after implementation of a water protocol for patients with cerebrovascular accident and dysphagia. *J Neurosci Nurs.* 2011; 43(3):165-171. doi: 10.1097/JNN.0b013e3182135adf

5. Frazier water protocol. KentuckyOne Health website. http://www.kentuckyonehealth.org/frazier-water-protocol Published 2015. Accessed September 7, 2015.

6. Carlaw C, Finlayson H, Beggs K, et al. Outcomes of a pilot water protocol project in a rehabilitation setting. *Dysphagia.* 2012; 27(3): 297–306.

7. Karagiannis MJP, Chivers L, Karagiannis TC. Effects of oral intake of water in patients with oropharyngeal dysphagia. *BMC Geriatrics.* 2011; 11:9 doi:10.1186/1471-2318-11-9

ADDITIONAL RESOURCES

Sharpe K, Ward L, Cichero J, Sopade P, Halley P. Thickened fluids and water absorption in rats and humans. *Dysphagia.* 2007; 22(3):193–203.

Can You Swallow This? A Practical Approach to Dysphagia. POGOe - Portal of Geriatrics Online Education website. 2014. https://pogoe.org/productid/21760

Clinical Corner: Oral Health. AMDA website. http://www.amda.com/tools/clinical/oralhealth.cfm

Study Guide Questions

    A. List three possible causes of dysphagia.

    B. Explain how various professional healthcare disciplines should be involved in the evaluation, treatment, and plan of care for individuals with dysphagia.

    C. Describe in detail four of the seven Principles of Consistency Alteration.

    D. List the four liquid consistencies served to individuals diagnosed with dysphagia.

    E. Using the previously planned general menu for the older adult, modify the menu to accommodate a Mechanical Soft diet requiring nectar-like liquids.

    F. Describe the method for determining accuracy of portion sizes of consistency altered foods after measuring the final volume. Why is this important?

    G. Discussion question: What can be done to make sure foods offered on consistency altered diets are as palatable and eye-appealing as possible?

Study Guide Suggested Responses can be found in Appendix 15.

Liquid Diets and Modifications

4

CLEAR LIQUID DIET

Use

The Clear Liquid Diet has been used to prevent dehydration in the following situations:

- In gastrointestinal illness, including abdominal distention, nausea, and vomiting.
- In conditions when it is necessary to minimize fecal residue, such as bowel preparation for surgery or a gastrointestinal procedure.
- To reintroduce foods following a period with no oral intake when poor tolerance or aspiration is anticipated.

Research has shown that, for postoperative[*] patients, there was no difference in tolerance whether provided a Clear Liquid Diet or Regular (General) Diet. (1)

Adequacy

This diet is inadequate in all nutrients for persons of all ages. It is used only when absolutely necessary. It should not be used more than 3 days without supplementation. Commercial clear liquid oral supplements may provide a source of protein and additional vitamins and minerals, but they are not intended as a sole source of nutrition. Some facilities allow hard candy on a clear liquid diet because it provides variety, flavor, and dissolves to sugar and water at body temperature. (4) However, sugar-free hard candies sweetened with sugar alcohols (e.g., sorbitol) should be used with caution because these ingredients have a laxative effect.

Note: A commercial elemental or semi-elemental formula may be useful if a clear liquid regimen is necessary for more than 3 days or if the patient has digestion or malabsorption problems.

Diet Principles

This diet is composed of clear liquids, traditionally that are transparent and liquid at body temperature, and largely composed of water, sugar, and/or salt. It is designed to provide fluids without stimulating extensive digestive processes, to relieve thirst, and to initiate oral feedings that will promote a gradual return to a normal intake of food. Small servings may be offered every 2 or 3 hours and at mealtime. See Chapter 6 for information on liquid diets for persons with diabetes mellitus.

---

[*] The Post-surgical Diet has been removed from the diet manual. It was traditionally prescribed when it is decided the post-surgical patient was ready to have some whole foods but was not yet ready for a routine diet. With decrease in length of hospital stays, and tendency toward early postoperative discharge, a step-wise progression from liquid diets to solid food is no longer practical or necessary. However, diet progression should be carefully evaluated in patients with significant bowel resections, strictures, fistula, or motility disorders (2). In addition, some patients were excluded from some studies (e.g., those undergoing emergent surgery, those with prior intestinal resections, and those with perforation or abscess with associated sepsis) (3). See Diet Progression for Gastroparesis in Chapter 6.

Table 4.1 Clear Liquid

Food for the Day	
Fruits	Strained fruit juices: apple, cherry, cranapple, cranberry, crangrape, grape, orange, grapefruit, lemon, lime.
Soup	Fat-free clear broth and bouillon.
Added Sugars	Flavored and unflavored gelatin; Popsicles®; fruit ice made without milk; sugar, honey, syrup; hard candy; sugar substitutes*.
Fluids	Coffee, tea, carbonated beverages, clear fruit beverage drinks, clear liquid nutritional supplement beverage drinks, sports drinks.

* Sugar alcohols (e.g., sorbitol) should be used with caution because these ingredients have a laxative effect.

Table 4.2 Sample Menu for Clear Liquid Diet

Breakfast	Supper
½ c. fruit juice	½ c. fruit juice
6 oz broth	6 oz broth
4 oz gelatin	4 oz gelatin
8 oz tea or coffee	1 Popsicle®
	8 oz tea or coffee
Lunch	**Snack Ideas**
½ c. fruit juice	½ c. fruit juice
6 oz broth	4 oz gelatin
4 oz gelatin	Popsicle®
1 Popsicle®	Clear liquid nutritional supplement
8 oz tea or coffee	

FULL LIQUID DIET

Use

The Full Liquid Diet may be prescribed for short-term use after oral surgery or for persons with gastroparesis (see Chapter 6). The Full Liquid Diet has traditionally been prescribed for short-term use as a transition step for the postoperative patient between the clear liquid and general diet. However, a review of the literature reveals there is no data to support the use of a full liquid diet as part of a postoperative diet progression, and it is not even mentioned in a recent literature review. (1) For patients with chewing or swallowing difficulties, consistency altered diets are recommended (see Chapter 3).

Adequacy

Depending on the amount and choice of food eaten, this diet can be adequate in energy, protein, and fat but may be inadequate in vitamins, minerals, and fiber. It is recommended for temporary use only. A daily multivitamin/mineral supplement or commercial nutritional supplement is recommended if the diet continues for more than 5 days.

Diet Principles

1. The Full Liquid Diet includes foods that are liquid at body temperature and tolerated by the patient. It includes all of the foods allowed on the clear liquid diet with the addition of milk and dairy products, strained soups, refined thin cooked cereal, and pureed fruit without seeds.

2. Because the diet typically includes many milk-containing foods, it may need modification for individuals who do not tolerate lactose. Acidophilus milk, buttermilk, lactose-free milk, other lactose-free dairy products, soymilk, or plain yogurt may be tolerated, and lactose-free medical nutritional supplement beverages can be useful.

3. Low-fat or fat-free dairy products should be considered for individuals' not tolerating fat. Modifications in carbohydrate levels may also be necessary for people with diabetes mellitus or hypoglycemia (see Chapter 6).

Table 4.3 Full Liquid

Food for the Day	
Vegetables *1 cup or more*	Potato, strained in cream soups; other mild-flavored vegetables, such as asparagus, beets or carrots, strained and combined with clear broth, cream soup, plain or flavored gelatin; vegetable juices.
Fruits *1 cup or more*	Fruit juices and nectars; pureed fruit without seeds.
Grains *1 or more servings*	Refined or strained cooked cereals that have been thinned with hot milk or hot half-and-half.
Dairy Products *2-3 servings*	As a beverage and in cooking; milk in milk drinks, such as eggnog, milk shake, malted milk or hot cocoa; in strained cream soups; yogurt without fruit pieces or seeds.
Protein Foods *2–7 ounce-equivalents*	Eggs* in eggnog, soft custard; pureed meat added to broth or cream soup.
Added Sugars	Sugar, honey, sugar substitutes**, syrup.
Fluids	Coffee, tea, carbonated beverages, flavored waters, sports drinks.
Other	Broth or strained cream soup combined with allowed strained vegetables; soft or baked custard, flavored and unflavored gelatin, plain ice cream, pudding, sherbet, Popsicles®, fruit ices, flavorings and mild spices in moderation; nutritional supplement beverages.

* Do not serve raw egg. Use blended baked custard, soft custard with added milk, or a commercial mixture that is pasteurized.

** Sugar alcohols (e.g., sorbitol) should be used with caution because these ingredients have a laxative effect.

Table 4.4 Sample Menu for Full Liquid Diet

Breakfast	Supper
½ c. fruit juice	6 oz soup*
8 oz thinned, cooked cereal with cream, sugar	½ c. pureed fruit
8 oz milk or milk beverage	½ c. pureed vegetable
6 oz tea or coffee	½ c. fruit or vegetable juice
	½ c. pudding or custard
	8 oz milk or milk beverage
Lunch	**Snack Ideas**
6 oz soup*	½ c. fruit juice
½ c. pureed fruit	½ c. pureed fruit
½ c. pureed vegetable	6 oz yogurt, smooth
½ c. fruit or vegetable juice	8 oz milk or milk beverage
½ c. strawberry ice cream, smooth	Nutritional supplement
8 oz milk or milk beverage	

*Soups may be fortified with dry milk, pureed meat and vegetables, and a fat serving. Note: canned soups are higher in sodium.

REFERENCES

1. Warren J, Bhalia V, Cresci G. Postoperative diet advancement: surgical dogma vs evidenced-based medicine. *Nutr Clin Pract.* 2011; 26(2):115-125.

2. Toulson Davisson Correia MI, Costa Fonseca P, Machado Cruz GA. Perioperative nutritional management of patients undergoing laparotomy. *Nutr Hosp.* 2009; 24(4):479-484.

3. Willcutts K. Pre-op NPO and traditional post-op diet advancement: time to move on. *Pract Gastroenterol.* 2010; December:16-27.

4. Academy of Nutrition and Dietetics. Nutrition Care Manual. Clear Liquids. https://www.nutritioncaremanual.org/topic.cfm?ncm_category_id=1&ncm_toc_id=255536&ncm_heading=Nutrition%20Care&ncm_content_id=110846#ClearLiquidDietInformation. Accessed September 21, 2015.

ENTERAL NUTRITION

Use

Enteral nutrition (tube feeding) may be prescribed for persons who are physically or psychologically unable to take food by mouth in amounts that will meet nutrient requirements. Enteral nutrition can either supplement a person's inadequate oral intake or it can provide the sole source of nutrition. Enteral nutrition must be closely monitored by a Registered Dietitian Nutritionist (RDN).

Adequacy

Most enteral feedings will be nutritionally adequate when given in recommended amounts, but it is important to evaluate each person individually.

Diet Principles

1. **Selection.** Choice of an enteral feeding product depends on the medical and nutritional needs of the individual as determined by the physician and dietitian. The individual's condition and nutritional status and requirements must be identified and then compared to formulas available. Choose the enteral formula which most closely meets the person's requirements.

   There are four general types of enteral formulas: standard, elemental (predigested), specialized, and modular.

   - Standard formulas are also called polymeric formulas. They contain unaltered (intact) proteins, carbohydrates, and fat. They are for people who can digest and absorb nutrients without difficulty. The calories usually range from 1.0-2.0 calories per milliliter (mL). The higher calorie formulas may be used for persons on fluid restrictions. Some standard formulas have no fiber and others have added fiber.

   - Elemental formulas are also called hydrolyzed formulas. These contain predigested carbohydrate, protein, and fat. These are for persons with digestion and/or absorption problems who cannot tolerate a standard formula.

   - Specialized formulas are designed to meet the needs of persons with specific medical problems such as kidney, liver, or lung disease.

   - Modular formulas usually consist of a single nutrient (carbohydrate, protein, or fat). These do not provide complete nutrition.

2. **Administration.** Access to the stomach or small intestine is gained via a small diameter, flexible feeding tube. The tube may be placed (a) through the nose into the stomach or bowel for short-term use, or (b) directly through the skin into the stomach or bowel for long-term use. Formula is delivered through the tube by gravity flow (bolus) or by use of an enteral feeding pump. The rate and volume of formula given depend on individual factors, such as nutritional status, body size, tolerance, and type of formula. The feeding is usually initiated at a slow rate and then advanced as tolerated to the goal rate. Formula does not require dilution. Even though formulas are typically more than 80% water, this is not sufficient to meet fluid requirements. Water flushes are necessary to meet hydration needs as well as to avoid clogged feeding tubes. Flushes must be given before and after feedings and each medication, and when the feeding is interrupted for any reason.

3. **Complications.** There are four major areas of complications associated with enteral nutrition: mechanical (tube obstruction, suspected inaccurate pump administration, tube displacement), metabolic (hyperglycemia, electrolyte imbalance, dehydration), gastrointestinal (diarrhea, nausea and vomiting, cramping, constipation), and respiratory (labored breathing, aspiration). Causes and contributing factors to these complications are many and varied. Careful observation and assessment are required to treat them. Some very basic preventative strategies are: elevate head of bed to 30 to 45 degrees and maintain strict sanitary practices when storing, handling, and administering feedings. Frequent monitoring of hydration status, lab work, weight status, and physical signs is important to identify complications early.

4. **Information** about specific enteral feeding formulas can be obtained from company representatives or company websites.

ADDITIONAL RESOURCES

Bankhead R, Boullata J, Brantley S, et al. A.S.P.E.N. Board of Directors. Enteral Nutrition Practice Recommendations. *J Parenter Enteral Nutr.* 2009; 33:122–167. doi: 10.1177/0148607108330314

Bourgault AM, Ipe L, Weaver J, Swartz S, O'Dea PJ. Development of evidence-based guidelines and critical care nurses' knowledge of enteral feeding. *Crit Care Nurse.* 2007; 27(4):17–29. http://ccn.aacnjournals.org/content/27/4/17.full.pdf+html

Parrish CR, McCray S. Enteral feeding: dispelling myths. *Pract Gastroenterol.* 2003; September: 33–50.

Parrish CR. Enteral feeding: The art and the science. *Nutr Clin Pract.* 2003; 18(1):76–85. doi: 10.1177/011542650301800176

Fisher C, Blalock B. Clogged feeding tubes: A clinician's thorn. *Pract Gastroenterol.* 2014; March:16-22.

Study Guide Questions

A. List three reasons why a Clear Liquid Diet may be prescribed.

B. List at least six fluids which can be included on a Clear Liquid Diet.

C. Plan a full one-day menu for an individual on a Full Liquid Diet.

D. What is the likely cause a person may be required to receive nutrition exclusively through an enteral route?

E. Discussion question: Is it possible for an individual to remain on a full liquid diet long term and maintain their nutritional status? Why or why not?

Study Guide Suggested Responses can be found in Appendix 15.

Diets for Weight Management

5

There are a record number of overweight adults and children in the United States today. In fact, one of the health initiatives for Healthy People 2020 is to reduce the prevalence of obesity among adults to less than 30.5%. (1) As of 2012, one out of three adults in the United States is obese and one out of six adolescents is obese. (1) Because of this epidemic, healthcare teams will be faced with caring for an increased number of overweight and obese residents. Poor diet and physical inactivity are the most important factors contributing to an epidemic of overweight and obesity. (2)

Being overweight or obese is described as having an excess of body weight according to standards for height. A more specific measurement would be body mass index (BMI), refer to Appendix 1. A BMI of 25 to 29.9 kg/m² is considered overweight. Obesity is defined as a BMI of greater than 30 kg/m².

In older adults, maintaining a higher BMI has been associated with lower mortality rates. (3) The best BMI for subjects greater than 60 years of age has been shown to be greater than 27. In a study of body weight in older subjects aged 84 to 88 years it was observed that mortality is increased when BMI is less than 22, but did not increase when BMI is greater than 30. (4) For healthy older adults living in their own home, intentional weight loss may improve physical function, quality of life and reduce the complications associated with obesity. For adults >70 years of age living in care facilities, avoiding weight fluctuations and maintaining usual body weight may be the goal. (5)

The economic impact of obesity has been estimated at near $147 billion per year when all health effects are taken into consideration. (6) Being overweight or obese are known risk factors for over 30 health conditions including type 2 diabetes, cardiopulmonary disease, stroke, hypertension (high blood pressure), gallbladder disease, osteoarthritis, sleep apnea, and some forms of cancer. It affects quality of life and limits mobility. (7) Obesity is also associated with hyperlipidemia (high blood cholesterol), complications associated with pregnancy, irregular menses, stress incontinence, depression, and increased risk for complications if surgical procedures are needed.

Treatment for being overweight or obese includes diet and behavior therapy. Exercise is a key part of the treatment and should be customized to the patient's ability. Patient motivation and readiness to make changes should also be evaluated as well as the individual's understanding of the causes of obesity and how obesity contributes to disease. Patients' own personal goals must always be considered prior to the initiation of a weight management program.

WEIGHT MANAGEMENT DIET

Use

The use of calorie-controlled diets for weight management follow the principles of the General Diet, except that the portion sizes are decreased based on the patient's nutritional needs, physical activity, and behavior therapy. People who are most successful at achieving and maintaining a healthy weight do so through continued attention to consuming only enough calories from foods and beverages to meet their needs, and by being physically active. (2) Medications may be used in treatment for individuals who meet criteria established by National Heart, Lung, and Blood Institute (NHLBI). (8)

Medical nutrition therapy for weight loss should last at least 6 months or until the individual reaches his or her goal weight, at which time a weight maintenance plan should be implemented. Positive outcomes include:

- Promoting weight loss by reducing calorie needs by 500 to 1,000 calories/day. Resting metabolic rate may be estimated using the Mifflin-St. Jeor equation using actual body weight. (9)

- Promoting weight maintenance by providing adequate calories based on expenditure once a weight loss goal is met.

- Achieving optimal serum lipid levels (total cholesterol, HDL and LDL cholesterol, and triglycerides).

- Preventing long-term complications such as hypertension (high blood pressure), cardiovascular disease, and diabetes.

- Improving overall health through optimal nutrition and long-term behavior changes.

Weight loss with the elderly population should be evaluated based on benefit for long-term outcomes. Weight loss with children should be evaluated and monitored by a healthcare team.

Adequacy

Very low calorie diets do not meet energy requirements or nutrient requirements and should only be used under medical supervision. Calorie levels less than 1,200 for most women and 1,500 for most men should be discouraged. These levels lack adequate intake to meet Dietary Reference Intakes (DRIs) and a multivitamin or mineral supplement should be considered. The diet should be based on the individual's nutritional needs and anticipated energy output.

Diet Principles

1. Maintain a healthy weight either by weight loss or weight maintenance. A 5 to 10% loss of current body weight is a reasonable goal to promote a lower blood sugar, blood cholesterol, and blood pressure.

2. Prevent additional weight gain which is critical for health goals.

3. Establish a pattern of safe weight loss of an average of 1 to 2 pounds per week. When rapid weight loss occurs, the chance of regaining is greater.

4. Support lifestyle, behavior modification, exercise, and diet changes that are an ongoing process that last indefinitely.

5. Monitor food intake and weight with a food diary or electronic application.

6. Include a minimum of 30 minutes of moderate-intensity physical activity (e.g., brisk walking) at least 5 days a week to help promote weight loss. To maintain weight loss, more than 250 minutes per week of moderate-intensity physical activity is recommended. (10) More information on specific physical activity recommendations for various age groups and persons with chronic medical conditions is available from The Office of Disease Prevention and Promotion. (11) Monitor exercise with a pedometer or electronic application.

7. Choose foods that are moderate to small in portion size to meet weight loss goals. See the USDA Food Patterns in Chapter 1, the Small Portions Diet in Chapter 12, and the Heart Healthy Diet in Chapter 7. See Table 5.1 for a comparison of sample menus for these meal plans.

8. Calorie-controlled diets may include a calorie range, such as 1,200 to 1,500 calories per day. For more information and tools, go to ChooseMyPlate.gov website which includes personalized daily food plans and weight loss information. (12)

9. Calories may also be reduced by offering "free foods," (e.g., sugar-free or reduced calorie condiments) to allow for calories to come primarily from nutrient-dense food sources. Use Appendix 14, "Choose Your Foods," for reference in meal planning.

10. Reduce intake of sugar sweetened beverages and replace with water or non-nutritive sweetened (diet) beverages to reduce calorie intake.

11. Spread meals and snacks throughout the day to prevent hunger periods.

12. Individuals with diabetes should continue to monitor carbohydrate, refer to Diets for Diabetes in Chapter 6.

Table 5.1 Sample Menus for Weight Management

Meal	Healthy U.S.-Style Eating Pattern – 1500 Calories	Small Portions Diet	Heart Healthy Diet
Breakfast	½ c. orange juice	½ c. orange juice	½ c. orange juice
	1 egg	1 egg	1 egg
	½ c. oatmeal	½ c. oatmeal	½ c. oatmeal
	1 slice whole wheat toast	½ slice whole wheat toast	1 slice whole wheat toast
	1 tsp. soft margarine	1 tsp. soft margarine	1 tsp. margarine (*trans* fat-free)
	2 tsp. sugar-free jelly	1 tsp. jelly	2 tsp. jelly
	1 c. fat-free milk	1 c. fat-free milk	1 c. fat-free milk
	Sugar substitute	1 Tbsp. sugar	1 Tbsp. sugar
	Hot beverage	Hot beverage	Hot beverage
Lunch	2 oz. roasted chicken breast	2 oz. roasted chicken breast	2 oz. baked chicken breast
	½ c. mashed potato with 2 oz. fat-free gravy	¼ c. mashed potatoes with 1 oz. fat-free gravy	½ c. mashed potatoes with 2 oz. fat-free gravy
	½ c. mixed vegetables	⅓ c. mixed vegetables	½ c. mixed vegetables
	½ oz. whole wheat roll	½ oz. whole wheat roll	1 oz. whole wheat roll
	1 tsp. soft margarine	1 tsp. soft margarine	1 tsp. margarine (*trans* fat-free)
	1 c. fat-free milk	1 c. fat-free milk	1 c. fat-free milk
Supper	2 oz. tuna on 2 slices whole wheat bread, 2 tsp. mayonnaise	2 oz. tuna on 1 slice whole wheat bread, 2 tsp. mayonnaise	2 oz. tuna on 2 slices whole wheat bread, 2 tsp. mayonnaise
	2 tomato slices	2 tomato slices	2 tomato slices
	1 cup leafy greens salad	½ c. leafy greens salad	1 c. leafy greens salad
	1 Tbsp. oil and vinegar dressing	1 Tbsp. oil and vinegar dressing	1 Tbsp. oil and vinegar dressing
	½ c. fruit cocktail	½ c. fruit cocktail	½ c. fruit cocktail
	1 c. fat-free milk	1 c. fat-free milk	1 c. fat-free milk

Continued on next page

Table 5.1 Sample Menus for Weight Management Continued from previous page

Meal	Healthy U.S.-Style Eating Pattern – 1500 Calories	Small Portions Diet	Heart Healthy Diet
Snacks	½ c. cantaloupe	½ c. cantaloupe	½ c. cantaloupe
	½ c. carrot sticks	½ c. carrot sticks	½ c. carrot sticks
	1 ½ c. popcorn	1 c. popcorn	3 c. popcorn, *trans* fat-free

REFERENCES

1. Office of Disease Prevention and Promotion. HealthyPeople2020. Nutrition and Weight Status. http://www.healthypeople.gov/2020/topics-objectives/topic/nutrition-and-weight-status/objectives Updated August 25, 2015. Accessed August 25, 2015.

2. U. S. Department of Health and Human Services and U. S. Department of Agriculture. *2015 – 2020 Dietary Guidelines for Americans,* 8th ed. http://health.gov/dietaryguidelines/2015/guidelines/ Published December 2015. Accessed January 13, 2016.

3. Janssen I, Katzmarzyk P, Ross R. Body mass index is inversely related to mortality in older people after adjustment for waist circumference. *J Am Geriatric Soc.* 2005; 53 (12):2112–2118.

4. Cook Z, Kirk S, Lawrenson S, Sanford S. Use of BMI in the assessment of undernutrition in older subjects: reflecting on practice. *Proc Nutr Soc.* 2005; 64(3):313–317.

5. Academy of Nutrition and Dietetics. Nutrition Care Manual. Older Adult Nutrition: Obesity. https://www.nutritioncaremanual.org/content.cfm?ncm_content_id=111285&ncm_category_id=1 Accessed August 31, 2015.

6. Finkelstein EA, Trogdon JG, Cohen JW, Dietz W. Annual medical spending attributable to obesity: payer-and service-specific estimates. *Health Affairs.* 2009; 28(5):w822-w831. doi:10.1377/hlthaff.28.5.w822

7. Vincent HK, Vincent KR, Lamb KM. Obesity and mobility disability in the older adult. *Obes Rev.* 2010; 11(8):568-579.

8. National Institutes of Health, National Heart, Lung, and Blood Institute and North American Association for the Study of Obesity. *The Practical Guide: Identification, Evaluation, and Treatment of Overweight and Obesity in Adults.* www.nhlbi.nih.gov/guidelines/obesity/prctgd_c.pdf Published October 2000. Accessed August 25, 2015.

9. Frankenfield D, Roth-Yousey L, Compher C. Comparison of predictive equations for resting metabolic rate in healthy nonobese and obese adults: a systematic review. *J Am Diet Assoc.* 2005; 105(5):775-789.

10. Donnelly, J.E., Blair, S.N., Jakicic, J.M., Manore, M.M., Rankin, J.W., and Smith, B.K. American College of Sports Medicine Position Stand: Appropriate physical activity intervention strategies for weight loss and prevention of weight regain for adults. *Med Sci Sports Exerc.* 2009; 41: 459–471.

11. 2008 Physical Activity Guidelines for Americans. Office of Disease Prevention and Promotion website. http://www.health.gov/paguidelines Published October 2008. Updated December 15, 2015. Accessed December 15, 2015.

12. U.S. Department of Agriculture Choose My Plate.gov website. http://www.choosemyplate.gov/ Published June 2, 2011. Accessed August 5, 2015.

ADDITIONAL RESOURCES

Mifflin MD, St. Jeor ST, Hill LA, et al. A new predictive equation for resting energy expenditure in healthy individuals. *Am J Clin Nutr*. 1990; 51(2):241–247. http://ajcn.nutrition.org/content/51/2/241.long

Raynor, HA, Champagne CM. Position of the Academy of Nutrition and Dietetics: Interventions for the treatment of overweight and obesity in adults. *J Acad Nutr Diet*. 2016; 116(1):129-147. http://dx.doi.org/10.1016/j.jand.2015.10.031

Websites

Academy of Nutrition and Dietetics: www.eatright.org

The Obesity Society: www.obesity.org

National Center for Health Statistics: www.cdc.gov/nchs

President's Council on Fitness, Sports and Nutrition: www.fitness.gov

Office of Disease Prevention and Promotion. HealthyPeople2020. Nutrition and Weight Status: http://www.healthypeople.gov/2020/topics-objectives/topic/nutrition-and-weight-status

BARIATRIC DIET

This diet is used for weight loss surgery procedures, generally performed laparoscopically, including roux-en-y gastric bypass, laparoscopic adjustable band, and sleeve gastrectomy.

Use

The Bariatric Diet is for the individual who has met the criteria and has undergone weight loss surgery. The two most common bariatric surgeries are the roux-en-y gastric bypass (RYGB), and the sleeve gastrectomy (SG) which are a combination of malabsorption and restrictive procedures (stomach and intestine). A purely restrictive procedure (stomach only), the laparoscopic adjustable gastric band (LAGB) is performed less often. It is important to determine what type of bariatric surgery was performed as the diet and nutrition plan could vary, depending on the program.

Adequacy

This diet is not adequate in any nutrient without proper supplementation. The postoperative diet for all types of bariatric surgeries should be started with water, ice chips, and clear unsweetened, diluted beverages that are sipped very slowly, with no carbonated or caffeinated beverages allowed. Patients then advance on postoperative day 2 or 3 to a Full and Clear Liquid Diet for approximately the next 14 days. A whey protein supplement maybe used to provide 60 to 80 grams protein per day. Full liquids need to be low in sugar (less than 25 grams of total sugar per serving), with up to 25 to 30 grams of protein per serving but not greater than 30 grams at one meal. Different programs have set their own restrictions and limitations with the use of protein shakes.

The Pureed Diet can be introduced around postoperative weeks 2 and 3, beginning with 1 Tablespoon of protein rich food. Protein food choices are encouraged three to six times per day with no more than 2 Tablespoons at a meal. Some programs continue with puree texture for as long as a month.

Soft solid foods are introduced around postoperative week 4 to 6. Foods are added one at a time and should be well-chewed, moist, and consumed very slowly. Some individuals may take as long as an additional 6 months before they are able to tolerate regular textured foods. A minimum of 2 ounces of protein at each meal is recommended and some may be able to tolerate 3 ounces of protein at a meal. Total volume of food at a meal should be no more than ½ to 1 cup. Liquids should not be consumed with solids. Liquids should not be consumed for at least 10 minutes before a meal, with some programs recommending to avoid liquids 30 minutes prior to the meal, and no sooner than 30 minutes or up to an hour after a meal. Liquids consumed too quickly after a meal may increase the risk of dumping syndrome and cause solid food to pass too quickly leading to early hunger. Fluid intake of 48 to 64 ounces of low-calorie, noncarbonated, and caffeine-free beverages is encouraged to prevent dehydration. Alcohol consumption is not advised.

A healthy diet with a structured meal and snack plan that focuses on protein food with each meal is recommended after weight loss surgery. Complications such as a gastrointestinal bleed or ulcer and vitamin and mineral deficiencies should be followed up on an outpatient basis.

Diet Principles

1. Eat three "meals" per day and maintain adequately spaced protein.

2. Consume protein foods first.

3. Consume a minimum of 60 grams of protein per day.

4. Consume no liquids with meals, 10 to 30 minutes before and 30 to 60 minutes after eating solids.

5. Consume 48 to 64 ounces of low-calorie, noncarbonated, and caffeine- free beverages per day.

6. Supplement with a chewable complete multivitamin for band and sleeve procedures and use a chewable multivitamin supplement developed for roux-en-y; petite or chewable calcium citrate 1200 to 1500 mg/day, taken in divided doses of 500 to 600 mg at least two hours apart from multivitamin with iron or iron supplement; 3,000 IU Vitamin D3; 45 to 60 mg of elemental iron such as ferrous fumarate or ferrous gluconate taken with 250 to 500 mg chewable Vitamin C to aid absorption; and 1000 mcg Vitamin B_{12} for roux-en-y and sleeve.

7. Daily exercise to maintain and build muscle; and to promote and maintain weight loss.

8. All surgical candidates should be screened for vitamin and mineral deficiency preoperatively and treated if a vitamin and mineral deficiency is present.

Table 5.2 Diet Progression Following Bariatric Surgery

Day 1–2	• Clear liquids only (water, broth, diet gelatin, sugar-free Popsicle®, protein infused water). Make sure upper gastrointestinal series (UGI) is cleared before advancing diet. Sip very slowly and no gulping.
Days 3–14	• Full liquid diet, low sugar (less than 25 grams total sugar) and less than 30 grams of protein per serving.
	• Whey protein supplements to provide a minimum of 60 grams protein/day.
Days 15–45	• Pureed diet.
	• Whey protein supplements to provide a minimum of 60 grams protein/day (only if difficulty meeting protein goal).
Day 45 and beyond	• Soft/regular texture. Chew food thoroughly, eat slowly, and stop eating when starting to feel full.
	• Avoid doughy breads, dried meat, sticky pasta and rice, high fat, and high sugar foods.
	• Continue goal of 60 grams protein and 48 to 64 ounces low-calorie, noncarbonated, caffeine-free beverages.

Continued on next page

Table 5.2 Diet Progression Following Bariatric Surgery Continued from previous page

Supplement Suggestions	• Whey protein (whey isolate is preferred; lactose-free maybe desirable) – only per surgery centers recommendations and if difficulty meeting protein goal.
	• Immediately postoperatively: Chewable multivitamin complete, chewable calcium citrate 1200 to 1500 mg/day, 3000 IU Vitamin D3 for LAGB, and additional 1000 mcg Vitamin B_{12} and 45 mg elemental iron taken with 250 to 500 mg chewable Vitamin C for SG.
	• Chewable multivitamin designed for RYGB taken in multiple doses; chewable calcium citrate 1200 to 1500 mg/day; 3,000 IU Vitamin D3; 45 mg elemental iron taken with 250 to 500 mg chewable Vitamin C; and 500 mcg Vitamin B_{12}.
	• All surgical candidates should be screened for vitamin and mineral deficiency preoperatively. If vitamin deficiency is present then treatment is needed to restore levels to normal.
Dietitian visits	• Preoperatively, postoperatively, 1 to 2 weeks postoperatively, 2, 3, 6, and 9 months, and then annually.
	• Vitamin and mineral levels should be monitored annually.

Please NOTE: Diet prescriptions vary among practitioners. The exact time of advancement and serving size is dependent on patients' tolerance, facility guidelines, and practitioners' preferences.

ADDITIONAL RESOURCES

Aills L, Blankenship J, Buffington C, et al. ASMBS Allied Health Nutritional Guidelines for the surgical weight loss patient. *Surgery for Obesity and Related Diseases*. 2008; 55:S73–S108.

Parkes E. Nutritional management of patients after Bariatric surgery. *Am J Med Sci*. 2006; 331:207–213.

Weight Management Dietetic Practice Group, Cummings S, Isom K. *Pocket Guide to Bariatric Surgery*, 2nd ed. Chicago, IL: Academy of Nutrition and Dietetics; 2015.

Websites

Academy of Nutrition and Dietetics: www.eatright.org

American Society for Metabolic and Bariatric Surgery: http://www.asmbs.org/

Study Guide Questions

A. What body mass index (BMI) ranges are adults in the United States considered overweight? What BMI levels are adults in the United States considered obese?

B. List at least six health-related problems associated with overweight and obesity.

C. List at least five sensible food and beverage choices that could be kept on hand to offer patients on a Weight Management Diet.

D. For individuals on a bariatric diet, what are three diet principles that should be considered in menu planning?

E. Discussion question: How can you make a Weight Management Diet in long-term care customer-oriented for the resident?

Study Guide Suggested Responses can be found in Appendix 15.

Diets for Diabetes

6

According to the National Diabetes Statistics Report, there are more than 29 million Americans with diabetes mellitus. (1) Of this population, 90 to 95% has type 2 diabetes and the remaining 5 to 10% has type 1 diabetes. Diabetes is a disease in which the body does not produce and/or properly use insulin. Insulin is a hormone that is needed for blood glucose (sugar) to get into the body and provide energy needed for daily life. Carbohydrates (sugars and starches) are digested into blood glucose. If the glucose is unable to be transported into the cell, the glucose remains in the blood stream and produces a state of hyperglycemia (high blood sugar). Prolonged high blood sugars may cause macrovascular (large vessel) and microvascular (small vessel) damage increasing a person's risk for other health complications.

Type 1 diabetes (previously known as juvenile diabetes or insulin-dependent diabetes or IDDM) is an autoimmune disease that affects the pancreas so that it does not make insulin. Insulin is required for a person with type 1 diabetes to survive. Insulin may be given by injections or by an insulin pump. Currently, there is no known cure for type 1 diabetes, although research is consistently underway.

Type 2 diabetes (previously known as adult onset diabetes or noninsulin dependent diabetes or NIDDM) is a disease that usually begins with insulin resistance, a condition in which the cells do not use insulin properly. As diabetes progresses, the pancreas gradually loses its ability to make insulin. Type 2 diabetes may require medication to control blood glucose. This could include oral medications, GLP-1 receptor agonists, or insulin. A person with type 2 diabetes taking insulin does not have type 1 diabetes; the description for this is Type 2 diabetes requiring insulin.

There are another 86 million people with prediabetes. (1) They have blood glucose levels that are higher than normal but not high enough to be diagnosed with diabetes. Diet, exercise, and weight management may prevent or delay the onset of type 2 diabetes.

Another type of diabetes is called gestational diabetes. This type of diabetes only occurs during pregnancy. After delivery of the baby, blood glucose usually returns to normal. Women who have gestational diabetes are at a higher risk for type 2 diabetes and developing gestational diabetes again with a future pregnancy. Meal planning, exercise, and possibly medication are used to control blood glucose during pregnancy.

DIABETES MEAL PLANNING PRINCIPLES

The following goals and principles are based on the Nutrition Therapy Recommendations for the Management of Adults with Diabetes. (2) The goals of nutrition therapy for adults with diabetes are:

- To encourage healthy eating in order to:
  - Achieve personalized blood glucose, blood pressure, and lipid goals.
  - Reach and maintain body weight goals.
  - Prevent or postpone complications of diabetes.
- To take into account individual needs including personal and ethnic preferences, math and reading ability, access to healthy foods, readiness to make changes, and other barriers to change.

- To maintain the enjoyment of eating by discussing foods in a positive manner and discouraging foods only when supported by science.

- To provide practical resources for meal planning instead of focusing on specific nutrients, or single foods.

1. **Individualization.** Individualization of treatment for patients with diabetes is essential. The effect of medical nutrition therapy on blood glucose and serum lipid levels must be evaluated and modified, if necessary. The dietary program and self-management plan must take into consideration the ability and willingness of the client with diabetes to follow through with recommendations. The plan should be sensitive to cultural, ethnic, and financial considerations. Reinforcement of teaching and encouragement are usually necessary over an extended period of time.

2. **Energy.** The caloric value of meal plans must provide adequate energy to achieve and maintain a desirable or reasonable weight. Weight reduction of 5 to 10% of initial body weight (approximately 10–20 pounds) may improve blood glucose and/or lipid levels as well as blood pressure in many people with type 2 diabetes who are also overweight/obese. For individuals with diabetes that are within a desirable weight range, caloric intake must match energy expenditure to maintain normal weight. For the person below desirable weight, caloric intake must allow for appropriate weight gain.

3. **Carbohydrate.** Carbohydrates include sugars and starches. They are always broken down and digested into glucose (blood sugar) for energy. In a person that does not have diabetes, the pancreas releases insulin based on the amount of carbohydrate that is consumed. There is no ideal amount of carbohydrate for persons with diabetes. For good health, carbohydrates from fruit, milk, whole grains, vegetables, and legumes should be encouraged over foods with added sugars, fats, and/or sodium. The DRIs (3) recommend 45 to 65% of total calories from carbohydrates. The Recommended Dietary Allowance (RDA) is a minimum of 130 grams of carbohydrate daily for children and adults. The RDA for pregnant women is a minimum of 175 grams daily, and the RDA during lactation is a minimum of 210 grams of carbohydrate daily. (3) Carbohydrates are found in four main groups of food: (a) starch, (b) fruits, (c) milk and milk substitutes, and (d) sweets, desserts, and other carbohydrates. These foods affect blood glucose in the same manner. The total amount of carbohydrate consumed is more important than the source of the carbohydrate. Research shows that sugars such as sucrose (table sugar), syrup, and honey have no more effect on blood glucose levels than other carbohydrates. Monitoring blood glucose after meals can help evaluate an individual's response to that meal and determine if the carbohydrate level needs to be adjusted, or for those who require medication, if the dose of medication needs to be adjusted.

   When foods containing added sugars are included, that carbohydrate content is counted as part of the total carbohydrate consumed at the meal or snack. See the Sweets, Desserts and Other Carbohydrates List in Appendix 14 for carbohydrate content per serving. Many of these foods were traditionally avoided before research revealed that these foods do not raise blood glucose more than other carbohydrates. Many of these foods also contain added fat and should be consumed in moderation if weight management is a goal. For persons managing diabetes with insulin secretagogues (i.e., sulfonylureas, glinides) or fixed doses of insulin, a consistent intake of carbohydrate is desirable and often achieved in a healthcare setting.

   For persons on flexible insulin doses (i.e., insulin-to-carbohydrate ratios), insulin doses are adjusted based on the amount of carbohydrate consumed at each meal. Therefore, a General Diet containing regular food is acceptable for diabetes meal planning. For persons using an insulin-to-carbohydrate ratio, having a knowledge of carbohydrate counting is necessary. *Choose Your Foods: Food Lists for Diabetes* was prepared by the Academy of Nutrition and Dietetics and the American Diabetes Association (refer to Appendix 14). Use the food list for reference in carbohydrate counting.

4. **Protein and Fat.** Protein and fat do not affect the blood glucose directly like carbohydrates do. The amount of protein and fat servings do not need to be consistent from day to day to achieve blood glucose control. For persons without diabetic kidney disease, there is insufficient evidence to recommend an ideal amount of protein. (2) See Chapter 9 for protein recommendations for persons with diabetic kidney disease. The evidence is inconclusive for an ideal fat intake for persons with diabetes. (2) The amount of protein and fat that is provided in the General Diet is appropriate for the individual with diabetes in healthcare institutions.

5. **Exercise.** Most people with diabetes benefit from regular exercise. Exercise improves the body's response to insulin, helps lower blood glucose levels, and is a key factor in the success of clients achieving and maintaining a desirable or reasonable body weight. Individuals using insulin may need adjustments to their meal pattern or insulin regimen to prevent hypoglycemia during or after strenuous activity.

6. **Reducing Cardiovascular Risk.** Because the diagnosis of diabetes is a single risk factor for cardiovascular disease, controlling blood lipid levels is an important treatment goal. Current recommendations support eating patterns that encourage intake of fruits, vegetables, legumes, whole grains, and low-fat dairy products as well as substituting monounsaturated and polyunsaturated fats in place of saturated and *trans* fat. Limiting alcohol intake and added sugars and losing excess weight are also recommended. (4) The recommendation for the general population to reduce sodium to less than 2,300 mg/day is also appropriate for people with diabetes. (2) Making medication changes to control lipids and blood pressure rather than using food restrictions may prevent malnutrition in the elderly.

7. **Meal Patterns.** Food, exercise, and diabetes medicines (insulin, GLP-1 receptor agonists and oral hypoglycemic agents) influence blood glucose concentration. These three influences need to be considered in various ways in the treatment of diabetes. When insulin therapy is used, the activity curve of the insulin determines the times of the day when needs for food are greatest. Exercise reduces the need for insulin and increases the need for carbohydrate. Usually a regular pattern for taking insulin injections, meals and snacks, and exercise can be worked out so that both hyperglycemia and hypoglycemia can be minimized. This is more important for the person taking insulin.

8. **Measuring Food.** Food should be measured with standard measuring equipment (8-ounce cup, measuring spoons, small food scale, ruler) until the amounts can be estimated accurately. To make certain measurements remain accurate, periodically use measuring equipment to recheck portions served. Foods are measured after they are cooked.

9. **Special Foods.** Special foods are not necessary and may be expensive. Foods labeled "sugar-free," "no sugar," "reduced sugar," or "lower sugar" may be high in calories, fat, and even carbohydrates. If these products are used, read nutrition labels carefully. Sugar-free does not mean carbohydrate-free. However, many sugar-free products are also low calorie and may be used as free foods or aid in weight management goals.

10. **Consistent Carbohydrate Diets in Institutions.** Many healthcare facilities use a consistent carbohydrate meal planning system. (5) For persons taking insulin secretagogues or fixed doses of insulin, a consistent carbohydrate meal plan is appropriate. The following diets are obsolete as they do not reflect current diabetes recommendations: no sugar added, no concentrated sweets, limited concentrated sweets, and low sugar. Long-term care facility residents eat better when they are given liberalized diets. Making medication changes to control blood glucose rather than restricting food can reduce malnutrition. The specific nutrition recommendations will depend upon treatment goals, the patient's clinical condition, medication usage, and patient preferences.

CONSISTENT CARBOHYDRATE DIET

Use

The Consistent Carbohydrate Diet is an outline for meal planning for the person with diabetes mellitus. This diet follows the principles of the General Diet but provides consistent carbohydrate intake at meals.

Adequacy

The suggested food plan includes foods in amounts that will provide the Dietary Reference Intakes (DRIs) recommended by the National Academy of Sciences for adults. Meal plans with less than 1,200 calories may be low in vitamins and minerals and are generally not recommended. In the elderly, under-nutrition is likely and weight loss diets should be prescribed with caution. The need for a daily multivitamin supplement should be evaluated.

Diet Principles

The Consistent Carbohydrate Diet implies that the amount of carbohydrates consumed is consistent and the time of the meals and snacks are consistent as well. This pattern will help promote optimal blood glucose control and is recommended for persons on insulin secretagogues and fixed doses of insulin. In most healthcare settings, acute or long-term care, meal times are consistent. The menu can be adjusted to be consistent with carbohydrates for all populations and therefore eliminate therapeutic diets.

Carbohydrate counting is based on choices or grams of carbohydrates. The individual is given a carbohydrate allowance that has been individualized to their nutrition therapy and blood glucose goals. One carbohydrate choice equals 15 grams of carbohydrate. Snacks are optional for many individuals with diabetes. However, in many institutions the length of time between the evening meal and breakfast is great and most individuals need an evening snack. Those who use carbohydrate counting may use the following conversion chart (Table 6.1).

Table 6.1 Conversion Guide for Carbohydrate Counting

Total Carbohydrate Grams	Carbohydrate Choices
0–5	0
6–10	½
11–20	1
21–25	1 ½
26–35	2
36–40	2 ½
41–50	3
51–55	3 ½
55–65	4
66–70	4 ½
71–80	5
81–85	5 ½
85–95	6
96–100	6 ½
101–110	7

Carbohydrate allowances may be "spent" at the discretion of the patient; however, not all choices have the same nutritional value and may alter overall nutrition status of the individual.

Menu portion sizes should be adjusted to reflect goals of nutritional management for individuals in a facility. Patients in healthcare settings may be offered a standard diet for diabetes that is consistent in carbohydrate or they may be given a General Diet menu with the carbohydrate choices or grams listed on the menu to facilitate carbohydrate counting. Traditionally, diabetic diets were ordered as "ADA" with the calorie level indicated. The American Diabetes Association does not have standard diets nor endorse standardized diets. The term *ADA* diet was attached to calorie levels and over time has been interpreted as a diabetic diet. The American Diabetes Association discourages the use of the term *ADA diet*. (6)

The following meal plan and sample menu shows an example of adapting a General Diet to a Consistent Carbohydrate Diet providing about 2,000 calories per day (Table 6.2).

Table 6.2 Sample Meal Plan and Sample Menu for Consistent Carbohydrate Diet

Meal Plan	Consistent Carbohydrate Diet	General Diet
Breakfast	½ c. orange juice (1 choice)	½ c. orange juice
5 carbohydrate choices equal to ~75 grams carbohydrate	½ c. oatmeal (1 choice)	½ c. oatmeal
	1 slice toast (1 choice)	1 slice toast
	1 egg	1 egg
	1 c. fat-free milk (1 choice)	1 c. fat-free milk
	1 Tbsp. regular jelly (1 choice)	1 Tbsp. jelly
	1 tsp. soft margarine	1 tsp. soft margarine
	coffee	coffee
Lunch	2 oz. roasted chicken breast	2 oz. roasted chicken breast
5 carbohydrate choices equal to ~75 grams carbohydrate	½ c. mashed potatoes with 2 oz. fat-free gravy (1 choice)	½ c. mashed potatoes with 2 oz. fat-free gravy
	½ c. mixed vegetables (without corn or peas)	½ c. mixed vegetables
	1 dinner roll (1 choice)	1 dinner roll
	1 tsp. soft margarine	1 tsp. soft margarine
	2 × 2 brownie/frosting (2 choices)	2 × 2 brownie/frosting
	1 c. fat-free milk (1 choice)	1 c. fat-free milk
	coffee	coffee
Supper	Tuna salad sandwich with 2 slices bread (2 choices)	Tuna salad sandwich with 2 slices bread
5 carbohydrate choices equal to ~75 grams carbohydrate	1 cup tomato soup with 2 crackers (1 choice)	1 cup tomato soup
		2 crackers
	½ c. fruit cocktail (1 choice)	½ c. fruit cocktail
	1 c. fat-free milk (1 choice)	1 c. fat-free milk
	coffee	coffee

Continued on next page

Table 6.2 Sample Meal Plan and Sample Menu for Consistent Carbohydrate Diet
Continued from previous page

Meal Plan	Consistent Carbohydrate Diet	General Diet
Snack	½ c. carrots	½ c. carrots
1–2 carbohydrate choices equal to 15–30 grams carbohydrate	½ c. cubed cantaloupe (½ choice)	½ c. cubed cantaloupe
	3 cups popcorn (1 choice)	3 cups popcorn

Gestational Diabetes Meal Plan

The meal plan for a woman with gestational diabetes follows the same principles as the Consistent Carbohydrate Diet. Traditionally, total carbohydrate intake is usually 40 to 45% of total calories. (7, 8) Some researchers advocate lower carbohydrate intakes, however, the minimum amount of carbohydrate recommended daily in pregnancy is 175 grams. (3) Emerging research using a higher fiber meal plan (enriched in complex carbohydrates coming from grains, vegetables, and fruits) with mainly low to moderate glycemic index foods has shown that higher carbohydrate intakes may be tolerated. (9, 10) This diet contained 60% of the total calories from carbohydrates at each meal and snack, and resulted in blood glucose levels within current therapeutic targets. (9, 10) Another study compared a diet containing 40% calories from carbohydrates to a diet containing 55% calories from carbohydrates; the carbohydrate amount did not influence insulin need or pregnancy outcome. (11) Generally, the meal pattern for breakfast is reduced in carbohydrates due to hormonal surges and insulin resistance in the morning hours. The carbohydrate allowance for breakfast is limited to two choices (30 grams) to help promote optimal blood glucose levels (Table 6.3). Once the meal plan is in place, blood glucose is checked on a regular basis. If the blood glucose levels show a trend of acceptable readings, the meal plan may be adjusted to a higher carbohydrate allowance.

Care must be taken to provide enough calories in the meal plan to promote proper weight gain and prevent starvation ketosis; extra protein and fat foods at each meal and snack time can aid in meeting calorie needs. An evening snack is necessary to prevent ketosis. Women are advised to check ketones before breakfast.

Table 6.3 Sample Meal Plan and Sample Menu for Gestational Diabetes ~2000 Calories

Breakfast: Two carbohydrate choices (30 grams)

- 1 slice whole wheat toast (1 choice)
- 1 egg or 1 Tbsp. peanut butter
- 1 tsp. soft margarine
- 8 oz. low-fat milk (1 choice)

Snack: Two carbohydrate choices (30 grams)

- 3 graham cracker squares (1 choice)
- 8 oz. low-fat milk (1 choice)

Lunch: Three to four carbohydrate choices(45–60 grams)

- 2 slices whole wheat bread (2 choices)
- 2-3 oz. roast beef
- 2 tsp. soft margarine
- ½ medium banana (1 choice)
- 6 oz. light yogurt (1 choice)
- 1 c. carrot and celery sticks

Continued on next page

Snack: Two carbohydrate choices (30 grams)

- 3 c. popcorn, lower fat (1 choice)
- 1 c. cantaloupe (1 choice)
- 1 unsweetened beverage

Supper: Three to four carbohydrate choices (45–60 grams)

- 3 oz. chicken breast
- 1 small baked potato (1 choice)
- ½ c. broccoli
- ½ c. peaches (1 choice)
- 1 small dinner roll (1 choice)
- 8 oz. low-fat milk (1 choice)
- 1 tsp. margarine

Snack: Two carbohydrate choices (30 grams)

- 6 whole wheat crackers (1 choice)
- 1 oz. cheese
- 8 oz. low-fat milk (1 choice)

Full and Clear Liquid Substitutions

When an individual with diabetes cannot eat solid food, it may be necessary to offer the Clear Liquid or Full Liquid Diet. Carbohydrate counting still plays a role with meal planning. The use of regular products is acceptable to maintain the level of carbohydrate in the meal plan. Sugar-free products should be limited on a liquid diet due to the decreased caloric value. Table 6.4 shows carbohydrate values for selected foods that could be offered on a Full or Clear Liquid Diet.

Table 6.4 Carbohydrate Content of Selected Foods for Clear or Full Liquid Diets

Food - 15 gram carbohydrate portions	Amount
Carbonated regular soda	½ cup
Cooked cereal	½ cup
Cream soup	1 cup
Custard, soft	½ cup
Eggnog	½ cup
Flavored gelatin, regular	½ cup
Ice cream, regular	½ cup
Light ice cream, vanilla	½ cup
Pudding, sugar-free	½ cup
Pudding, regular	¼ cup
Sherbet	¼ cup
Sugar	1 Tbsp
Yogurt, flavored low-fat, sugar sweetened	⅓ cup

Hypoglycemia

Hypoglycemia or low blood sugar can be caused by taking too much diabetes medication, eating too few carbohydrates at meal time, skipping meals, drinking alcohol, or getting more exercise than usual. For persons on mealtime insulin who have an inconsistent dietary intake, one strategy to reduce hypoglycemia is to administer mealtime insulin immediately after meals to match carbohydrate intake. (12) Symptoms of hypoglycemia may vary among individuals. Common signs are feeling shaky, sweaty, tired, hungry, irritated or confused, rapid heart rate, blurred vision or headaches, and numbness or tingling in the mouth and lips. In severe cases, the person may lose consciousness.

The treatment for low blood sugar is the "Rule of 15." This means once a low blood sugar is recognized, 15 grams of carbohydrate is given. Pure glucose is the preferred treatment but any carbohydrate food containing glucose may be used. It is recommended to use only carbohydrate to treat hypoglycemia and not to use foods high in protein or fat. Protein can stimulate the pancreas to release insulin and does not prevent a repeat low blood sugar. Fat slows down the absorption of carbohydrate leading to a delay in raising blood glucose. See Table 6.5 for carbohydrates commonly used to treat hypoglycemia.

Table 6.5 Treatment of Low Blood Sugar "Rule of 15"

Good Choices 15 gram carbohydrate portions	Not recommended due to high protein and/or fat content
4 glucose tablets or 1 tube glucose gel	Donuts
½ cup fruit juice	Ice cream, milkshakes
½ cup regular soda	Candy bars
1 Tbsp. sugar	Sandwiches
1 Tbsp. honey	Pies, cakes, cookies

The blood sugar should be rechecked in 15 minutes. If the blood sugar remains low, then retreat with 15 grams of carbohydrate. Recheck the blood sugar again in 15 minutes and repeat as necessary until the blood sugar is within normal limits. If the next meal is more than one hour away, serve a snack consisting of 30 grams of carbohydrate. If the next meal is less than one hour away, continue to monitor blood glucose levels until mealtime. A repeat low blood sugar may occur if not treated properly.

Effective treatment for hypoglycemia in the healthcare setting is essential. Historically the addition of table sugar to juice or other liquids has been used to elevate blood glucose levels. This is not recommended as it may over treat the low blood sugar. A high blood sugar may be the result, causing a roller coaster effect.

Herbal Therapy and Vitamin or Mineral Supplementation

Herbal therapy is becoming more common to aid in the treatment of disease states. The herbal industry is not regulated by the Food and Drug Administration (FDA) and therefore does not uphold the same standards as other conventional therapies. There is insufficient evidence to support the use of cinnamon and other herbal products for persons with diabetes. Persons with diabetes need to exercise extreme caution with herbal therapies because some may interfere with diabetes medication or may cause the body to become more insulin resistant. Contact a physician or pharmacist for more information.

There is no clear data that shows benefit from the use of any vitamin or mineral supplement for persons with diabetes who do not have underlying deficiencies. In fact, regular supplementation with antioxidants, such as vitamins A, C, or E, is not recommended due to safety concerns associated with long-term use. Certain populations may need supplementation for reasons unrelated to diabetes including the elderly, pregnant and lactating women, and those on low calorie diets.

Gastroparesis

Gastroparesis (delayed stomach emptying) is a complication of diabetes that may require diet modification. Offer individuals four or more small meals daily as large meals slow stomach emptying. (13, 14) Fat, fiber, and solid foods slow down stomach emptying. (14) If a person has severe nausea and vomiting, then a Clear Liquid Diet (see Chapter 4) is recommended. Once clear liquids are tolerated, the next step is a Full Liquid Diet (see Chapter 4). Some people do not tolerate high fat liquids such as whole milk, cream soup, and milkshakes. However, liquids high in fat should be allowed unless they worsen symptoms. Some people will need liquid nutrition supplements to meet their nutrition needs. Once full liquids are tolerated, a low-fat, low-fiber diet is the next step (Table 6.6). Some high fiber foods may cause bezoar formation (indigestible material that collects in your digestive tract) and may need to be avoided (13). Alcohol should be avoided as it can modify gastric emptying. Carbonated beverages may cause gastric distention and should be minimized. (15) If solid foods are not tolerated, pureed foods are also an option (see Chapter 3).

Symptoms of gastroparesis can change or come and go, therefore, an individual's ability to tolerate foods may change over time.

Table 6.6 Low-Fat, Low-Fiber Diet for Gastroparesis

Food for the Day	Recommended	Restrict if not tolerated
Vegetables *1–4 cups*	Choose cooked or canned vegetables without skins or seeds except those not recommended. May have potatoes without skins; tomato juice, sauce, and paste.	Raw, deep-fried and lightly cooked vegetables; creamed vegetables; tomato seeds and skins; avocado, broccoli, Brussels sprouts, corn, green beans, peas, potato skins, sauerkraut, dried beans and peas; cooked spinach and greens.
Fruits *1–2.5 cups*	Choose cooked or canned fruits without skin or seeds (e.g., applesauce, peaches, or pears); ripe banana or melons; fruit juice without pulp.	Fresh fruit except ripe banana or melon; dried fruits; canned fruit with skin or seeds; juice with pulp; jam and marmalade.
Grains *3–10 ounce-equivalents*	White bread, rolls, pasta and rice; refined cereals including cream of wheat and crispy rice; soda crackers.	Whole grain breads, cereals, pasta; wild and brown rice; graham crackers; bran; high fat breads including biscuits, cornbread, croissants, donuts, muffins, pancakes, and waffles.
Dairy Products *2–3 cups*	Fat-free or low-fat milk, low-fat yogurt, fat-free or low-fat cheese; fat-free or low-fat cottage cheese. *If tolerated:* Whole or reduced-fat milk.	Whole or reduced-fat milk *if not tolerated*; cheese or cottage cheese made with whole or reduced fat milk.

Continued on next page

Food for the Day	Recommended	Restrict if not tolerated
Protein Foods *2–7 ounce-equivalents*	Choose tender lean meats which are baked, broiled or grilled and trimmed of fat. Beef (round, flank and loin cuts), pork (loin), ham, skinless chicken and turkey, fish, canned tuna in water, eggs, egg substitutes, 97% fat-free deli meats. If not tolerated, try ground meat. Smooth peanut butter or nut butters (2 Tbsp/day).	Tough, gristly or deep fried meats, bacon, hot dogs, luncheon meats, pork steak, prime rib, ribs, sardines, sausage; dried beans and peas. Crunchy peanut butter or nut butters.
Oils/Solid Fats *May need to limit to 1 serving per meal or snack if not tolerated.*	Butter, margarine, mayonnaise, oil (1 teaspoon). Reduced-fat margarine or mayonnaise (1 Tbsp). Cream, salad dressing, cream cheese (1 Tbsp). Sour cream (2 Tbsp). May use fat-free condiments as desired.	Avocado, bacon, coconut, and nuts.
Added Sugars/ Miscellaneous	Plain pudding made with skim milk, gelatin, fat-free ice cream, sherbet, Popsicles®, angel food cake, sugar, brown sugar, clear jelly, honey, syrup, marshmallows, hard candy, coffee, tea, soft drinks, catsup, mustard, lemon juice, and vinegar.	High fat desserts (cake, pie, cookies, pastries), desserts with coconut, nuts, raisins; seeds, popcorn, pickles, and whole spices.
Fluids	Clear sports drinks, clear fruit drinks, coffee, and tea (hot and iced). *If tolerated:* Clear carbonated beverages.	Juice with pulp; smoothies with pieces of fruit not allowed. Carbonated beverages *if not tolerated.* Alcohol.
Soup	Fat-free broth or bouillon, soups made with skim milk, broth soup made with allowed vegetables and pasta.	Soups made with whole milk or cream; soups made with vegetables not allowed.

REFERENCES

1.   Centers for Disease Control and Prevention. *National Diabetes Statistics Report: Estimates of Diabetes and Its Burden in the United States, 2014.* Atlanta, GA: U.S. Department of Health and Human Services; 2014.

2.   Evert AB, Boucher JL, Cypress M, et al. Nutrition therapy recommendations for the management of adults with diabetes. *Diabetes Care.* 2013; 36(11): 3821-3842.

3.   Institute of Medicine, Food and Nutrition Board. *Dietary Reference Intakes for Energy, Carbohydrate, Fiber, Fat, Fatty Acids, Cholesterol, Protein, and Amino Acids (Macronutrients).* Washington DC: The National Academies Press, 2002/2005.

4. Fox CS, Golden SH, Anderson C, et al. AHA/ADA Scientific Statement: Update on prevention of cardiovascular disease in adults with type 2 diabetes mellitus in light of recent evidence: a scientific statement from the American Heart Association and the American Diabetes Association. *Circulation.* 2015; 132: 691-718. doi:10.1161/CIR.0000000000000230

5. Umpierrez GE, Hellman R, Korytkowski MT, et al. Management of hyperglycemia in hospitalized patients in non-critical care setting: an endocrine society clinical practice guideline. *J Clin Endocrinol Metab* 2012; 97(1):16–38. doi: http://dx.doi.org/10.1210/jc.2011-2098

6. American Diabetes Association. Diabetes care in the hospital, nursing home, and skilled nursing facility. Sec. 13. *In* Standards of Medical Care in Diabetes – 2015. *Diabetes Care* 2015; 38(Suppl. 1):S80–S85.

7. Academy of Nutrition and Dietetics Evidence Analysis Library. *GDM macronutrient and micronutrient intake.* http://www.andeal.org/topic.cfm?menu=5288 Published 2008. Accessed June 21, 2015.

8. Setji TL, Brown AJ, Feinglos MN. Gestational diabetes mellitus. *Clinical Diabetes.* 2005; 23 (1):17–24.

9. Hernandez TL, Van Pelt RE, Anderson, MA et al. A higher-complex carbohydrate diet in gestational diabetes mellitus achieves glucose targets and lowers postprandial lipids: A randomized crossover study. *Diabetes Care.* 2014; 37:1254–1262.

10. Hernandez TL, Van Pelt RE, Anderson, MA et al. Women with gestational diabetes mellitus randomized to a higher–complex carbohydrate/low-fat diet manifest lower adipose tissue insulin resistance, inflammation, glucose, and free fatty acids: a pilot study. *Diabetes Care.* 2016; 39:39–42.

11. Moreno-Castilla C, Hernandez M, Bergua M, et al. Low-carbohydrate diet for the treatment of gestational diabetes mellitus: a randomized controlled trial. *Diabetes Care.* 2013; 36(8):2233-2238. doi:10.2337/dc12-2714

12. Munshi MN, Florez H, Huang ES, et al. Management of diabetes in long-term care and skilled nursing facilities: A position statement of the American Diabetes Association. *Diabetes Care.* 2016; 39(2):308-318. doi: 10.2337/dc15-2512

13. Parrish CR, McKray S. Gastroparesis and nutrition: The art. *Pract Gastroenterol.* 2011; September: 26-41. https://med.virginia.edu/ginutrition/wp-content/uploads/sites/199/2014/06/ParrishGastroparesisArticle.pdf Accessed January 24, 2016.

14. Parkman HP, Yates K, Hasler WL, et al. Dietary intake and nutritional deficiencies in patients with diabetic or idiopathic gastroparesis. *Gastroenterology.* 2011; 141(2): 486–498. e7. doi:10.1053/j.gastro.2011.04.045

15. Camilleri M, Parkman HP, Shafi MA, Abell TL, Gerson L. Clinical guideline: management of gastroparesis. *Am J Gastroenterol..* 2013; 108(1):18-38. doi:10.1038/ajg.2012.373

ADDITIONAL RESOURCES

American Association of Diabetes Educators. *The Art and Science of Diabetes Self-Management Education Desk Reference,* 3rd edition. 2014. www.diabeteseducator.org.

American Diabetes Association. *Therapy for Diabetes Mellitus and Related Disorders,* Sixth Edition. 2014. www.diabetes.org.

International Diabetes Center. *Staged Diabetes Management, Third edition.* 2012. www.idcpublishing.com.

Websites

American Association of Diabetes Educators: www.diabeteseducator.org

American Diabetes Association: www.diabetes.org

Diabetes Prevention Program Outcomes Study: https://dppos.bsc.gwu.edu/web/dppos/lifestyle

JDRF: www.jdrf.org

National Diabetes Education Program: http://ndep.nih.gov/

Study Guide Questions

    A. Differentiate between the following:

- Type 1 diabetes
- Type 2 diabetes
- Gestational diabetes
- Prediabetes

    B. List three factors which can prevent or delay the onset of type 2 diabetes.

    C. List at least three goals of nutrition therapy in treating diabetes.

    D. What are the differences between the sample menu in comparing the Consistent Carbohydrate and General diet?

    E. One carbohydrate choice is equal to how many grams of carbohydrate per serving?

    F. List at least four symptoms of hypoglycemia.

    G. What is the Treatment of Low Blood Sugar "Rule of 15?"

    H. Discussion question: Why is it important to liberalize diets for persons with diabetes in a long-term care setting?

Study Guide Suggested Responses can be found in Appendix 15.

Fat Modified Diets

7

HEART HEALTHY DIET

As new research is published, the Heart Healthy Diet continues to evolve. This diet no longer restricts total fat. (1) While one group still recommends limiting dietary cholesterol (1), many others no longer consider it a nutrient of concern. (2, 3, 4)

Saturated fats are limited, however, when reducing them in the diet they should not be replaced with refined carbohydrates. Instead, it is recommended that saturated fats be replaced with polyunsaturated fats first, followed by monounsaturated fats. (1, 2, 3, 4, 5, 6) *Trans* fats from partial hydrogenation should be avoided. (4, 5) It is recommended persons consume fish (preferably oily) to obtain omega-3 fat in their diet. (1, 4, 5, 7)

Weight loss (5-10% of body weight) is important for persons who are overweight or obese. (1) Refer to Chapter 5, Diets for Weight Management. Sodium restriction is important for persons with high blood pressure. (3) Refer to Chapter 8, Sodium Restricted Diets.

Lastly, focusing on a healthy eating pattern (e.g., DASH in Chapter 8, Mediterranean-Style in Chapter 1, Healthy U.S.-Style in Chapter 1, Vegetarian in Chapter 12) is recommended instead of focusing on single nutrients. (1, 2, 3, 4, 5, 6) The dietary pattern should be individualized based on the patient's specific lipid levels and food preferences.

Use

This diet is prescribed to reduce cholesterol or lipids in the blood. The purpose in following this diet is to reduce total blood cholesterol, "bad" low-density lipoprotein (LDL) cholesterol, and triglycerides; and to increase "good" high-density lipoprotein (HDL) cholesterol. This diet is intended to be a therapeutic diet and may not be appropriate for elderly residents living in a long-term care facility. The elderly population living in a long-term care facility should be on the most liberalized diet possible. Refer to "Meeting the Nutritional Needs of Older Adults" in Chapter 2.

Adequacy

The suggested food plan includes food in the amounts that will provide the Dietary Reference Intakes (DRIs) recommended by the National Academy of Sciences for adults.

Diet Principles

1. Follow a healthy eating pattern that includes fruits, vegetables, legumes, whole grains, low-fat dairy foods, fish, poultry, nontropical vegetable oils, and nuts. Limit intake of sweets, sugar-sweetened beverages, and red meats.

2. Include at least two servings of fish/seafood weekly (preferably fatty fish such as halibut, herring, mackerel, salmon, sardines, trout, and albacore tuna). One serving equals 4 ounces of fish.

3. Reduce saturated fats and avoid *trans* fats. Replace saturated fat with polyunsaturated fats (first choice) or monounsaturated fats (second choice). Refer to *Choose Your Foods*, Appendix 14, for a list of foods that have significant amounts of monounsaturated fats, polyunsaturated fats, and saturated fats. See Table 7.2 for a list of foods with significant amounts of *trans* fats.

If blood lipids are not in goal range after following the Heart Healthy Diet for at least 3 months, consideration of the use of supplemental plant sterols/stanols (~2 g/day) and soluble fibers (5 to 10 g/day from foods and/or supplemental sources) is recommended. (1) See Table 7.3 for food sources of plant sterols/stanols. See Table 7.4 for sources of soluble fiber.

Table 7.2 *Trans*-Fat Foods Sources

Food Sources
• Food prepared with partially hydrogenated vegetable oils (baked goods such as cookies, crackers, and snack cakes)
• Commercially prepared fried foods
• Some margarines with *partially hydrogenated oil* in the ingredients list
• Fried foods served in restaurants and fast food restaurants such as French fries, chicken nuggets, fish patties, and fried pies
• Look for the words *partially hydrogenated oil* in the ingredients list

Table 7.3 Food Sources of Plant Sterols and Stanols (nutrition information from respective companies)

Food Sources*	Amount (grams)
Smart Balance® Heart Right Fat Free Milk, (Cow's Milk) 8oz	0.40
Benecol® Spread, Regular and Light, 1 Tbsp	0.50
Rice Dream® Heart Wise Rice Milk, 8oz	0.65
Lifetime® Low-Fat Cheese Slices, variety flavors, 1 slice	0.65
Corazonas™ Heartbars, 1 bar	0.80
Benecol® Smart Chews, 2 chews	0.80
Minute Maid HeartWise®, 8oz	1.00

*Natural foods rarely have levels of sterols/stanols to be considered a significant source.

Table 7.4 Food Sources of Soluble Fiber

Food Sources	Amount (grams)
Peanut Butter, 1 Tbsp	0.3
Cheerios®, 1 cup	1.0
Kashi® Heart to Heart cereal, 1 cup	1.0
Flaxseed, 1 Tbsp	1.1
Oat flakes, 1 cup	1.5
Asparagus, ½ cup	1.7
Oranges, 1 small	1.8
Apricots, 4 with skin	1.8
Sweet Potato with skin	1.8

Continued on next page

Table 7.4 Food Sources of Soluble Fiber Continued from previous page

Food Sources	Amount (grams)
Brussels sprouts, ½ cup	2.0
Cooked oat bran cereal, ¾ cup	2.2
Oatmeal, regular or steal cut, ¾ cup dry	3.0
Beans (e.g. navy, kidney, black), 1 cup	4.0-4.8

Source: Thalheimer, JC. A Soluble Fiber Primer — Plus the Top Five Foods That Can Lower LDL Cholesterol. *Today's Dietitian*. 2013; 15(12):16. http://www.todaysdietitian.com/newarchives/120913p16.shtml Accessed August 21, 2015

Table 7.5 Heart Healthy Diet

Food for the Day	Recommended	Choose Less Often
Vegetables *1–4 cups*	All fresh, frozen, or canned vegetables, and 100% vegetable juice.	Commercial fried vegetables, vegetables in butter, cream sauce, or cheese sauce, fried potatoes, French fries, chips.
Fruits *1–2.5 cups*	Any fresh, frozen, dried, or canned fruits or 100% fruit juice.	Fried fruit, fruit served with added fat.
Grains *3–10 ounce-equivalents* *At least half of which are whole grains*	Whole-grain breads, cereals, pasta, crackers, and tortillas; brown rice, quinoa, whole wheat couscous, barley, and oats.	Fried rice; refined grains and grains made with saturated or trans fats (e.g., commercial muffins, biscuits, doughnuts, sweet rolls, croissants, cheese breads, party crackers); regular granolas, regular granola bars, or sweets made with partially hydrogenated oils.
Dairy Products *2–3 cups*	Fat-free or low-fat (1%) milk, fat-free dry milk, evaporated fat-free milk, buttermilk made from fat-free milk, fat-free soy milk or milk substitutes such as almond milk; fat-free or low-fat yogurt including Greek yogurt; fat-free or low-fat cheese and cottage cheese.	Whole or reduced-fat milk, regular evaporated milk, whole or reduced-fat yogurt, whole milk cheese, whole milk ice cream.
Protein Foods *2–7 ounce-equivalents*	Lean beef and pork (loin, leg, round, 97% extra lean hamburger), lamb, veal, skinless poultry, 95–99% fat-free lunch or deli meats, fish, dried beans, nuts and nut butters, eggs, meat alternatives / substitutes.	High fat cuts of beef, pork, lamb: ground meat that is 75-80% lean, bacon, salt pork, ribs, hot dogs, sausage, regular cold cuts, skin of chicken or turkey, fish canned in oil. Protein foods fried in saturated or *trans* fats.
Oils, Solid Fats	Unsaturated oils (e.g., canola, corn, flaxseed, olive, peanut, safflower, soybean, sunflower); low-fat or nonfat salad dressings or those made with unsaturated oil; see Fat List in Appendix 14.	Butter, margarine containing *trans* fat, solid shortening, lard, salt pork, chicken fat, cocoa butter, coconut milk, coconut oil, palm oil, palm kernel oil, creamy salad dressings; nondairy creamers, partially hydrogenated oils (*trans* fat).

Continued on next page

Table 7.5 Heart Healthy Diet Continued from previous page

Food for the Day	Recommended	Choose Less Often
Oils, Solid Fats (Continued)	Avocado, olives, margarine (*trans* fat-free), mayonnaise Fat-free or low-fat sour cream and cream cheese.	Coconut. Cream, half and half, sour cream, cream cheese.
Added Sugars *Limit added sugars*	Cakes, cookies or other desserts made with unsaturated oils. Fat-free sweets such as gelatin, angel food cake; fat-free or low-fat sherbet, ice cream, frozen yogurt, or pudding. Honey, jelly, sugar, pancake syrup.	Any cakes, cookies, pies, or other desserts made with butter, shortening, cream, or other saturated or trans fats. Puddings, custards, and ice creams made with whole milk or reduced-fat milk.
Seasonings/Condiments	Herbs, spices, seasonings, and flavorings. Vinegar.	Cream sauces and gravies unless fat free or low-fat.
Fluids	Water and other fluids, such as coffee, tea, and sugar-free beverages.	High sugar beverages including sweetened fruit juices and soft drinks (soda).

Table 7.6 Sample Menu for Heart Healthy Diet

Breakfast	Supper
½ c. orange juice	2 oz. tuna salad made with
1 egg	2 tsp. mayonnaise on
½ c. oatmeal	2 slices whole wheat bread
1 slice whole wheat toast	2 tomato slices
2 tsp. jelly	1 c. leafy greens salad
1 tsp. margarine (*trans* fat-free)	1 Tbsp. oil and vinegar dressing
1 c. fat-free milk	½ c. fruit cocktail
Hot beverage	1 c. fat-free milk
Sugar, pepper (optional)	Water
Lunch	**Snack Ideas**
2 oz. baked chicken breast	½ c. cantaloupe
½ c. mashed potatoes with 2 oz. fat-free gravy	½ c. carrot sticks
½ c. mixed vegetables	3 c. popcorn, *trans*-fat free
1 oz. whole wheat roll	
1 tsp. margarine (*trans* fat-free)	
1 c. fat-free milk	
Water	

LOW-FAT DIET

Use

The Low-Fat Diet may be prescribed to reduce fat intake due to diseases of the gallbladder, liver, or pancreas, or if disturbances in digestion and absorption of fat occur. For diet management of high blood cholesterol and other blood lipids, see the Heart Healthy Diet.

Adequacy

The suggested food plan includes foods in amounts that will provide the DRIs recommended by the National Academy of Sciences for adults. Restriction of fat may result in a diet low in calories. When additional calories are needed, they should be added in the form of complex carbohydrates. Medium chain triglycerides (MCT) may also be useful in meeting energy needs.

Diet Principles

1. Less than 30% total calories from fat. (8, 9, 10)
2. The specific grams of fat allowed will vary depending upon the medical condition and will be identified by the provider or registered dietitian nutritionist.

Table 7.7 Low-Fat Diet

Food for the Day	Recommended	Choose Less Often
Vegetables *1–4 cups*	All fresh, frozen, or canned vegetables; vegetables juice. Any fat used in preparation must be taken from the fat allowance.	Fried vegetables such French fries and potato chips. Vegetables in a cream or cheese sauce such as creamed potatoes.
Fruits *1–2.5 cups*	Any fresh, frozen, dried, or canned fruits; fruit juice.	Fruit prepared with fat.
Grains *3–10 ounce-equivalents* *At least half of which are whole grains.*	Whole-grain breads, cereals, rice, pasta, crackers, and tortillas; brown rice, quinoa, whole wheat couscous, barley, oats, pretzels.	High-fat breads such as muffins, croissants, biscuits, waffles, pancakes, popovers, rich rolls, sweet rolls, and doughnuts; party crackers; granola; fried rice; buttered popcorn.
Dairy *2–3 cups*	Fat-free milk, buttermilk made from fat-free milk, fat-free dry milk, nonfat yogurt. Any low-fat dairy substitute (rice, soy or almond). Fat-free or low-fat cottage cheese. Fat-free or low-fat cheese.	Whole milk, reduced-fat and low-fat milk; ice cream; whole milk yogurt, whole milk cheese, whole milk cottage cheese, coconut milk.
Protein Foods *2–7 ounce-equivalents*	Lean beef, pork, lamb, veal, poultry; 95–99% fat-free luncheon meats, fish. Egg whites, egg substitutes or eggs; hard-cooked, poached or scrambled.	Ribs, regular luncheon meat, hot dogs, corned beef, sausages, processed meats; fried meat, poultry or fish; fish packed in oil; poultry with skin. Fried eggs.

Continued on next page

Table 7.7 Low-Fat Diet Continued from previous page

Food for the Day	Recommended	Choose Less Often
Oils, Solid Fats *These foods must count towards daily fat allowance.* See Fat List in Appendix 14.	Unsaturated oils (e.g., canola, corn, flaxseed, olive, peanut, safflower, soybean, sunflower), non-hydrogenated margarines. Fats from seeds and nuts, nut butters, olives, and avocados. Fat-free or low-fat salad dressing, cream cheese, sour cream, mayonnaise.	Butter, stick margarine; solid shortening, lard, bacon, salt pork, chicken fat, coconut oil, palm oil, palm kernel oil; creamy salad dressings; nondairy creamers, partially hydrogenated oils. Coconut. Cream, cream cheese, sour cream, and mayonnaise.
Added Sugars *Limit added sugars*	Fat-free sweets such as gelatin, angel food cake; fat-free or low-fat desserts such as sherbet, ice cream, frozen yogurt or pudding. Honey, jelly, sugar, pancake syrup.	Any high fat dessert such as cakes, cookies, or pies. Puddings, custards, and ice creams made with whole milk or reduced-fat milk.
Seasonings/Condiments	All spices, seasonings, and flavorings. Vinegar.	Cream sauces and gravies unless fat free.
Fluids	Water and other fluids, such as milk, coffee, tea, fruit or vegetables juice.	

Table 7.8 Sample Menu for Low-Fat Diet

Breakfast	Supper
½ c. orange juice	2 oz. tuna salad (water packed) made with
1 scrambled egg	2 tsp. reduced-fat mayonnaise on
½ c. oatmeal	2 slices bread
1 slice whole wheat toast	2 tomato slices
2 tsp. jelly	1 Tbsp. low-fat vinaigrette dressing
1 tsp. soft margarine	½ c. fruit cocktail
1 c. fat-free milk	1 c. fat-free milk
Hot beverage	Water
Sugar, pepper (optional)	
Lunch	**Snack Ideas**
2 oz. roasted chicken breast	½ c. cantaloupe
½ c. mashed potatoes with 2 oz. fat-free gravy	½ c. carrot sticks
½ c. mixed vegetables	3 c. popcorn, no fat added
1 oz. whole wheat roll	
1 tsp. soft margarine	
1 c. fat-free milk	
Water	

REFERENCES

1. Jacobson TA, Maki KC, Orringer C, et al. National Lipid Association recommendations for patient-centered management of dyslipidemia: part 2. *J Clin Lipidol.* Published Online:September 18, 2015. DOI: http://dx.doi.org/10.1016/j.jacl.2015.09.002

2. Fuller NR, Sainsbury A, Caterson ID, Markovic TP. Egg consumption and human cardio-metabolic health in people with and without diabetes. *Nutrients.* 2015; 7(9):7399-7420. doi:10.3390/nu7095344.

3. Eckel RH, Jakicic JM, Ard JD, et al. 2013 AHA/ACC Guideline on lifestyle management to reduce cardiovascular risk. *Circulation.* 2014; 129:S76-S99. doi: 10.1161/01.cir.0000437740.48606.d1

4. US Department of Health and Human Services. *Scientific Report of 2015 Dietary Guidelines Advisory Committee.* Washington, DC: US Department of Health and Human Services; 2015. http://health.gov/dietaryguidelines/2015-scientific-report/pdfs/scientific-report-of-the-2015-dietary-guidelines-advisory-committee.pdf

5. Willett WC. Dietary fats and coronary heart disease. *J Intern Med.* 2012; 272:13–24. doi:10.1111/j.1365-2796.2012.02553.x

6. Fox CS, Golden SH, Anderson C, et al. AHA/ADA Scientific Statement: Update on prevention of cardiovascular disease in adults with type 2 diabetes mellitus in light of recent evidence: a scientific statement from the American Heart Association and the American Diabetes Association. *Circulation.* 2015; 132: 691-718. doi:10.1161/CIR.0000000000000230

7. Maehre HK, Jensen I, Elvevoll EO, and Eilertsen K. ω-3 fatty acids and cardiovascular diseases: effects, mechanisms and dietary relevance. *Int J Mol Sci.* 2015; 16(9): 22636–22661. doi: 10.3390/ijms160922636

8. Academy of Nutrition and Dietetics. Nutrition Care Manual. Pancreatitis Nutrition Therapy. https://www.nutritioncaremanual.org/client_ed.cfm?ncm_client_ed_id=127 Accessed November 16, 2015.

9. Academy of Nutrition and Dietetics. Nutrition Care Manual. Gallbladder Nutrition Prescription. https://www.nutritioncaremanual.org/topic.cfm?ncm_toc_id=18679 Accessed November 16, 2015.

10. Duggan SN, Conlon KC. A practical guide to the nutritional management of chronic pancreatitis. *Pract Gastroenterol.* 2013; June: 24-32. https://med.virginia.edu/ginutrition/wp-content/uploads/sites/199/2014/06/Parrish_June_13.pdf

ADDITIONAL RESOURCES

Pancreatitis. National Institute of Diabetes and Digestive and Kidney Diseases website. http://www.niddk.nih.gov/health-information/health-topics/liver-disease/pancreatitis/Pages/facts.aspx

Parrish CR, DiBaise JK. Short bowel syndrome in adults – part 2. Nutrition therapy for short bowel syndrome in the adult patient. *Pract Gastroenterol.* 2014; October: 40-51. https://med.virginia.edu/ginutrition/wp-content/uploads/sites/199/2014/06/Parrish-October-14.pdf

Websites

American Heart Association: www.heart.org

National Institute of Diabetes and Digestive and Kidney Diseases. http://www.niddk.nih.gov/health-information/health-topics/Pages/default.aspx

Study Guide Questions

A. What are the recommendations for total fat, cholesterol, saturated fat and *trans* fats for a person following a Heart Healthy diet?

B. List 3 examples of foods with significant amounts of *trans* fats? List 3 examples of good food sources of soluble fiber?

C. List at least three diseases for which a Low-Fat Diet may be prescribed.

D. The Low-Fat diet limits fat consumption to approximately what % of total calories from fat per day?

E. Discussion question: How can recipes be modified to reduce the overall fat in that food?

Study Guide Suggested Responses can be found in Appendix 15.

Sodium Restricted Diets

8

NO ADDED SALT DIET

The No Added Salt diet limits sodium to 3,000 and 4,000 mg [130–174 mEq] sodium.

Use

The No Added Salt (NAS) diet averages less than 4,000 mg sodium per day and is a more palatable moderate sodium restricted diet while still providing benefits toward lowering cardiovascular events. (1, 2) The NAS diet is an appropriate diet for the elderly who have increased risk of weight loss. (3) For management of fluid restrictions, see Fluid Restrictions in Chapter 9.

Adequacy

The suggested food plan provides foods in amounts that will provide the DRIs recommended by the National Academy of Sciences for adults.

Diet Principles

1. Table salt (sodium chloride) is made up of about 40% sodium and should be limited in the diet. One teaspoon of table salt is the equivalent of 2,300 mg of sodium. Foods processed with salt are limited. Other foods that contain liberal amounts of natural sodium or sodium compounds may be limited.

2. The General Diet (including lightly salted foods in cooking) is served without a salt packet or client is counseled to avoid use of salt shaker. Limit foods with visible salt including chips, salted pretzels, salted nuts, salted crackers, and salted popcorn.

3. Some higher sodium foods may be served during the week, but they should be limited so that the daily average of sodium over the week is less than 4,000 mg sodium. Foods high in sodium are listed in the *Food for the Day* in Table 8.5.

4. The lower 3000 mg range of the NAS diet may be met by using mostly fresh or frozen vegetables, allowing no cured meats like ham or sausage, no high sodium breakfast meats, no high brine foods like sauerkraut or deli pickles, and avoidance of salty snacks between meals. See *Tips to Reduce Salt and Sodium* in Table 8.4.

5. Salt substitutes may promote acceptance of sodium-restricted diets but should be used only if permitted by the physician as they may contain potassium.

6. Sea salt is not a suitable 'salt substitute' for the table. It is available in many particle sizes and used for specific culinary purposes. Sea salt is 97 to 100% sodium chloride. It may have other beneficial nutrients like calcium and magnesium but is not a significant source of these minerals. (4)

Table 8.1 Sample Menu for No Added Salt Diet

(3000–4000 mg sodium [130–174 mEq])

Breakfast	Supper
½ c. orange juice	2 oz. tuna on 2 slices whole wheat bread
1 egg	2 tsp. mayonnaise
½ c. oatmeal	2 tomato slices
1 slice whole wheat toast	1 c. leafy greens salad
2 tsp. jelly	1 Tbsp. oil and vinegar dressing
1 tsp. soft margarine	½ c. fruit cocktail
1 c. milk	1 c. milk
Hot beverage	Water
Sugar, pepper (optional)	*NO SALT PACKET*
NO SALT PACKET	
Lunch	**Snack Ideas**
2 oz. roasted chicken breast	½ c. cantaloupe
½ c. mashed potatoes with 2 oz. gravy	½ c. carrot sticks
½ c. mixed vegetables	3 c. popcorn, no salt added
1 oz. whole wheat roll	
1 tsp. soft margarine	
1 c. milk	
Water	
NO SALT PACKET	

DASH DIET

Use

The DASH (dietary approaches to stop hypertension) Diet emphasizes foods high in nutrients such as potassium, magnesium, calcium, and fiber that have been linked to antihypertensive effects. (5) This diet is high in fruits, vegetables, low-fat dairy products, and reduced in saturated and total fat to lower blood pressure. (5) See Table 8.2. The DASH Diet is adopted by the American College of Cardiology/American Heart Association 2013 Task Force for reduction of cardiovascular risk. (6)

Adequacy

The suggested food plan provides foods in amounts that will provide the Dietary Reference Intakes (DRIs) recommended by the National Academy of Sciences for adults.

Diet Principles

Excessive intake of sodium chloride (table salt) is a major factor in elevating blood pressure and is a risk factor for cardiovascular and renal disease. In addition to reducing sodium chloride intake, other factors that can decrease blood pressure include weight loss, moderation of alcohol intake, and consuming a diet based on the DASH diet. (7)

The DASH diet has two levels of daily sodium consumption: 2,300 mg and 1,500 mg. (8) The 2300 mg sodium diet is the lowest sodium restriction recommended by the Institute of Medicine to improve health outcomes in certain populations. (9) The 2015 – 2020 Dietary Guidelines for Americans states adults with prehypertension and hypertension would benefit from further reduction to 1500 mg sodium per day. (10) However, analysis of the 1500 mg sodium diet reveals it cannot meet 27 key nutrients. (11) For this reason, only the 2,300-mg sodium DASH diet is included in this chapter.

Table 8.2 Daily Nutrient Goals Used in the DASH Studies

Total Fat	27% of calories	Sodium	2,300 mgs
Saturated Fat	6% of calories	Potassium	4,700 mgs
Protein	18% of calories	Calcium	1,250 mg
Carbohydrate	55% of calories	Magnesium	500 mg
Cholesterol	150 mg	Fiber	30 g

Adapted from NIH Publication No. 06-4082, Your Guide to Lowering Your Blood Pressure with DASH. Revised April 2006, p. 5. (8)

The 2,300-mg sodium DASH diet should be used with caution in the following circumstances:

1. The DASH diet is high in potassium and increases risk of hyperkalemia for elderly with one or more of these diagnoses: diabetes, chronic renal (kidney) insufficiency, end-stage renal (kidney) disease, severe heart failure, and adrenal insufficiency. (7)

2. The DASH diet may increase risk of hyperkalemia if one or more medications are taken that impair potassium excretion. (7) These drugs include oral potassium supplements, beta β-adrenergic blockers, nonsteroidal anti-inflammatory drugs, angiotensin-converting enzyme (ACE) inhibitors, angiotensin receptor blockers (ARBs), and potassium-sparing diuretics. (12, 13)

3. Older adults may limit their caloric intake and increase their risk of nutritional deficiencies. (14, 15)

4. The DASH diet is not recommended for people with stage 3 or 4 chronic kidney disease due to the high potassium and phosphorus content of the diet. (7)

The DASH diet reduces blood pressure with an eating plan low in saturated fat, cholesterol, and total fat; and high in fruits, vegetables, fat-free or low-fat (1% milk) and low-fat milk products. The DASH diet can be adapted for weight loss if needed, which will also decrease blood pressure.

Table 8.3 DASH Diet

Food for the Day	Serving Sizes
Vegetables	1 c. raw leafy vegetable
4–5 servings	½ c. cut-up raw or cooked vegetables
	½ c. vegetable juice
Fruits	1 medium fruit
4–5 servings	¼ c. dried fruit
	½ c. fresh, frozen, or canned fruit
	½ c. fruit juice

Continued on next page

Table 8.3 DASH Diet Continued from previous page

Food for the Day	Serving Sizes
Grains *6–8 servings* *Aim for whole grains for most of grain servings per day*	1 slice bread ½ c. cooked rice or pasta ½ c. cooked cereal 1 oz. dry cereal (or check serving size on box)
Dairy products *2–3 cups*	1 c. skim or 1% milk 1 ½ oz. fat-free, low-fat or reduced fat cheese 1 c. fat-free or low-fat regular yogurt 1 c. fat-free or low-fat frozen yogurt
Meats, poultry and fish *6 servings or less*	1 oz. cooked lean meats, poultry or fish (trim visible fats; broil, roast or poach; remove skin from poultry) 1 egg – limit to 4 egg yolks per week 1 oz. low sodium ham
Nuts, seeds, and legumes *4–5 servings per week*	⅓ c. or 1 ½ oz. unsalted nuts 2 Tbsp. peanut butter 2 Tbsp. or ½ oz. unsalted seeds ½ c. cooked legumes (dry beans and peas)
Oils/Fats *2–3 servings* *Use soft margarine or liquid margarines, vegetable oil such as canola, corn, olive, or safflower*	1 tsp. soft margarine 1 tsp. vegetable oil 1 Tbsp. mayonnaise 1 Tbsp. regular salad dressing 2 Tbsp. low-fat dressing Fat-free gravy
Sweets and Added Sugars *5 or less per week*	1 Tbsp. sugar 1 Tbsp. jelly, jam or regular syrup ½ c. sorbet, gelatin 1 c. lemonade

ALCOHOL: Limit alcohol to ≤2 alcoholic drinks per day for men and ≤1 alcoholic drink per day for women and lighter-weight persons.

1 drink = 12 oz regular beer; 5 oz wine (12% alcohol); 1.5 oz. of 80-proof distilled spirits.

Moderate drinking is recommended for those who drink alcohol as alcohol can negatively influence blood pressure.

Adapted from NIH Publication No. 06-4082, Your Guide to Lowering Your Blood Pressure with DASH. Revised April 2006, p. 8–9 (8)

*Based on 2,000 calories daily.

Table 8.4 Tips to Reduce Salt and Sodium

- Choose 'low or reduced' sodium, or 'no salt added' versions of foods and condiments when available.
- Choose fresh, frozen, or canned ('low or reduced sodium' or 'no salt added') vegetables.
- Use fresh poultry, fish, and lean meat, rather than canned, smoked or processed types.
- Choose ready-to-eat breakfast cereals that are lower in sodium.
- Limit cured foods (such as bacon and ham), foods packed in brine (such as pickles, pickled vegetables, olives, and sauerkraut); and condiments (such as mustard, horseradish, ketchup, and barbecue sauce). Limit even lower sodium versions of soy sauce and teriyaki sauce. Treat these condiments sparingly as you do table salt.
- Cook rice, pasta, and hot cereals without salt. Limit or avoid on instant or flavored rice, pasta, and cereal mixes, as these products usually have added salt.
- Choose 'convenience' foods that are lower in sodium. Limit or avoid on frozen dinners, mixed dishes such as pizza, packaged mixes, canned soups or broths, and salad dressings—these often have a lot of sodium.
- Rinse canned foods, such as tuna and canned beans, to remove some of the sodium.
- Use spices instead of salt. In cooking and at the table, flavor foods with herbs, spices, lemon, lime, vinegar, or salt-free seasoning blends. Start by cutting salt in half.
- On Nutrition Facts labels, aim for foods that are less than 5% of the daily value of sodium. Foods with 20% or more daily value of sodium are considered high.

Adapted from NIH Publication No. 06-4082, Your Guide to Lowering Your Blood Pressure with DASH. Revised April 2006, pp. 17, 19. (8)

LOW SODIUM DIET or 2300 mg Sodium Diet

This diet restricts sodium intake to 2,300 mg [100 mEq] daily.

Use

The 2300 mg Low Sodium diet is the lowest sodium restriction recommended by the Institute of Medicine to improve health outcomes in certain populations. (9) This diet is useful in preventing or controlling edema or hypertension (high blood pressure). This diet is appropriate for persons with ascites (see Chapter 9). Caution is required for use with frail elderly because weight loss may occur as a result of palatability concerns. (15, 16, 17) Elderly require higher levels of salt to detect salt flavor in their diet. (18, 19, 20) For management of fluid restrictions, see Fluid Restrictions in Chapter 9.

Adequacy

The suggested food plan provides foods in amounts that will provide the DRIs recommended by the National Academy of Sciences for adults.

Diet Principles

1. Prepare all foods without salt and do not add salt at the table. Avoid all processed and prepared foods and beverages high in sodium. One teaspoon of table salt is the equivalent of 2,300 mg of sodium.

2. Limit the amounts of milk, meat, ready-to-eat cereals, and breads and desserts made with salt and baking powder or soda.

3. Some medications, including over-the-counter preparations for treatment of indigestion or excess acid, contain large amounts of sodium.

4. Salt substitutes may promote acceptance of sodium-restricted diets, but they should be used only if permitted by physician. One teaspoon of salt substitute (usually potassium chloride) contains between 2,240 mg (57 mEq) and 3,180 mg (81 mEq) of potassium. The

high potassium levels can be harmful for some patients with renal (kidney) concerns or receiving certain medications. (12) See Dash Diet 'cautions' no. 2 on p. page 89 for list of medications.

Table 8.5 Low Sodium Diet

Food for the Day	Recommended – Low in sodium	Choose Less Often – High in sodium
Vegetables *1–4 cups*	Vegetables may be raw or cooked; fresh, frozen, or no added salt canned vegetables. Low sodium* tomato or vegetable juices.	Canned vegetables (unless labeled "no added salt"); sauerkraut; tomato juice or vegetable juices canned with salt.
Fruits *1–2.5 cups*	Fresh, frozen, canned, dried or 100% fruit juice.	Dried fruits with sodium sulfite.
Grains *3–10 ounce-equivalents* *At least half of which are whole grains.*	Bread, rolls, buns, bagels, English muffins, oatmeal, farina, shredded wheat, puffed wheat or rice cereal, tortillas, rice, pasta, couscous, quinoa; unsalted popcorn, unsalted pretzels, unsalted top crackers.	Breads, rolls, or crackers with salted toppings; chips, pretzels or other high sodium snacks; packaged rice, macaroni, or noodle mixtures; salted popcorn, instant hot cereals, and commercial bread stuffing.
Dairy Products *2–3 cups*	Milk, nondairy milks (soy, almond, rice), yogurt or Greek yogurt. Swiss cheese.	Buttermilk, cottage cheese, or other aged cheeses. Processed cheese, cheese spreads or sauces.
Protein Foods *2–7 ounce-equivalents*	Fresh beef, pork, poultry, fish, lamb, veal, venison, wild game; dry beans or legumes, eggs, nuts, and seeds.	Smoked, salted, cured, koshered meats, or fish such as bacon, bologna, chipped beef, corned beef, hot dogs, ham, lunch or deli meats, Canadian bacon, pickled meats, salt pork, sausage. Canned tuna, salmon, sardines; imitation crab or lobster. Most commercial entrees. Salted nuts and seeds. Canned beans (unless labeled 'no salt added')
Oils, Solid Fats	Vegetable oils (canola, flaxseed, olive, peanut, sesame, and soybean oil). Butter, cream, cream cheese, sour cream, margarine, mayonnaise.	Salted gravy, bacon, salt pork, seasoned dips. Limit regular salad dressing to 1 tablespoon per day.
Added Sugars	Sugar, honey, jelly, jam, pancake syrup.	
Fluids	Water and other fluids, such as coffee, tea, 100% fruit juice.	Commercially canned soups, bouillon, broths, dehydrated soup mixes; bouillon cubes, granules, or packets.

Continued on next page

Table 8.5 Low Sodium Diet Continued from previous page

Food for the Day	Recommended – Low in sodium	Choose Less Often – High in sodium
Seasonings/Condiments	Salt substitute, approved by physician or dietitian. Herbs and spices with no salt added. Vinegar.	Salt and salt-based seasonings. Prepared condiments such as steak sauce, soy sauce, teriyaki sauce, barbecue sauce, salsa, ketchup, and mustard. Olives, pickles, relishes.

*Low sodium foods contain no more than 140 mg of sodium per serving.

Table 8.6 Sample Menu for Low Sodium Diet

(2300 mg sodium [100 mEq])

Breakfast	Supper
½ c. orange juice	2 oz. tuna (low sodium) on
1 egg	2 slices whole wheat bread
½ c. oatmeal	2 tsp. mayonnaise
1 slice whole wheat toast	2 tomato slices
2 tsp. jelly	1 c. leafy greens salad
1 tsp. soft margarine	1 Tbsp. oil and vinegar dressing
1 c. milk	½ c. fruit cocktail
Hot beverage	1 c. milk
Sugar, pepper (optional)	Water
NO SALT PACKET	*NO SALT PACKET*
Lunch	**Snack Ideas**
2 oz. roasted chicken breast	½ c. cantaloupe
½ c. mashed potatoes (cooked from fresh)	½ c. carrot sticks
½ c. mixed vegetables (cooked from fresh or frozen)	3 c. popcorn, no added salt
1 oz. whole wheat roll	
2 tsp. soft margarine	
1 c. milk	
Water	
NO SALT PACKET	

REFERENCES

1. O'Donnell MF, Mente A, Rangarajan S, et al. Urinary sodium and potassium excretion, mortality and cardiovascular events. *New Engl J Med.* 2014; 371: 612-623.

2. Heaney, RP. Making sense of the science of sodium. *Nutr Today.* 2015; 50(2):63–66.

3. Morley JE. Hypertension: Is it overtreated in the elderly? *J Am Med Dir Assoc.* 2010; 11(3):147–152.

4. Antman EM, Appel LJ, Balentine D, et al. Stakeholder discussion to reduce population—wide sodium intake and decrease sodium in the food supply: a conference report from the American Heart Association Sodium Conference 2013 Planning Group. *Circulation.* 2014; 129(25):e660-e679.

5. Appel LJ, Moore TJ, Obarzanek E, et al. A clinical trial of the effects of dietary patterns on blood pressure. *New Engl J Med.* 1997; 336(16):1117–1124.

6. Eckel RH, Jakicic JM, Ard JD, et al. 2013 AHA/ACC Guideline on lifestyle management to reduce cardiovascular risk. *Circulation.* 2014; 129:S76-S99. doi: 10.1161/01. cir.0000437740.48606.d1

7. Appel LJ, Brands MW, Daniels SR, Karanja N, Elmer PJ, Sacks FM. Dietary approaches to prevent and treat hypertension. A scientific statement from the American Heart Association. *Hypertension.* 2006; 47(2):296–308.

8. US Department of Health and Human Services, National Institutes of Health, National Heart, Lung, and Blood Institute. *Your Guide to Lowering Your blood Pressure with DASH,* 2006. https://www.nhlbi.nih.gov/files/docs/public/heart/new_dash.pdf

9. Committee on the Consequences of Sodium Reduction in Populations: Food and Nutrition Board; Board on Population Health and Public Health Practice; Institute of Medicine; *Sodium Intake in Populations: Assessment of Evidence.* Washington,DC: National Academies Press (US); 2013.

10. U. S. Department of Health and Human Services and U. S. Department of Agriculture. *2015 – 2020 Dietary Guidelines for Americans,* 8th ed. http://health.gov/dietaryguidelines/2015/guidelines/ Published December 2015. Accessed February 3, 2016.

11. Maillot M, Drewnowski A. A conflict between nutritionally adequate diets and meeting the 2010 dietary guidelines for sodium. *Am J Prev Med.* 2012; 42(2):174–179.

12. Perazella MA, & Mahnensmith RL. Hyperkalemia in the elderly, drugs exacerbate impaired potassium homeostasis. *J Gen Intern Med.* 1997; 12:646–656.

13. Tyson, CC, Nwankwo, C, Lin, Pao-Hwa, Svetkey, LP. The Dietary Approaches to Stop Hypertension (DASH) eating pattern in special populations. *Curr Hypertens Rep.* 2012; 14(5):388–396.

14. Lichtenstein AH, Appel LJ, Brands M, et al. Diet and lifestyle recommendations revision 2006: a scientific statement from the AHA nutrition committee. *Circulation.* 2006; 114:82–96.

15. Franz MJ, Bantle JP, Beebe CA, et al. Position statement: Evidence-based nutrition principles and recommendations for the treatment and prevention of diabetes and related complications. *Diabetes Care.* 2002; 25(1):170.

16. Kohrs M. A rational diet for the elderly. *Am J Clin Nutr.* 1982; 36:796–802.

17. Buckler DA, Kelber ST, Goodwin JS. 1994. The use of dietary restrictions in malnourished nursing home patients. *J Am Geriatr Soc.* 1994; 42:1100–1102.

18. Nordin S, Razani LJ, Markison S, Murphy, C. Age-associated increases in intensity discrimination for taste. *Exp Aging Res.* 2003; 29(3):371–381.

19. Stevens JC, Cain WS. Changes in taste and flavor in aging. *Crit Rev Food Sci Nutr.* 1993; 33(1):27–37.

20. Mojet J, Christ-Hazelhof E, Heidema J. Taste perception with age: Generic or specific losses in threshold sensitivity to the five basic tastes? *Chem Senses.* 2001; 26:845-860.

Websites

SNAP-ed Connection: https://snaped.fns.usda.gov/resource-library/foods/information-sodiumsalt

Tips to Eat Less Salt and Sodium: http://www.nhlbi.nih.gov/health/educational/healthdisp/pdf/tipsheets/Tips-to-Eat-Less-Salt-and-Sodium.pdf

United States Department of Agriculture: http://www.nutrition.gov/whats-food/salt-sodium

Study Guide Questions

A. What micronutrients are included in the DASH diet guidelines?

B. What is the purpose of following a DASH diet?

C. What is the sodium range of the No Added Salt diet in milligrams as compared to a Low Sodium diet?

D. Why is a No Added Salt recommended for elderly clients rather than a Low Sodium diet?

E. Discussion question: To promote food palatability on a sodium restricted diet, how can flavors be enhanced?

Study Guide Suggested Responses can be found in Appendix 15.

Diets for Renal and Liver Disease

9

MODIFIED RENAL DIET

Use

The Modified Renal Diet may be prescribed for individuals with end-stage renal disease (ESRD) who are on dialysis and reside in a healthcare setting. These individuals often have other medical conditions and a high incidence of malnutrition related to poor appetite and gastrointestinal intolerances such as nausea and vomiting. (1) Many individuals with renal disease in long-term care will not need a strict therapeutic diet because their appetite is already so limited. The use of the Modified Renal Diet in this setting can allow the person to enjoy the main menu with relatively few changes, a key factor in satisfaction and diet adherence. (2)

The diet principles that follow should be implemented on initiation of the diet. The registered dietitian nutritionists' in the facility and in the dialysis unit should collaborate to individualize nutrition therapy and promote consistency for the best overall health outcome for the individual. (3, 4)

Adjustments to the renal diet will depend on the person's individual laboratory results and tolerance of dialysis treatments. (5) If the individual is transported from the facility to a dialysis unit for treatments, a nourishing snack or sack meal may need to be planned and sent along with the individual, depending on the timing of meals, see "Carry-Out Meals and Snacks" below.

Adequacy

The suggested diet plan may not provide adequate quantities of B vitamins, calcium, and vitamin D as recommended by the National Academy of Sciences for adults. The Dietary Reference Intakes (DRIs) for phosphorus and potassium intake may not be met. The kidney's impairment affects the levels of these nutrients and the interactions between them. (6, 7) The dialysis unit dietitian will need to recommend appropriate vitamins and minerals. As a result of the kidney's impaired function, any over-the-counter nutritional supplements such as glucosamine, multivitamins, minerals, and amino acids should be used only with the approval of the physician and registered dietitian nutritionist (RDN) providing care related to dialysis treatment.

Diet Principles

The Modified Renal Diet is limited in sodium, phosphorus, and potassium with emphasis on adequate protein and calories; however, the least restrictive menu should be used. The following modifications should be made in addition to the No Added Salt Diet (see Chapter 8) to create the Modified Renal Diet. These principles should be done initially, then, with input from the dialysis unit RDN and client, further substitutions may be necessary.

1. **Energy**. Adequate caloric intake of 35 calories per kilogram (kg) is essential. Individuals over 60 may require fewer calories: 30 to 35 calories per kg. (8, 9) When calorie intake is inadequate, the body will break down protein for energy instead of using it for essential growth and repair of body tissues. Individuals receiving peritoneal dialysis receive up to 30% of calories from the dialysate infusion and may require modification in calorie intake to prevent weight gain (10). Consult the dialysis unit or facility RDN for an individualized meal plan.

2. **Carbohydrates**. The addition of refined carbohydrates and simple sugars (i.e., desserts) can be useful in achieving adequate protein-sparing calories. If the person with ESRD has diabetes, refer to the Diets for Diabetes in Chapter 6. Carbohydrates low in potassium should be used to treat hypoglycemia (i.e., glucose tablets, cranberry juice cocktail, lemonade, non-cola carbonated beverages).

3. **Protein.** Patients on dialysis require more protein (1.2 to 1.4 grams per kg per day) due to dialysate loss. (8, 9) A minimum of 6 ounces of meat or meat alternative should be encouraged. Protein of high biological value is preferable; at least half of the protein intake should come from animal-derived foods including meat, poultry, fish, milk, yogurt, cheese, and eggs. Soybeans provide an alternative complete protein.

   Suggestions for increasing protein include:

   • Double egg portion at breakfast

   • Large portion of meat at midday and evening meal

   • Meat or egg sandwich for snack

   For vegetarians, the phosphorus content of beans and legumes means alternative special protein supplements may be needed. However, recent research indicates that the effect on serum phosphorus may be less than previously believed. (11) Diets should be individualized based on serum phosphorus values. A serving of beans and legumes may be included daily if desired.

4. **Sodium.** Sodium (Na+) restriction may be needed to control fluid, especially between dialysis treatments, and to manage blood pressure. (12) The No Added Salt Diet principles apply to the Modified Renal Diet along with the following:

   • Substitute lower sodium plain meats to replace high sodium meats (e.g., ham, sausage). Remove the breading found on prepared meat items such as breaded fish or chicken.

   • Substitute all soup with either appropriately made lower sodium soups or a lower potassium vegetable (Table 9.1). Fluid in soup must be counted as part of fluid restriction (Table 9.5).

   • Choose fresh, frozen, or canned ("low sodium," "no salt added," or "reduced sodium") vegetables.

   • Avoid salt substitutes, seasoning mixes, and low sodium broths or bouillons that contain potassium.

   • Avoid foods with visible salt such as chips, pretzels, salted nuts and popcorn, and salted crackers.

   • Avoid foods in a brine including sauerkraut and pickles.

5. **Potassium.** Potassium (K+) is usually limited for persons receiving hemodialysis to avoid dangerous levels that could cause heart problems. People on Continuous Ambulatory Peritoneal Dialysis (CAPD) often experience low levels of potassium and usually do not need a potassium restriction. (10) The following steps will decrease potassium for the Modified Renal Diet:

   • Substitute citrus, prune, tomato, and vegetable juices with cranberry, apple, or other lower potassium juice (vitamin C-fortified).

   • Substitute citrus fruit, bananas, tomatoes, and prunes with lower potassium fruits. Fresh tomatoes can be allowed in small amounts (one to two slices per meal). Star fruit (carambola) is toxic for the person with kidney disease and should not be served. (13)

- Typically, small amounts of tomato sauce are tolerated (i.e., half portion of spaghetti sauce with regular portion of noodles); the meat provided still needs to be a regular or double portion.

- No baked potatoes or potato chips, even if low salt. Allow mashed or boiled potatoes if serving size does not exceed ¼ cup per day.

- Do not use salt substitutes, seasoning mixes, and low sodium broths or bouillons containing potassium.

- See Appendix 7 "Potassium Content of Selected Foods."

- See Potassium Content in Selected Foods (Table 9.1) for more substitution ideas.

Table 9.1 Potassium (K+) Content in Selected Foods*

Food Group	Foods High in Potassium (≥250 mg K+/ Serving)	Foods Lower in Potassium (120–250 mg K+/Serving) *Lowest K+ sources are bolded (≤120 mg K+/Serving)*
Vegetables	Artichoke	**Bamboo Shoots**
	Asparagus	**Bean sprouts**
	Beans, dried, cooked, (includes baked beans, lentils and lima beans)	Beets, canned, drained
		Broccoli
	Beet greens, cooked	**Cabbage**
	Beets	Carrots
	Brussels sprouts	Cauliflower
	Collards, cooked	**Celery**
	Kale	Corn
	Kohlrabi	Cucumber, peeled
	Parsnips	Eggplant
	Potato, baked, boiled or prepared from frozen	**Green Beans**
		Green/Red Peppers
	Potato, mashed, from homemade	**Lettuce, iceberg**
	Spinach, cooked	Mixed Vegetables, canned or frozen
	Pumpkin, canned	Mushrooms, ¼ cup
	Salsa	Mustard greens, cooked
	Squash, winter, cooked	Okra
	Sweet potato, cooked	**Onions**
	Swiss chard, cooked	**Peas**
	Tomato (whole, juice or sauce)	Potatoes, mashed, made with water, boxed flakes or granules
	Vegetable juice	Radishes
		Spinach, fresh
		Turnips

Continued on next page

Food Group	Foods High in Potassium (≥250 mg K+/ Serving)	Foods Lower in Potassium (120–250 mg K+/Serving) *Lowest K+ sources are bolded (≤120 mg K+/Serving)*
Vegetables *(Continued)*		Turnip Greens, cooked
		Water Chestnuts
		Wax (Yellow) Beans
		Zucchini/Summer Squash
Fruits	Avocado	Apple (including juice)
	Banana	**Applesauce**
	Cantaloupe	Apricots
	Dried fruit, raisins	Blackberries
	Honeydew melon	**Blueberries**
	Kiwifruit	Cherries
	Mango	Cranberries (juice and all forms)
	Nectarine	**Fruit Cocktail**
	Orange (fruit and juice)	**Grapes (including juice)**
	Papaya	Grapefruit, ½ medium
	Pomegranate	Peaches, raw and canned
	Prunes (fruit and juice)	Pear, raw
		Pears, canned
		Pineapple (including juice)
		Plums, raw and canned
		Raspberries
		Strawberries
		Tangerines (Mandarin Oranges)
		Tropical Fruit Mix, canned
		Watermelon
Dairy Products	Milk, fresh or canned	Cottage cheese
	Yogurt	
Protein Foods	Dried beans and peas such as pork and beans, refried beans, split peas, kidney beans, lentils.	Peanut butter, 1 Tbsp.
	Soybeans, cooked	
Others	Salt substitutes (containing potassium chloride).	2 Tbsp. Ketchup, chili sauce, taco sauce or salsa.
	Low sodium broth and bouillon (may contain potassium chloride; check nutrient analysis before using).	

*Unless otherwise noted, portions are ½ cup; or if whole, 1 medium piece.

Nutrient values from (15) U.S. Department of Agriculture, Agricultural Research Service, Nutrient Data Laboratory. USDA National Nutrient Database for Standard Reference, Release 22: 2009. http://www.ars.usda.gov/Services/docs.htm?docid=20960

6. **Phosphorus**. Phosphorus needs to be limited in the diet and treated with physician-ordered phosphate binders, which are given with each meal and snack. If phosphorus is uncontrolled, painful bone loss and calcium deposits in tissue can occur as well as extreme itching. (15) The phosphate binders are necessary to allow enough protein to be consumed.

Emerging research indicates that 40 to 100% of phosphorus from food additives may be absorbed and increase serum levels more than from the organic phosphorus present in food. Check food labels of packaged and processed foods and avoid/limit the use of foods with phosphorus in the ingredient list. (10, 11) By comparison, only about 50% of the phosphorus found in plant sources is absorbed. See Table 9.2 for foods high in phosphorus.

Table 9.2 High Phosphorus Foods

Food Category	Foods High in Phosphorus
Vegetables	Lima beans, cooked legumes (dry beans and peas).
Fruits	None
Grains	Whole wheat bread, corn tortillas, corn bread, whole wheat bread, biscuits, brown rice, pancakes, waffles, muffins.
	Cereals made with bran or whole grains (shredded wheat, oats).
Dairy Products	Milk, cheese, pudding, yogurt, cottage cheese, eggnog.
Protein Foods	Beef, pork, lamb, veal, poultry, fish, egg yolks.
	Legumes (dry beans and peas) such as pork and beans, refried beans, split peas, kidney beans.
	Nuts and seeds, peanut butter.
	Soybeans, tofu.
Oils, Solid Fats	None
Added Sugars	Desserts containing >1 ounce chocolate.
	Cake doughnuts.
	Ice cream.
	Cream pies.
Others	Breads and desserts made with baking powder, processed foods listing phosphorus compounds in the ingredient list, some non-dairy creamers, bottled iced tea, and colas.

Nutrient values from (15) U.S. Department of Agriculture, Agricultural Research Service, Nutrient Data Laboratory. USDA National Nutrient Database for Standard Reference, Release 22: 2009. http://www.ars.usda.gov/Services/docs.htm?docid=20960

The following steps will decrease phosphorus for the Modified Renal Diet:

- Limit or avoid for whole grain or bran-containing breads and cereals. Use refined carbohydrates such as white bread and white rice.

- Avoid or limit the use of processed foods, packaged foods that list phosphorus compounds in the ingredient list.

- Restrict dairy products to 1 to 2 servings per day. This includes milk, half-and-half, yogurt, custard, pudding, ice cream, frozen yogurt, cheese, and cottage cheese. See Table 9.3 for dairy serving sizes. Almond milk is low in phosphorus and may be used in place of milk. See Table 9.4 for more substitution ideas.

Table 9.3 Dairy Serving Sizes

Food	Serving Size
Milk	½ cup
Half and half	½ cup
Cheese	1 ounce
Cottage cheese	⅓ cup
Yogurt (not Greek)	½ cup
Custard	⅓ cup
Pudding	½ cup
Ice cream or frozen yogurt	½ cup
Eggnog	½ cup

Table 9.4 Phosphorus Substitutions

Instead of:	Replace with:
Milk	Almond milk
Hard cheese	Cream cheese
Ice cream	Sherbet, sorbet
Baked beans, lima beans	Mixed vegetables or green beans
Nuts or seeds	Unsalted pretzels or popcorn
Peanut butter (2 Tbsp. serving)	Limit to 1 Tbsp. with jelly
Chocolate	Graham crackers, animal crackers, hard or jellied candy
Whole grain bread	White or rye bread, enriched, plain white bagel
Whole grain cereals	Rice or corn cereal
Cola and pepper-type carbonated drinks, beer, or bottled beverages with added phosphorus	Root beer, orange, lemon-lime, ginger ale, coffee, tea, lemonade, punch

7. **Fluids.** All foods contain some fluid; however, only foods liquid at room temperature (including soup) or foods that become liquid when swallowed, such as gelatin, need to be counted. Fluid restriction, when ordered, must be individualized. (12) See the Sample Menu Plan for Fluid Restrictions in Table 9.5

Table 9.5 Fluid Restrictions

Foods that are considered liquids (1 fluid ounce = 30 mL):
• ½ Cup Gelatin or 1 cup of Crushed Ice = 120 mL
• ½ Cup Ice Cream or Sherbet = 90 mL
• Popsicles® (Double) = 80 mL
• ⅔ cup soup = 120 mL liquid (remainder is solids)

SAMPLE MENU PLAN FOR FLUID RESTRICTIONS

Fluid Restriction	Breakfast	Lunch	Dinner	Nursing or Snacks
1000 mL	240 mL	240 mL	240 mL	280 mL
1200 mL	360 mL	240 mL	240 mL	360 mL
1500 mL	360 mL	360 mL	360 mL	420 mL
1600 mL	480 mL	360 mL	360 mL	400 mL
1800 mL	480 mL	480 mL	360 mL	480 mL
2000 mL	480 mL	480 mL	480 mL	560 mL

To increase compliance with the Modified Renal Diet, the practice of providing half-portions of desired, but restricted, foods is appropriate as then only half the carbohydrate, sodium, phosphorus, and potassium has been consumed. The RDN in the dialysis unit can also provide recommendations regarding the volume of desired foods that could be consumed either the night before or the morning of dialysis treatments to assist with diet satisfaction.

Table 9.6 Sample Menu for Modified Renal Diet for individuals **receiving hemodialysis treatment**

Breakfast	Supper
½ c. vitamin C-fortified apple juice	2 oz. tuna on 2 slices enriched white bread with 2 tsp mayonnaise
2 eggs	
¾ c. puffed rice cereal	1 tomato slice
1 slice white toast	1 c. leafy greens salad
2 tsp. jelly	1 Tbsp. oil and vinegar dressing
2 tsp. soft margarine	½ c. fruit cocktail canned in heavy syrup
½ c. reduced-fat or whole milk	*NO MILK*
Sugar, pepper *(optional)*	½ c. cranberry juice cocktail
NO SALT PACKET	*NO SALT PACKET*

Lunch	Snack Ideas
4 oz. roasted chicken breast	½ c. watermelon
¼ c. mashed potatoes	½ c. carrot sticks
½ c. mixed vegetables	1 roast beef sandwich
1 oz. white roll	

Continued on next page

2 tsp. soft margarine

1 cookie

NO MILK

½ c. vitamin C-fortified apple juice

NO SALT PACKET

Carry-Out Meals and Snacks for Dialysis

Individuals with renal disease may need to be away during the day for dialysis or other appointments. Sending along an appropriate meal will make their day easier and more comfortable. Perishable foods should be well-chilled and packed in insulated containers with appropriate utensils. Note: regulations at the dialysis unit may limit what is appropriate for that meal's time frame and convenience (i.e., lunch needs to be consumed after dialysis is over).

The following are suggestions for simple, portable meals:

- Sandwiches on bread, pocket bread or flour tortillas: Meat (roast beef, pork, poultry) with margarine or mayonnaise or egg salad, chicken/turkey salad, or tuna salad.

- Chef salad and bread: Cubed meat, tuna, and/or egg with lettuce and low potassium raw vegetables; salad dressing; dinner roll, muffin, unsalted crackers, unsalted popcorn, or unsalted pretzels.

- Low or medium potassium fruit: Small apple, blueberries, grapes, applesauce, pineapple, or canned, drained fruit such as peaches, pears, fruit cocktail.

- Low or medium potassium raw vegetable: Cucumber slices, green pepper strips, lettuce, broccoli, carrots, cauliflower, celery, radishes, turnips.

- Beverage (regular or sugar-free depending upon diet requirements): Apple juice, grape juice, cranberry juice cocktail, lemonade, punch, non-cola carbonated beverages including ginger ale, lemon-lime, and root beer.

  Note: be sure to check for sodium on the nutrition label of all canned and bottled beverages. Check the ingredient list for phosphorus additives.

- Snacks suggestions: To add calories to a meal or for a midmorning or midafternoon snack: Bagel with cream cheese, graham crackers, unsalted crackers, unsalted tortilla chips, rice cakes, vanilla wafers, animal crackers, approved cookies, sweetened gelatin cup.

- DO NOT SEND: Bologna, cheese, peanut butter, ham, ham salad, banana, melon, fresh orange, dried fruit, tomato, milk, orange juice, grapefruit juice, tomato juice, or cola beverages.

Individuals who have end stage renal disease but are not on dialysis also may require diet modification, refer to low protein modified renal diet information.

LOW PROTEIN MODIFIED RENAL DIET

Use

The purpose of a low protein diet is to slow the progression to end stage renal disease. The Low Protein Modified Renal Diet may be prescribed for individuals with chronic kidney disease (CKD) stages 3, 4, and 5, and end-stage renal disease (ESRD) who are *not* on dialysis. These individuals often have other medical conditions such as hypertension, cardiovascular disease, and diabetes. As CKD progresses, they may have a high incidence of malnutrition related to poor appetite and gastrointestinal intolerances such as nausea and vomiting. (1) Many people with renal disease in long-term care will not need a strict therapeutic diet because their appetite is already so limited. The use of the Low Protein Modified Renal Diet in this setting can allow the person to enjoy the main menu with relatively few changes, a key factor in satisfaction and diet adherence. (2)

Adequacy

The suggested diet plan may not provide adequate quantities of B vitamins, calcium, and vitamin D, as recommended by the National Academy of Sciences for adults. The Dietary Reference Intakes (DRIs) for protein, phosphorus, and potassium intake may not be met. The kidney's impairment affects the levels of these nutrients and the interactions between them. (5) The diet principles that follow should be implemented on initiation of the diet. The registered dietitian nutritionist (RDN) in the facility will need to recommend necessary vitamin and mineral supplementation, and individualize nutrition therapy for the best overall health outcome for the individual.

Diet Principles

The Low Protein Modified Renal Diet is similar to the Modified Renal Diet but is more limited in protein. Sodium and phosphorus guidelines are similar. Potassium restriction may not be indicated, but should be initiated when hyperkalemia is present. (16) Calorie needs are based on weight status. Energy requirements may be less in the overweight individual. The following modifications should be made in addition to the No Added Salt Diet (see Chapter 8) to create the Low Protein Modified Renal Diet. These principles should be done initially, then, with input from the facility RDN and client, further substitutions may be necessary.

1. **Protein.** Individuals with CKD stages 3, 4, and stage 5 not on dialysis may benefit from a lower protein intake of 0.8 grams per kilogram (kg) per day. (17) For people with diabetic kidney disease, protein intake of 0.8 grams per kg per day is recommended. (18) Protein of high biological value is preferable; at least half of the protein intake should come from animal-derived foods, including meat, poultry, fish, milk, yogurt, cheese, and eggs. Soybeans provide an alternative complete protein. (9)

2. **Energy**. Adequate calorie intake of 30 to 35 calories per kg is essential. The lower end of the range estimate is suggested for overweight and obese individuals and individuals over 60 years of age with CKD who are not on dialysis (16). For the individual with BMI >30 consult with the facility RDN to further individualize diet and/or refer to Diets for Weight Management in Chapter 5.

3. **Carbohydrates**. The addition of refined carbohydrates and simple sugars can be useful in achieving adequate protein–sparing calories. If the individual with CKD stages 3, 4, and 5 not on dialysis has diabetes, refer to the Diets for Diabetes in Chapter 6. As CKD advances, diabetes medicines may need to be adjusted to prevent hypoglycemia. (19)

4. **Sodium.** Restriction of sodium similar to the Modified Renal Diet are also recommended.

5. **Phosphorus**. Phosphorus restriction similar to the Modified Renal Diet is suggested. A phosphorus binder may be prescribed by the medical provider.

6. **Potassium.** Potassium is liberalized to follow the general diet menu for fruits and vegetables. Restriction is indicated if the patient has hyperkalemia. (16)

7. **Fluids**. Fluid restriction must be individualized based on medical status, edema status, blood pressure control, and urine output.

Table 9.7 Sample Menu for Low Protein Modified Renal Diet for individuals with CKD stages 3, 4, and stage 5 **NOT** receiving dialysis treatment

Breakfast	Supper
½ c. orange juice (or ½ c. vitamin C-fortified apple juice for low K+)	2 oz. tuna on 2 slices enriched white bread with 2 tsp. mayonnaise
1 egg	2 tomato slices (1 slice for low K+)
¾ c. puffed rice cereal	1 c. leafy greens salad
1 slice white toast	1 Tbsp. oil and vinegar dressing
2 tsp. jelly	½ c. fruit cocktail canned in heavy syrup
2 tsp. soft margarine	Almond milk
½ c. reduced-fat or whole milk	(or Fruit Punch for low K+)
Sugar, pepper *(optional)*	*NO SALT PACKET*
NO SALT PACKET	
Lunch	**Snack Ideas**
2 oz. roasted chicken breast	½ c. watermelon
½ c. mashed potatoes (¼ c for low K+)	½ c. carrot sticks
½ c. mixed vegetables	Crisped Rice Marshmallow Bar
1 oz. white roll	
2 tsp. soft margarine	
1 cookie	
Almond milk (or Lemonade for low K+)	
NO SALT PACKET	

Emergency Dialysis Diet

Emergencies such as snowstorms, floods, or illness may cause someone to miss a scheduled dialysis treatment. The guidelines in Table 9.8 can help prevent complications.

Table 9.8 Emergency Dialysis Diet

Potassium	Choose only the lowest potassium fruits, vegetables, and juices.
	Limit fruits to 1 ½ c. daily.
	Limit vegetables to ½ c. daily.
	Limit juice to ½ c. daily.
Phosphorus	Limit dairy products to one serving daily.
Protein Foods	Limit meat, poultry, fish, and eggs to a total of 4 oz. daily.
	Avoid high sodium items like peanut butter, ham, bacon, sausage, hot dogs, and processed lunchmeats.

Continued on next page

Table 9.8 Emergency Dialysis Diet Continued from previous page

Fluids	Limit salty foods to avoid drinking too much water or other beverages.
	Drink only half the amount of fluids usually allowed.
Carbohydrates	Eat more buttered white bread or rolls, rice, buttered pasta, cereal (without nuts and fruit), low salt crackers, vanilla wafers, bagels, English muffins, tortillas, angel food cake, unsalted pretzels and popcorn, rice cakes or animal crackers to satisfy hunger.

Adapted from "Iowa Snowstorm Diet" by Debra Hassebrock, RD, LD. Used with permission.

REFERENCES

1. Lopes AA, Elder SJ, Ginsberg N, et al. Lack of appetite in haemodialysis patients-associations with patient characteristics, indicators of nutritional status and outcomes in the international DOPPS. *Nephrol Dial Transplant.* 2007; 22(12):3538–3546. doi: 10.1093/ndt/gfm453

2. Niedert KC, American Dietetic Association. Position paper of the American Dietetic Association: Liberalization of the diet prescription improves quality of life for older adults in long-term care. *J Am Dietetic Assoc.* 2005; 105(12):1955–1965.

3. Hutson, B. & Stuart, N. Nutrition management of the adult hemodialysis patient. In: Byham-Gray L., Stover, J. & Wiesen K, eds. *Renal Dietitians Dietetic Practice Group of the Academy of Nutrition and Dietetics and the Council on Renal Nutrition of the National Kidney Foundation. A Clinical Guide to Nutrition Care in Kidney Disease,* 2nd ed. Chicago, IL: Academy of Nutrition and Dietetics; 2013:55-56.

4. Renal Practice Group of the American Dietetic Association. *National Renal Diet, Professional Guide,* 2nd ed. Chicago, IL: American Dietetic Association; 2002.

5. Brink BR, & Reams SM. Renal diets for nursing facilities: A team approach. *The Consultant Dietitian.* 1997; 21(1):4–6.

6. Chazot C, & Kopple JD. Vitamin metabolism and requirements in renal disease and renal failure. In: Kopple JD, & Massry SG, eds. *Kopple & Massry's Nutritional Management of Renal Disease* , 2nd ed. Philadelphia, PA: Lippincott Williams & Wilkins; 2004:315-356.

7. Moe SM. Calcium, phosphorus and vitamin D metabolism in renal diseases and chronic renal failure. . In: Kopple JD, & Massry SG, eds. *Kopple & Massry's Nutritional Management of Renal Disease* , 2nd ed. Philadelphia, PA: Lippincott Williams & Wilkins; 2004:261-285.

8. Hutson, B. & Stuart, N. Nutrition management of the adult hemodialysis patient. In: Byham-Gray L., Stover, J. & Wiesen K, eds. *Renal Dietitians Dietetic Practice Group of the Academy of Nutrition and Dietetics and the Council on Renal Nutrition of the National Kidney Foundation. A Clinical Guide to Nutrition Care in Kidney Disease,* 2nd ed. Chicago, IL: Academy of Nutrition and Dietetics; 2013:56.

9. National Kidney Foundation. K/DOQI nutrition in chronic renal failure. *Am J of Kidney Dis.* 2000; 35 (6)(Suppl 2). doi:10.1053/kd.2000.6669

10. McCann L. Nutritional management of adult peritoneal dialysis patient. In: Byham-Gray L., Stover, J. & Wiesen K, eds. *Renal Dietitians Dietetic Practice Group of the Academy of Nutrition and Dietetics and the Council on Renal Nutrition of the National Kidney Foundation. A Clinical Guide to Nutrition Care in Kidney Disease,* 2nd ed. Chicago, IL: Academy of Nutrition and Dietetics; 2013:77.

11. Sarathy S, Sullivan C, Leon JB, Sehgal AR. Fast Food, phosphorus-containing additives and the renal diet. *J Ren Nutr.* 2008; 18(5):466-470.

12. Sarkar SR, Kotanko P, & Levin NW. Fellows' Forum in Dialysis: Interdialytic weight gain: Implications in hemodialysis patients. *Semin Dial.* 2006; 19:429–433. doi: 10.1111/j.1525-139X.2006.00199_1.x

13. Yap HJ, Chen YC, Fang JT, Huang, CC. Star fruit: A neglected but serious fruit intoxicant in chronic renal failure. *Dial Transplant.* 2002; 31:564–567, 597.

14. U.S. Department of Agriculture, Agricultural Research Service, Nutrient Data Laboratory. USDA National Nutrient Database for Standard Reference, Release 22: 2009. http://www.ars.usda.gov/Services/docs.htm?docid=20960

15. Hutson, B, & Stuart N. Nutritional management of adult hemodialysis patient. In: Byham-Gray L., Stover, J. & Wiesen K, eds. *Renal Dietitians Dietetic Practice Group of the Academy of Nutrition and Dietetics and the Council on Renal Nutrition of the National Kidney Foundation. A Clinical Guide to Nutrition Care in Kidney Disease,* 2nd ed. Chicago, IL: Academy of Nutrition and Dietetics; 2013:58.

16. Harvey, K. Nutritional management in Chronic Kidney Disease Stages 1 through 4. In: Byham-Gray L., Stover, J. & Wiesen K, eds. *Renal Dietitians Dietetic Practice Group of the Academy of Nutrition and Dietetics and the Council on Renal Nutrition of the National Kidney Foundation. A Clinical Guide to Nutrition Care in Kidney Disease,* 2nd ed. Chicago, IL: Academy of Nutrition and Dietetics; 2013:31-33.

17. Kidney Disease Improving Global Outcomes. KDIGO 2012 Clinical Practice Guideline for the Evaluation and Management of Chronic Kidney Disease. *Kidney Int Suppl. 2013;* 3(1):75. http://www.kdigo.org/clinical_practice_guidelines/pdf/CKD/KDIGO_2012_CKD_GL.pdf

18. American Diabetes Association. Foundations of Care and Comprehensive Medical Evaluation. Sec. 3. *In* Standards of Medical Care in Diabetes – 2016. *Diabetes Care* 2016; 39(Suppl. 1):S23–S35. doi:10.2337/dc16-S006

19. Tuttle KR, Bakris GL, Bilous RW, et al. Diabetic kidney disease: a report from an ADA consensus conference. *Diabetes Care.* 2014;37(10):2864–2883 doi: 10.2337/dc14-1296

Websites

Academy of Nutrition and Dietetics: www.eatright.org/resource/health/diseases-and-conditions/kidney-disease/kidney-disease-and-diet

National Kidney Foundation: www2.kidney.org/professionals/KDOQI/guidelines_nutrition/nut_a25.html

National Kidney Center: www.nationalkidneycenter.org/chronic-kidney-disease

Centers for Disease Control and Prevention: www.cdc.gov/diabetes/programs/initiatives/kidney.html

National Kidney Disease Education Program: www.nkdep.nih.gov/identify-manage/ckd-nutrition/training-modules.shtml

NUTRITIONAL GUIDELINES FOR LIVER (HEPATIC) DISEASE

The goal of diet therapy for persons with liver disease is to manage their symptoms without causing protein calorie malnutrition (PCM) or further damage to the liver. The type of liver disease and their other medical conditions will affect what diet modifications are needed. The doctor might order a diet limiting fluid and sodium intakes and/or a diet for diabetes.

Hepatitis or liver inflammation from viral infections, cancer, medications, alcohol or gallstones causes abdominal pain and jaundice (yellowing of the eyes and skin). Hepatitis can be acute and last less than 3 months, however, some forms can become chronic and even lead to cirrhosis or liver cancer. (1) Acute hepatitis requires additional protein and calories to improve recovery. (1) Fulminant hepatitis is the most severe and life-threatening form, often from an overdose of acetaminophen with alcohol.

Cirrhosis is an advanced and chronic liver disease caused by loss of healthy liver tissue to fibrosis and permanent scarring. Cirrhosis leads to complications such as ascites (fluid collection in the abdomen), encephalopathy (a confused to comatose state), bone disease, malabsorption, injury to the kidneys (hepatorenal syndrome), and end-stage liver disease. (2) Albumin, prealbumin, cholesterol, clotting factors, glycogen, and Vitamin D levels drop as these require activation by the liver. (2, 3, 4) Blood glucose levels can vary from high to low with insulin resistance and poor fasting glycogen metabolism. (3, 4)

Edema and ascites can make people with cirrhosis appear to gain weight but further evaluation will show their upper bodies are very thin with loss of fat and muscle mass (a loss of "dry" weight masked by the fluid retention). Appetites and intakes are poor and calorie needs may be higher leading up to 75% of individuals to have malnutrition and up to 50% to have moderate to severe protein calorie malnutrition (PCM). (3, 4) PCM worsens their quality of life and increases mortality rates. Those with severe and end-stage liver disease could require a liver transplant.

Alcoholic liver disease (ALD) is caused by toxicity of alcohol to liver cells over several years. The amount of alcohol required to cause damage varies by age, gender, genetics, and other medical conditions such as gastric bypass surgery. Alcoholic liver disease starts as inflammation and fat deposits that injure the liver. Abstinence from alcohol and a healthful diet may initially slow or reverse the damage but often cirrhosis will develop. (1, 2, 4, 5)

Nonalcoholic fatty liver disease (NAFLD) or **nonalcoholic steatohepatitis** (NASH) are caused by fat deposits in the liver and can also progress over several years to cirrhosis. The main causes are obesity due to excessive calorie intake and inactivity, chronic use of total parenteral nutrition, poorly controlled diabetes, and infection. (6, 7) NAFLD is the most common chronic liver disease worldwide with a reported prevalence ranging from 6 to 33%. (6) More people will be affected by NAFLD and NASH due to increasing rates of obesity and type 2 diabetes. (6, 7) A reasonable weight, exercise, good blood glucose management, and a healthful diet are recommended.

Hepatic encephalopathy (HE) is a complication of severe liver disease. Fasting, gastrointestinal bleeding, constipation, renal failure, and excessive protein intake all increase the risk for HE. Older research suggested they could be helped by severely limiting protein, especially meat protein intake, but this is no longer recommended as protein restriction can worsen their risk of malnutrition. (2, 4, 7, 8) Moderate amounts of protein spread throughout the day may help those that are protein sensitive. (2, 3, 4) There are several medications to help treat or prevent this condition and some of these also cause loose stools.

Diet Principles

A healthy diet offering adequate calories, carbohydrates, fats, and protein to achieve an acceptable "dry" weight can improve their overall health. Usually 4 to 6 smaller meals or snacks per day will be the best tolerated and metabolized.

1. **Calories** from a variety of foods are needed to maintain a healthy weight and help the liver function as well as it can. If weight loss is needed, it should be done slowly and at not more than 1 to 2 pounds per week. Four to six smaller meals and snacks throughout the day may help ensure adequate calorie intake at 25 to 40 calories per kilogram (kg) ideal or a reasonable "dry" weight. (1, 2, 3, 4, 6)

2. **Protein** is important for liver cell repair and maintaining muscle mass. Strict protein restrictions should be avoided due to the risk of malnutrition. The goal should be 1 to 1.5 grams protein per kg of ideal or a reasonable "dry" weight or 60 to 90 grams per day for most people. Dairy, egg, soy, grain, and vegetable proteins may be easier for those with liver disease to tolerate than meat protein. (3) Offering the usual menu 2 to 4 ounces of meat or eggs at each meal meets the goal of adequate but not excessive protein intakes

and further restrictions are not recommended. Milk and yogurt should only be limited if they also have kidney disease. Branch-chain amino acids (BCAA) supplements may help treat or prevent PCM but the research remains unclear. (3, 4, 8)

3. **Carbohydrates.** Encourage complex carbohydrates from whole grain foods and fresh fruits and vegetables. Regular soda, juices, and sweet desserts should be used in limited amounts to avoid hyperglycemia and more fat deposits in the liver, especially for those with diabetes or NAFLD. A carbohydrate rich bedtime snack helps maintain energy and blood sugar levels throughout the night. (1, 2, 3, 4) Most people will benefit from a snack such as a half sandwich, ½ cup of a high calorie nutritional supplement, cereal or cookie with milk, or yogurt.

4. **Fat** intake should be adjusted to help maintain a healthy "dry" weight. Less than 30% of calories from fat is the usual goal, plus additional fat if needed for weight gain. (2, 4, 8, 9, 10) Some people with liver disease have problems digesting and absorbing fat and will get diarrhea if they eat fatty foods. See Chapter 7 for information on a Low-Fat Diet.

5. **Sodium** should be limited to maintain normal fluid and electrolyte balance. Those that have fluid retention and swelling in the abdomen (ascites) or the legs (peripheral edema) need a Low Sodium Diet of 2000 to 3000 mg sodium per day. (1, 2, 3, 11, 12, 13, 14) A more severe sodium restriction is unnecessary and may lead to malnutrition. (14, 15, 16) See Chapter 8 for information on a Low Sodium Diet.

6. **Fluids** may need to be limited (1,500 to 2,000 mL of fluid per day) if serum sodium levels are low or if fluid retention is not well controlled. Avoid fluid restriction if serum sodium is in the normal range. (14, 17) See Fluid Restrictions in Chapter 9.

7. Several vitamin and mineral deficiencies are common in persons with liver disease. (9, 10) Vitamin and mineral supplements may be ordered by the healthcare provider. Thiamin and folate supplements may be ordered for a few days for those with active alcoholism or severe malnutrition. Zinc and iron deficiencies are common. (1, 2, 3, 4) Vitamins A, D, E and K levels often drop with fat malabsorption and poor liver function. (2, 4)

8. Alcohol, certain medications, and some herbal supplements are quite toxic to the liver and should be avoided.

9. Malnourished individuals with poor oral intake of food and oral nutrition supplements may benefit from enteral nutrition support. (18)

REFERENCES

1. Academy of Nutrition and Dietetics. Nutrition Care Manual. Hepatitis. www.nutritioncaremanual.org/topic.cfm?ncm_toc_ID=18539. Accessed 6/30/2015.

2. Academy of Nutrition and Dietetics. Nutrition Care Manual. Cirrhosis. www.nutritioncaremanual.org/topic.cfm?ncm_toc_ID=18609. Accessed 6/30/2015.

3. Chadalavada R, Sappati Biyyani RS, Maxwell J, Mullen K. Nutrition in hepatic encephalopathy. *Nutr Clin Pract.* 2010; 25(3):257-264.

4. Mouzaki M, Ng V, Kamath BM, Selzner N, Pencharz P, Ling SC. Enteral energy and macronutrients in end-stage liver disease. *J Parenter Enteral Nutr.* 2014; 38(6):673-681.

5. Dugum M, McCullough A. Diagnosis and management of alcoholic liver disease. *J Clin Transl Hepatol.* 2015. 3(2):109-116.

6. Demir M, Lang S, Steffen HM. Nonalcoholic fatty liver disease: Current status and future directions. *J Dig Dis.* 2015, Sep 25. doi: 10.1111/1751-2980.12291. [Epub ahead of print]

7.   Ahmed A, Wong, RJ, Harrison SA. Nonalcoholic fatty liver disease review: Diagnosis, treatment, and outcomes. *Clin Gastroenterol Hepatol*. 2015 Jul 27. pii: S1542-3565(15)00988-X. doi: 10.1016/j.cgh.2015.07.029. [Epub ahead of print]

8.   Amodio P, Canesso F, Montagnese S. Dietary management of hepatic encephalopathy revisited. *Curr Opin Nutr Metab Care*. 2014; 17(5):448-452.

9.   Göktürk HS, Selçuk H. Importance of malnutrition in patients with cirrhosis. *Turk J Gastroenterol*. 2015; 26(4):291-296. doi: 10.5152/tjg.2015.0224

10. Cheung K, Lee SS, Raman M. Prevalence and mechanisms of malnutrition in patients with advanced liver disease, and nutrition management strategies. *Clin Gastroenterol Hepatol*.2012; 10(2):117-125.

11. Gu X, Yang X, Zhu H, Xu B. Effect of a diet with unrestricted sodium on ascites in patients with hepatic cirrhosis. *Gut and Liver*. 2012; 6(3):355-361. doi:10.5009/gnl.2012.6.3.355.

12. Pedersen JS, Bendtsen F, Møller S. Management of cirrhotic ascites. *Therapeutic Advances in Chronic Disease*. 2015; 6(3):124-137. doi:10.1177/2040622315580069.

13. Zhu YF, Gu XB, Zhu HY, Yang XJ, Wang D, Yu P. Influence of non-sodium restricted diet with diuretics on plasma rennin, renal blood flow and in patients with cirrhotic ascites. *Chinese Journal of Experimental and Clinical Virology* 2013; 27(1):50-53.

14. European Association for the Study of the Liver. EASL clinical practice guidelines on the management of ascites, spontaneous bacterial peritonitis, and hepatorenal syndrome in cirrhosis. *J Hepatol*. 2010; 53(3): 397 – 417.

15. Moore KP, Wong, F, Gines P, Bernardi M, Ochs A, Salerno F, et al. The management of ascites in cirrhosis: report on the consensus conference of the International Ascites Club. *Hepatology* 2003; 38(1): 258-266.

16. Morando F, Rosi S, Gola E, et al. Adherence to a moderate sodium restriction diet in outpatients with cirrhosis and ascites: a real-life cross-sectional study. *Liver Int*. 2015; 35(5):1508-1515. doi:10.1111/liv.12583

17. Purnak T, Yilmaz Y. Liver disease and malnutrition. *Best Pract Res Clin Gastroenterol*. 2013; 27(4):619-629. doi: 10.1016/j.bpg.2013.06.018

18. Plautha M, Cabre´b E, Riggioc O, et al. ESPEN guidelines on enteral nutrition: liver disease. *Clinical Nutrition*. 2006; 25(2):285-294.

Websites

Center for Disease Control and Prevention. Viral Hepatitis. http://www.cdc.gov/hepatitis/index.htm

Hepatitis B Foundations: http://www.hepb.org

MedicineNet.com. Liver Disease. http://www.medicinenet.com/liver_disease/article.htm

National Institutes of Health: www.nlm.nih.gov/medlineplus/liverdiseases.html

Study Guide Questions

A. What key nutrients are considered in the Modified Renal Diet?

B. Who is responsible for calculating and teaching individuals and caregivers about the client's diet restrictions?

C. List at least four sources of high biological value protein.

D. Why is adequate energy intake essential to individuals with end-stage renal disease?

E. Milk is usually limited in the Modified Renal Diet to _____ cup because it is high in the nutrient _____.

F. List four examples of common foods that would be considered "fluids" and should be included in a fluid restriction.

G. Use of salt substitute and low sodium broth and bouillon should only be used with the approval of the physician or dietitian. What component of these foods is of particular concern?

H. Discussion question: What interventions can be implemented to promote adequate energy intake for individuals with end-stage renal disease?

Study Guide Suggested Responses can be found in Appendix 15.

Fiber Modified Diets

HIGH FIBER DIET

Use

The High Fiber Diet may be useful in the treatment of many of the diseases of public health significance—obesity, cardiovascular disease, type 2 diabetes, and inflammatory diseases—as well as being associated with decreased constipation and improved intestinal health. These conditions can be prevented or treated by increasing the amounts and varieties of fiber-containing foods. (1, 2, 3) Additionally, a diet higher in fiber is likely to be less calorically dense and have a higher satiety value than a diet lower in fiber. (4)

Adequacy

The suggested food plan provides foods in amounts that will provide the Dietary Reference Intakes (DRIs) recommended by the National Academy of Sciences for adults.

Diet Principles

1. The High Fiber Diet contributes 25–38 grams of dietary fiber, defined as plant materials resistant to digestion. (5) Because fiber is found exclusively in plant foods, increase consumption of whole grains (e.g., whole wheat, bulgur, oatmeal, whole cornmeal, brown rice, buckwheat, wild rice, whole rye, whole-grain barley, amaranth, millet, quinoa, sorghum, and popcorn), fruits, vegetables, beans, nuts, and seeds. Increased fiber intake should come from a variety of food sources rather than from fiber supplements to ensure adequate nutrient intake. (6) See Appendix 2 "Fiber Content of Selected Foods."

2. High dietary fiber foods should be added gradually to prevent possible short-term side effects including abdominal discomfort, bloating, cramping, or diarrhea. If symptoms continue, reduce fiber intake.

3. A high fiber diet should be accompanied by a liberal intake of water or other fluids. Because fiber holds water, thereby softening the stool, at least 8 cups of liquids should be ingested daily. Inadequate fluid intake can lead to constipation or impaction in the colon because dietary fiber absorbs water from the intestinal tract.

4. Despite the popular notion that indigestible fiber from nuts, corn, popcorn, and seeds could lodge in the diverticula and cause inflammation and infection, no scientific data support this; so eliminating specific foods is not necessary. (7,8)

Table 10.1 High Fiber Diet

Food for the Day	Recommended – High in fiber
Vegetables *1–4 cups*	All vegetables except vegetable juice: asparagus, broccoli, Brussels sprouts, carrots, cabbage, cauliflower, celery, corn, green beans, greens, lima beans, okra, onions, parsnips, peas, peppers, potatoes (white or sweet, including skin), radishes, sauerkraut, spinach, squash, tomatoes, yams. Those with skins or seeds will contain more fiber.
Fruits *1–2.5 cups*	All fruits except fruit juice: apples, apricots, berries, cherries, figs, grapefruit, oranges, peaches, pears, pineapple, plums, prunes, and rhubarb. Those with skins or seeds will contain more fiber.
Grains *3–10 ounce-equivalents* *More than half of all grains eaten should be whole grains for extra fiber**	Whole grain breads, cereals, and pastas, listing whole-grain flour as the first ingredient; use whole-grain flours in cooking whenever possible (e.g., whole-wheat breads, whole-grain pasta, oatmeal, whole wheat or corn tortillas, brown or wild rice, popcorn, whole wheat couscous, quinoa, whole wheat crackers, whole wheat buns and rolls). Substitute whole wheat or oat flour for up to half of the flour in pancake, waffle, muffin or other flour-based recipes.
Dairy Products *2–3 cups*	Not a source of fiber.
Protein Foods *2–7 ounce-equivalents*	Cooked legumes (dried beans and peas), nuts, and soybeans. Use whole grains in mixed dishes, such as barley in vegetable soup or stews and bulgur wheat in casseroles or stir-fries. May also add flax seed, wheat germ, chia seed, or other whole grains.
Oils, Solid Fats, Added Sugars	Coconut, avocado.

*Many, but not all whole-grain products are good sources of dietary fiber. Use the Nutrition Facts label on whole-grain products to choose foods that are a good or excellent source of dietary fiber.

Table 10.2 Sample Menu for High Fiber Diet

Breakfast	Supper
1 small orange	2 oz. tuna on 2 slices whole wheat bread with 2 tsp. mayonnaise
1 egg	
½ c. oatmeal with up to 1 Tbsp ground flaxseed	2 tomato slices
1 slice whole wheat toast	1 c. leafy greens salad
2 tsp. jelly	1 Tbsp. oil and vinegar dressing
1 tsp. soft margarine	½ c. fruit cocktail
1 c. milk	1 c. milk
Hot beverage	Water
Sugar, pepper (optional)	

Continued on next page

Table 10.2 Sample Menu for High Fiber Diet Continued from previous page

Lunch	Snack Ideas
2 oz. roasted chicken breast	1 c. cantaloupe
3 oz. baked potato with skin	½ c. carrot sticks
½ c. mixed vegetables with corn and peas	3 c. popcorn
1 oz. whole wheat roll	
2 tsp. soft margarine	
1 c. milk	
Water	

LOW FIBER DIET

Use

The Low Fiber Diet is designed for use in patients receiving radiation therapy on or near the intestine; in partial bowel obstruction; in periods of disease flares or intestinal strictures in inflammatory bowel disease (Crohn's disease or ulcerative colitis); diverticulitis; and persons recovering from surgery on the gastrointestinal tract. (9, 10, 11) Long-term use of this diet is discouraged because it may contribute to constipation. (3)

Adequacy

The suggested food plan provides foods in amounts that will provide the DRIs recommended by the National Academy of Sciences for adults for all nutrients except fiber.

Diet Principles

The diet includes foods that will reduce frequency and volume of stools. It is smooth in texture and is mechanically and chemically nonirritating. The goal is to eat less than 10 to 15 grams of fiber daily. (11) Food tolerances vary greatly and patients should be encouraged to eat the most liberal diet possible and include adequate fluids. (10)

Table 10.3 Low Fiber Diet

Food for the Day	Recommended – Low in fiber	Not recommended – High in fiber
Vegetables *1–cups*	All strained vegetable juices; iceberg lettuce*; most well cooked or canned without seeds or skins; mashed potatoes without skins.	All raw vegetables except iceberg lettuce*; vegetables with skins or seeds, spinach and greens, winter squash, sweet potatoes, Brussels sprouts, peas, corn.
Fruits *1–2.5 cups*	Melons and ripe bananas; most well cooked or canned fruits without skins, seeds or membranes; pulp free juice.	Prune juice; any juice with pulp; most fresh fruits, berries, and other fruit with skin, seeds, or membranes; dried fruit.

*avoid lettuce with esophageal stricture

Continued on next page

Table 10.3 Low Fiber Diet Continued from previous page

Food for the Day	Recommended – Low in fiber	Not recommended – High in fiber
Grains *3–10 ounce-equivalents*	Enriched white bread without seeds; cornbread, biscuits, muffins, pancakes, waffles, plain sweet roll, saltines, graham crackers made with refined flours; enriched, cooked refined cereals, such as farina, grits, cornmeal; dry cereals such as puffed rice, rice flakes, cornflakes or others that are low in fiber; white pasta; white rice. Choose grains with less than 2 grams of fiber per serving.	Bread, crackers, pasta or cereals containing whole grains, bran, dried fruits, nuts, or seeds; brown or wild rice.
Dairy Products *2–3 cups*	All milk and milk drinks; smooth yogurt; mild cheese; cottage cheese.	Yogurt, if flavored with fruit containing small seeds or added fiber.
Protein Foods *2–7 ounce equivalents*	Ground or well-cooked meat, poultry, or fish; eggs; smooth nut butters, if tolerated; tofu.	Legumes (dried beans and peas), chunky nut butters; tough meats, soybeans.
Oils, Solid Fats	Vegetable oils, margarine, butter, cream, mayonnaise, mildly seasoned salad dressings.	Coconut, avocado; salad dressings with seeds or berries.
Added Sugars	Pudding, custard, flavored or frozen yogurt with allowed fruits, gelatin, plain sherbet, fruit ice, Popsicles®; plain cake and cookies; pie made with allowed fruits; honey, syrups, hard candy, marshmallows; jelly.	All desserts and candy containing coconut, nuts, seeds, or dried fruit; jams and preserves.
Fluids	Water and other fluids, such as milk, coffee, tea, fruit or vegetable juice, carbonated beverages.	Prune juice, any juice with pulp.
Others	Salt, pepper, ketchup, mustard, spices and herbs, vinegar.	Nuts and seeds, popcorn, pickles and relish with seeds.

Table 10.4 Sample Menu for Low Fiber Diet

Breakfast	Supper
½ c. grape juice	2 oz. tuna on 2 slices enriched white bread with 2 tsp. mayonnaise
1 egg	
½ c. puffed rice cereal	½ c. tomato juice
1 slice enriched white toast	½ c. green beans, canned
2 tsp. jelly	½ c. canned peaches
1 tsp. soft margarine	1 c. milk
1 c. milk	Water
Hot beverage	
Sugar, salt, pepper (optional)	
Lunch	**Snack Ideas**
2 oz. roasted chicken breast	½ c. applesauce
½ c. mashed potatoes with 2 oz. gravy	6 oz. yogurt, smooth
½ c. mixed vegetables (no peas or corn)	8 animal crackers
1 oz. enriched white roll	
1 tsp. soft margarine	
1 c. milk	
Water	

REFERENCES

1. Threapleton D, Greenwood D, Evans C, et al. Dietary fiber intake and risk of first stroke: A systematic review and meta-analysis. *Stroke*. Published online before print March 28, 2013. doi:10.1161/STROKEAHA.111.000151

2. Buil-Cosiales P, Zazpe I, Toledo E, et al. Fiber intake and all-cause mortality in the prevencion con dieta mediterranea (PREDIMED) study. *Am J Clin Nutr* 2014; 100(6):1498-1507.

3. Kim Y, Je Y. Dietary fiber intake and total mortality: a meta-analysis of prospective cohort studies. *Am J Epidemiol* 2014; 180(6):565-573.

4. Ning H, Van Horn L, Shay C, Lloyd-Jones, D. Associations of dietary fiber intake with long-term predicted cardiovascular disease risk and c-reactive protein levels (from the national health and nutrition examination survey data [2005-2010]). *Am J Cardiol* 2014; 113(2):287-291.

5. Dahl WJ, Stewart ML. Position of the Academy of Nutrition and Dietetics: Health Implications of Dietary Fiber. *J Acad Nutr Diet*. 2015; 115(11):1861 - 1870. doi. org/10.1016/j.jand.2015.09.003

6. The Academy of Nutrition and Dietetics. Evidence Analysis Library. Dietary Fiber. http://www.andeal.org/topic.cfm?menu=1586 Accessed June 20, 2015.

7. Marcason W. What is the latest research regarding the avoidance of nuts, seeds, corn, and popcorn in diverticular disease? *J Am Dietetic Assoc*. 2008; 108(11):1956.

8. Strate L, Liu Y, Syngal S, Aldoori,W, Giovannucci, E.. Nut, corn and popcorn consumption and the incidence of diverticular disease. *JAMA*. 2008; 300(8):907–914.

9. Academy of Nutrition and Dietetics. Nutrition Care Manual. Low Fiber Nutrition Therapy. https://www.nutritioncaremanual.org/client_ed.cfm?ncm_client_ed_id=3. Accessed May 31, 2015.

10. Diet and IBD. Crohn's and Colitis Foundation of America Web site. http://www.ccfa. org/resources/diet-and-ibd.html Published May 30, 2012.Updated 2015. Accessed May 30, 2015.

11. Low-fiber diet:MedlinePlus Medical Encyclopedia. http://www.nlm.nih.gov/ medlineplus/ency/patientinstructions/000200.htm Published October 28, 2014. Updated May 12, 2015. Accessed May 30, 2015.

ADDITIONAL RESOURCES

National Digestive Diseases Information (NIDDC): http://digestive.niddk.nih.gov/ ddiseases/pubs/diverticulosis/index.htm Updated September 19, 2013.

Peery A, Sandler R, Ahnen D, et al. Constipation and a low-fiber diet are not associated with diverticulosis. *Clin Gastroenterol Hepatol* 2013:11(12): 1622-1627.

Study Guide Questions

A. List at least three diseases for which a High Fiber Diet may be useful.

B. The High Fiber Diet contributes ___–___grams of dietary fiber.

C. List five examples of foods naturally high in fiber.

D. Fiber should be added gradually to prevent what four short-term side effects?

E. What are the potential complications of inadequate fluid intake?

F. Long-term use of a Low Fiber Diet is discouraged because it can contribute to _____.

G. Discussion question: What are dietary interventions that can be incorporated into the diet on a routine basis to reduce the use of bowel medications?

Study Guide Suggested Responses can be found in Appendix 15.

Food Allergies and Intolerances

FOOD ALLERGIES AND INTOLERANCES

Adverse food reaction is a general term for any abnormal reaction, allergic or nonallergic, resulting from the ingestion of food. (1) Food allergy is commonly suspected, yet healthcare providers diagnose it less frequently than most people believe. In many cases, it is a food intolerance—not a true allergy—that is causing the problem.

Food Allergy

Food allergies are currently estimated to affect approximately 5 percent of children under the age of five and 4 percent of teens and adults. (2) The National Institute of Allergy and Infectious Disease defines food allergy as "an adverse health effect arising from a specific immune response that occurs reproducibly to a given food."(2) Diagnosis of a food allergy can usually be made based on skin or lab tests and a detailed diet history. Symptoms may be immediate or delayed up to a few hours, and range from uncomfortable (e.g., hives, stomach upset) to life threatening (e.g., swelling of the tongue, closing of the throat). A severe type of reaction is called anaphylaxis, commonly known as anaphylactic shock. Anaphylactic shock can produce symptoms such as those listed in addition to a drop in blood pressure, unconsciousness, and even death.

Food Intolerance

A food intolerance presents when eating a certain food or foods triggers a negative physiological response but does not involve the immune system. Elimination diets, detailed diet history, and specialty tests are the most common methods for diagnosis. This is not life threatening, but symptoms may be severe and include gastrointestinal distress, and headaches. For some food intolerances, such as lactose intolerance, smaller portions (e.g., 4 ounces milk) or a modified version of the offending food (e.g., lactose-reduced or lactose-free milk, yogurt, or cheese) may be well tolerated.

Celiac Disease and Nonceliac Gluten Sensitivity

Celiac disease is an autoimmune disease. There are many different symptoms including diarrhea, constipation, anemia, and low bone density. At present, the only treatment is to follow a gluten-free diet. Gluten is the protein found in wheat, rye, barley, and oats (unless it is gluten-free oats). When eaten, gluten causes an immune system response that damages the lining of the small intestine. Continuous exposure to gluten can cause a wide variety of health problems.

Nonceliac gluten sensitivity is thought to be an immune system response to gluten. The treatment is to follow a gluten-free diet. Refer to the Gluten Restricted Diet in this chapter

Common Food Allergens in the United States

Eight foods account for 90% of food allergies. Wheat, milk, eggs, fish, crustacean shellfish, tree nuts, soy, and peanuts are the most common allergens. In adults, the most common foods that cause allergic reactions are shellfish (such as crayfish, lobster, shrimp, and crab), peanuts, tree nuts, fish, and eggs. The most common food allergens in children are eggs, milk, and peanuts. (2, 3)

Simplified Diet Manual, Twelfth Edition. Edited by Paula Watkins.
© 2016 Iowa Academy of Nutrition and Dietetics.

Treatment

Presently there are no medications that cure food allergies or food intolerances. Strict avoidance of the allergy-causing food is the only way to avoid a reaction. (4) Reading ingredient labels for all foods and good food safety/sanitation practices to prevent cross-contamination are the keys to maintaining control over the allergy.

Individuals with a history of systemic reaction/anaphylaxis or thought to be a risk for anaphylaxis should have an epinephrine kit on hand per medical prescription. Food allergic individuals with asthma are more likely to have a severe reaction. For individuals with mild symptoms (e.g., rash), considered **not** to be at risk for more severe symptoms or anaphylaxis, antihistamines (e.g., diphenhydramine) may be prescribed. (2, 4) A "Food Allergy and Anaphylaxis Emergency Care Plan" (5) provides individualized, easy to follow instructions for situations of suspected or known exposure to food allergens.

Food Allergen Labeling

Food Allergen Labeling and Consumer Protection Act (FALCPA) mandates that the eight most common food allergens—wheat, milk, eggs, fish, crustacean shellfish, tree nuts, soy, and peanuts— be declared in plain language in the ingredient list, or as part of a "Contains" statement (e.g., "Contains milk, wheat") or via parenthetical statement (e.g., whey (milk)) in the ingredients list. These eight food allergens must be listed on ingredient labels if they are present any amount; this includes spice blends, colors, and flavors. Additionally, manufactures must list the specific type of nut or seafood present in the product. (6)

Currently, there are not laws governing the use of advisory statements such as "made on equipment with," "processed in a facility with," or "may contain." If you suspect or are unsure if a product contains a food allergen you should always call the manufacturer. (6, 8)

FALCPA applies to all packaged foods, both domestic and imported, regulated under the Federal Food, Drug, and Cosmetic Act. (7) Foods exempt from FALCPA include raw agricultural products (fresh fruits and vegetables) and **highly** refined oils. (6, 7) Meat, poultry, and egg products are regulated by The Food Safety and Inspection Services (FSIS). For the eight most common food allergens FSIS encourages allergen statements and labeling consistent with FALCPA. (8) Labeling of most alcoholic beverages (alcoholic drinks, spirits, and beer) is regulated by the Alcohol, Tobacco Tax, and Trade Bureau (TTB).

The U.S. Food and Drug Administration (FDA) has defined the term "gluten-free" for voluntary use in the labeling of foods. Since 2014, any food product bearing a gluten-free claim label must meet the requirements of the agency's gluten-free labeling rule. It requires that, in order to use the term "gluten-free" on its label, a food must meet all of the requirements of the definition, including that the food must contain less than 20 parts per million of gluten. The rule also requires foods with the claims "no gluten," "free of gluten," and "without gluten" to meet the definition for "gluten-free." The rule excludes those foods whose labeling is regulated by the FSIS and the TTB as listed above. More information on gluten-free food labeling is available at the FDA website. (9)

Food Allergen Avoidance Diets

The following diets do not include a complete list of all foods that may contain the potential allergen and does not imply the allergen is always present in a food. Label reading and good food safety/sanitation techniques are essential steps for allergen free diets.

Remember to consider the steps involved in production and service of a food item as well. For example deep fried foods have a high risk for cross contamination and generally should be avoided by food allergic individuals. A deli slicer may be used to slice cheese as well as meats. The risk for cross contamination is also high in buffet style service related to spillage and "self-service" as multiple items may use the same utensil.

To promote safer dining experiences, SafeFARE (10) was developed in coordination with The Food Allergy Research and Education (FARE) organization, the National Restaurant Association (NRA) and MenuTrinfoo. It provides the restaurant industry, as well as food allergic diners, food allergen specific training and resources.

Dr. Ruchi Gupta, MD, MPH is an allergist and mother of a child with food allergies. Her book, *The Food Allergy Experience* and website (11), contain sample letters for communicating the needs of a food allergic child with schools and daycares.

Milk Allergy

Eliminating all milk and milk by-products from the diet is necessary. In addition, goat, sheep and other mammalian milk and their products must also be eliminated, due to the risk of cross reaction.

Milk is an important source of protein, calcium, vitamin A, vitamin D, riboflavin, pantothenic acid, and phosphorus. Enriched soy, almond, hemp, or rice milk beverages are good alternative sources of calcium, vitamin A, and vitamin D. These enriched beverages can also be used as a substitute for milk in recipes. Alternative sources of riboflavin, pantothenic acid, and phosphorus are found in legumes (such as peas, beans, or soy), nuts, and whole grains. Soymilk and foods from the protein group are alternative sources of protein.

Reading food labels is crucial. For a milk-free diet, you should avoid foods with the ingredients listed in Table 11.1.

Table 11.1 Milk Allergy (12, 13)

Avoid foods that contain the following ingredients:	
Artificial butter flavor	Ice cream
Butter, butter fat, butter acids, butter esters, butter oil	Lactoglobulin, lactalbumin, lactalbumin phosphate, lactoferrin
Buttermilk	Lactose
Casein	Lactulose
Caseinates (such as ammonium, calcium, magnesium, potassium, or sodium caseinate)	Milk (milk derivatives, powder, protein, solids, malted, condensed, evaporated, dry, whole, low-fat, nonfat, skimmed, and goat's milk)
Cheese (all forms) and cheese flavor	Nougat
Cottage cheese	Pudding
Cream	Recaldent™ (an ingredient in whitening chewing gum)
Curds	Rennet casein
Custard	Simplesse® (a fat substitute)
Diacetyl	Sour cream, sour cream solids
Ghee	Sour milk solids
Goat's milk	Tagatose
Half & half	Whey (in all forms, including sweet, delactosed, and protein concentrate)
Hydrolysates (listed as casein, milk protein, protein, whey, or whey protein hydrolysate)	Yogurt
Foods that may contain milk ingredients:	
Baked goods	Luncheon meat, hotdogs, sausages
Carmel candies	Margarine
Chocolate	Nisin
Culture and other bacterial cultures	Nondairy products

Egg Allergy

Eggs, all food products that contain egg or an egg derivative as an ingredient must be avoided completely, even if a diagnosis of allergy to only egg whites or egg yolks has been made. It is difficult to separate the egg white and yolk from each other completely, without having some cross contamination. Eggs provide the diet with vitamin B_{12}, pantothenic acid, riboflavin, selenium, and biotin. These nutrients can be easily provided by other foods in the diet, such as whole grains, legumes, and meat products.

Reading food labels is crucial. For an egg-free diet, you should avoid foods with the ingredients listed in Table 11.2.

Table 11.2 Egg Allergy (12, 13)

Avoid foods that contain the following ingredients:	
Albumin (may also be spelled albumen)	Lysozyme
Egg (white, yolk, dried, powdered, solids)	Mayonnaise
Egg substitutes	Meringue, meringue powder
Eggnog	Surimi
Globulin	Vitellin
Livetin	Ovalbumin, Ovomucin, Ovomucoid, Ovovitellin
Foods that may contain egg ingredients:	
Baked goods	Lecithin
Breaded items	Marzipan
Drink foam (alcoholic, specialty coffee)	Marshmallows
Egg substitutes	Meatloaf or meatballs
Fried rice	Nougat
Ice cream	Pasta

Peanut Allergy

Peanuts and peanut derivatives need to be avoided. Peanuts provide niacin, vitamin E, magnesium, chromium, and manganese. A diet with a variety of vegetables, whole grains, meats, and legumes will meet these needs as well.

Reading food labels is crucial. There is a risk of cross contamination and cross contact between tree nuts, peanuts, and seeds as they are often processed on shared equipment. For a peanut-free diet, you should avoid foods with the ingredients listed in Table 11.3.

Table 11.3 Peanut Allergy (12, 13)

Avoid foods that contain the following ingredients:	
Artificial nuts (Nu-Nuts®)	Ground nuts
Arachis oil (may contain peanut protein)	Lupine
Beer nuts	Mandelonas
Goobers	Mixed nuts

Continued on next page

Table 11.3 Peanut Allergy (12, 13) Continued from previous page

Avoid foods that contain the following ingredients:	
Monkey nuts	Peanut flour
Nut pieces	Peanut protein hydrolysate
Nutmeat	Peanut oil (cold pressed, expeller pressed, or extruded)
Peanuts	Pesto
Peanut butter	

Foods that may contain peanut ingredients:	
African, Asian, and Mexican dishes	Enchilada sauce
Baked goods	Marzipan
Candy (including chocolate)	Mole sauce
Egg rolls	Nougat

Tree Nut Allergy

An allergy to tree nuts is one of the most common food allergies in adults. Tree nuts include almonds, Brazil nuts, cashews, chestnuts, hazelnuts, hickory nuts, pecans, pine nuts, pistachios, walnuts, coconut, and macadamia nuts.

Tree nuts are added to many foods, so reading food labels is critical with this food allergy. There is a risk of cross contamination and cross contact between tree nuts, peanuts, and seeds as they are often processed on shared equipment. For a tree nut-free diet, you should avoid foods with the ingredients listed in Table 11.4.

Table 11.4 Tree Nut Allergy (12, 13)

Avoid foods that contain the following ingredients:	
Almonds and almond paste	Marzipan
Artificial nuts	Natural nut extract (e.g. almond)
Beechnut	Nougat
Brazil nuts	Nu-Nuts® artificial nuts
Cashews	Nut butters
Chestnuts	Nut distillates/alcohol extracts
Chinquapin nut	Nut hull extract
Coconut (FDA identified as a tree nut, October 2006)	Nut meal, nut meat, nut pieces
Filbert/hazelnut	Nut oil
Gianduja (creamy mixture of chocolate and chopped toasted nuts found in premium or imported chocolate)	Nut paste (such as almond paste)
Ginkgo nut	Pecans
Hickory nuts	Pesto
Litchi/lichee/lychee nut	Pili nut
Macadamia nuts	Pine nuts

Continued on next page

Table 11.4 Tree Nut Allergy (12, 13) Continued from previous page

Avoid foods that contain the following ingredients:	
Pistachios	Shea nut
Praline	Walnuts

Foods that may contain tree nut ingredients:	
Barbeque sauce	Energy bars
Baked goods	Flavored coffee
Cereal	Granola bars
Candy (including chocolate)	Marinades

Fish Allergy

All species of fish or products containing fish derivatives should be avoided if diagnosed with a fish allergy. Allergic reactions to vapors from cooking fish have been reported. Nutrients that are found in fish can also be found in meats, grains, legumes, and oils; therefore, substitution should be fairly easy.

For a fish free diet you should avoid the foods with the ingredients listed in Table 11.5.

Table 11.5 Fish Allergy (12, 13)

Avoid foods that contain the following ingredients:	
Caviar	Roe
Fish (all fish species for example: anchovies, bass, catfish, cod, flounder, grouper, haddock, hake, mahi mahi, perch, pollock, salmon, sardines, scrod, swordfish, sole, snapper, tilapia, trout, tuna)	Seafood flavoring, fish flavor, fish gelatin
Fish oil (may be added to milk, juice, or yogurt for omega-3 supplementation)	Shark (shark cartilage or shark fin)
Fish sauces (Asian fish sauce, nouc mam in Vietnamese)	Surimi or artificial crab or "sea legs"
Fish stock	Sushi, sashimi
Fishmeal, fish flour	Worcestershire sauce (contains anchovy)

Foods that may contain fish ingredients:	
Barbecue sauce	Salad dressing (Caesar usually contains anchovy)
Bouillabaisse	

Shellfish Allergy

All species of crustacean shellfish or products containing shellfish derivatives should be avoided if diagnosed with a shellfish allergy. Allergic reactions to handling shellfish or to vapors from cooking shellfish have been reported. Nutrients that are found in shellfish can also be found in meats, egg, whole grains, seed, and oils; therefore, substitution should be fairly easy.

For a shellfish free diet you should avoid the foods with the ingredients listed in Table 11.6.

Table 11.6 Shellfish Allergy (12, 13)

Avoid foods that contain the following ingredients:
All shellfish species
Barnacle
Crab
Crawfish (cherrystone, crayfish, ecrevisse)
Lobster (langouste, langoustine, Moreton, bay bugs, scampi, tomalley)
Prawns
Shrimp (crevette, scampi)
Follow your allergist's advice regarding these ingredients:
Mollusks such as abalone, clam, cockle, cuttlefish, limpet, mussel, oyster, octopus, periwinkle, scallops, sea cucumber, sea urchin, snails (escargot), squid (calamari), and whelk (Turban shell) are NOT considered major allergens by the FDA and may NOT be fully identified on the product label. If a food product has a vague ingredient term such as "natural flavor," call the manufacturer.
Foods that may contain shellfish ingredients:
Bouillabaisse
Cuttlefish ink
Glucosamine
Fish stock
Seafood flavoring
Surimi

Soy Allergy

Soy or products containing soy derivatives should be avoided if diagnosed with a soy allergy. Nutrients that are found in soy can also be found in meat, eggs, and enriched or fortified grains; therefore, substitution should be fairly easy.

For a soy free diet you should avoid the foods with the ingredients listed in Table 11.7.

Table 11.7 Soy Allergy (12, 13)

Avoid foods that contain the following ingredients:
Edamame
Miso
Natto
Soy (soy albumin, soy cheese, soy fiber, soy flour, soy grits, soy ice cream, soy milk, soy nuts, soy sprouts, soy yogurt)
Soya
Soybeans (cooked, raw, toasted, curd, granules)
Soy protein (concentrate, hydrolyzed, isolate)
Soybean oil (cold pressed, expeller pressed, or extruded soybean oil)
Shoyu

Continued on next page

Table 11.7 Soy Allergy (12, 13) Continued from previous page

Avoid foods that contain the following ingredients:
Soy sauce
Tamari
Tempeh
Textured vegetable protein (TVP)
Tofu

Follow your allergist's advice regarding these ingredients:

- Many soy allergic individuals can safely eat soy lecithin
- FDA exempts highly refined soybean oil from being labeled as an allergen

Foods that may contain soy ingredients:
Asian cuisine
Vegetable broth
Vegetable gum
Vegetable starch

Wheat Allergy

Eliminating all wheat, wheat flours and wheat by-products from the diet is necessary. Spelt, kamut, and triticale are closely related to wheat and should be avoided as well. This diet is designed to be wheat-free; for a gluten-free diet refer to the Gluten Restricted Diet in this chapter.

Wheat is an important source of thiamin, riboflavin, niacin, iron, selenium, and chromium. Flours and starches from rice, potato, buckwheat, tapioca, millet, corn, quinoa, and amaranth, can be used as alternatives for wheat and wheat products. Look for replacement flours and products that have been fortified with thiamin, riboflavin, niacin, and iron.

Reading food labels is crucial. For a wheat-free diet, you should avoid foods with the ingredients listed in Table 11.8.

Table 11.8 Wheat Allergy (12, 13)

Do not eat foods that contain the following ingredients:	
Bread crumbs	Flour (all purpose, bread, cake, durum, enriched, graham, high gluten, high protein, instant, pastry, phosphated, self-rising, soft wheat, steel ground, stone ground, unbleached, white, whole wheat)
Bran	
Bulgur	
Cereal extract	
Couscous	Hydrolyzed wheat protein
Cracker meal	Matzoh, matzoh meal
Durum	Seitan
Einkorn	Semolina
Emmer	Spelt
Farina	Triticale
	Wheat (wheat berries, wheat bran, wheat bran hydrolysate, wheat germ, wheat germ oil, wheat gluten, wheat grass, wheat starch, sprouted wheat)

Continued on next page

Table 11.8 Wheat Allergy (12, 13) Continued from previous page

Foods that may contain wheat ingredients:	
Glucose syrup	Malt
Grain coffee substitute	Oats
Granola	Soy sauce
Hydrolyzed plant protein (HPP)	Starch (gelatinized starch, modified starch, modified food starch, vegetable starch)
Hydrolyzed vegetable protein (HVP)	Surimi

REFERENCES

1. Clinical manifestations of food allergy: An overview. Burks, W. UptoDate Web site. http://www.uptodate.com/contents/clinical-manifestations-of-food-allergy-an-overview?source=search_result&search=food+allergy+children&selectedTitle=1%7E150 Updated Oct 6, 2014. Accessed July 10, 2015.

2. Boyce JA, Assa'ad A, Burks AW, et al. Guidelines for the diagnosis and management of food allergy in the United States: report of the NIAID-sponsored expert panel. *J Allery Clin Immunol* 2010; 126:S1- S58.

3. Food Allergy Facts and Statistics for the U.S. Food Allergy Research & Education (FARE) Web site. http://www.foodallergy.org/document.doc?id=194 Accessed July 15, 2015.

4. Food Allergy Treatment and Management. American Academy of Allergy, Asthma, and Immunology Web site. http://www.aaaai.org/conditions-and-treatments/allergies/food-allergies.aspx Accessed July 10, 2015.

5. Food Allergy & Anaphylaxis Emergency Care Plan. Food Allergy Research and Education (FARE) Web site. https://www.foodallergy.org/faap Published 2015. Accessed August 12, 2005.

6. Food Allergen Labeling And Consumer Protection Act of 2004 Questions and Answers. U.S. Food and Drug Administration Web site. http://www.fda.gov/Food/GuidanceRegulation/GuidanceDocumentsRegulatoryInformation/Allergens/ucm106890.htm Published December 12, 2005. Updated July 18, 2006. Accessed July 20, 2015.

7. Food Allergies: What You Need to Know. U.S. Food and Drug Administration Web site. http://www.fda.gov/Food/ResourcesForYou/Consumers/ucm079311.htm Published June 2010. Updated May 12, 2015. Accessed August 2, 2015.

8. Allergies and Food Safety. United States Department of Agriculture Food Safety and Inspection Services Web site. http://www.fsis.usda.gov/wps/wcm/connect/1e98f24c-d616-443f-8490-f7372476d558/Allergies_and_Food_Safety.pdf?MOD=AJPERES Published July 2011. Accessed August 3, 2015.

9. Questions and Answers: Gluten-Free Food Labeling Final Rule. U.S. Food and Drug Administration Website. http://www.fda.gov/Food/GuidanceRegulation/GuidanceDocumentsRegulatoryInformation/Allergens/ucm362880.htm Updated June 16, 2015. Accessed August 12, 2015.

10. Dining Out with Food Allergies. SafeFARE Website http://www.safefare.org/ Published 2014. Accessed August 12, 2015.

11. The Food Allergy Experience Website. http://www.foodallergyexperience.com/ Accessed August 12, 2015.

12. Tips for Avoiding Your Allergen. Food Allergy Research and Education (FARE) Web site. http://www.foodallergy.org/document.doc?id=133 Published 2014. Accessed July 21, 2015.

13. Academy of Nutrition and Dietetics. Nutrition Care Manual. Multiple Food Allergies Nutrition Therapy. https://www.nutritioncaremanual.org/client_ed.cfm?ncm_client_ed_id=29 Accessed July 25, 2015.

Websites

Allergen Saf-T-Zone™ System http://www.sanjamar.com/product/allergen-saf-t-zone-system/

GLUTEN RESTRICTED DIET

Use

The Gluten Restricted Diet is used for people with celiac disease, non-celiac gluten sensitivity, or dermatitis herpetiformis. Celiac disease and dermatitis herpetiformis are conditions in which eating gluten triggers an immune response in the body that causes tissue inflammation in the gut or on the skin. (1) Celiac disease is diagnosed with a blood test that must be done while the person is eating gluten. It may also be diagnosed from tissue biopsy of the small intestine. Avoiding all gluten is the only treatment available to relieve symptoms and heal the gut and/or skin.

Some patients may request a gluten-free diet for perceived symptom relief. More research is needed. (2) In 2012, an international group of celiac experts classified non-celiac gluten sensitivity as a distinct condition. There are no clinical tests to identify non-celiac gluten sensitivity. (1) Diagnosis relies on ruling out celiac disease and wheat allergy and how the individual feels after avoiding gluten. A trial of a low FODMAP diet (see page page 134) may be beneficial for persons with non-celiac gluten sensitivity. Gastrointestinal symptoms improved on this diet. (2)

Adequacy

The suggested food plan includes foods in amounts that will provide the quantities of nutrients recommended by the National Academy of Sciences for adults. Patients may have malabsorption problems; therefore, calorie, protein, vitamin, and mineral intake should be monitored with optimal energy and nutrient intake provided. (3)

While many highly acceptable gluten-free alternatives are now available in grocery stores, few are enriched or fortified. This could contribute to lower than expected nutritional value of meals, especially for the nutrients added in grain enrichment: thiamin, niacin, riboflavin, folate, and iron. Also, many gluten-free grain substitutes contain little dietary fiber.

Planning for and providing a variety of menu items for individuals in assisted living and long-term care contributes to nutritional quality as well as quality of life.

Diet Principles

1. This diet restricts gluten by avoiding foods, beverages, and medications containing wheat, rye, and barley. Gluten-free oats may be used if tolerated. (3) A pharmacist can determine if medications contain gluten.

2. Grains and starches that may be used include corn, rice, potato, soy, tapioca, bean, sorghum, amaranth, buckwheat, quinoa, teff, millet, Montina™, and nut flours. Oats must be certified from a gluten-free source.

3. It is important to carefully read ingredient labels on all prepared foods to determine possible gluten content. Ingredients such as modified food starch, hydrolyzed or texturized vegetable proteins, soy sauce or soy sauce solids, and malt or malt flavoring may indicate gluten content from an unacceptable source. The source of food starch and modified starch is corn unless the label indicates it was made from wheat. Common

recipe ingredients that often contain gluten include canned cream soups, sauces and gravies, and frozen entrees. Cornstarch works well as a substitute for wheat flour in homemade gravy.

4. Care to avoid cross contamination in food preparation is essential.

    a. Train food service staff to prepare and serve gluten-free meals and snacks. Require that they wear clean aprons/coats and gloves when preparing gluten-free foods. Keep all outside food and beverages out of the production area.

    b. Designate a set of preparation and serving utensils, including measuring utensils and cutting boards, to be used only for gluten-free foods. Mark them clearly for gluten-free use only.

    c. Thoroughly wash and rinse work surfaces and utensils to remove gluten from them.

    d. Use only pans and skillets without non-stick coatings.

    e. Store all gluten-free ingredients in sealed, marked packages and containers. Store gluten-free foods above other foods in the pantry.

    f. Purchase a toaster to be used only for gluten-free bread.

    g. Cooking meat on foil on a grill protects it from cross-contamination.

    h. Use squeeze bottles for condiments such as mayonnaise, ketchup, pickle relish, and jam. Or, provide these in single-serve packets to be opened at the table.

5. When first diagnosed with celiac disease, many people are also lactose intolerant to some degree. This usually goes away as they avoid gluten and the gut heals. Refer to the Lactose Restricted Diet, which may greatly decrease symptoms. These patients can be encouraged to try lactose-containing foods after a few weeks of following a Gluten Restricted Diet.

6. Plan for new gluten-restricted admissions by having a written menu and ingredients on hand that can be safely prepared and served. Stock gluten-free frozen entrees, gluten-free breads, hard corn taco shells, single-serving rice bowls, soups, or gluten-free cereals. Train staff to use only designated preparation equipment.

7. A registered dietitian nutritionist familiar with gluten restrictions can assist in diet planning and education to assure nutritional adequacy.

Table 11.9 Gluten Restricted

Food for the Day	Recommended	Avoid
Vegetables *1–4 cups*	Vegetables may be raw or cooked; fresh, frozen, canned, dried/dehydrated, or 100% vegetable juices.	Creamed or breaded vegetables; some canned baked beans.
Fruits *1–2.5 cups*	Fruits may be fresh, frozen, canned (in own juices or light syrup), dried (with no sugar added) or 100% fruit juice.	Any fruit containing wheat flour used as a thickener.
Grains *3–10 ounce-equivalents*	Rice, wild rice; gluten-free breads, cereals, quick breads; gluten-free pasta and noodles; corn tortillas.	Any made with wheat, rye, barley; triticale, spelt, wheat germ, graham, durum, semolina, couscous.
	Buckwheat, cornmeal, cornstarch, millet, gluten-free oats, quinoa, tapioca.	Oats containing gluten.
	Gluten-free communion wafers.	Communion wafers containing gluten.

Continued on next page

Table 11.9 Gluten Restricted Continued from previous page

Food for the Day	Recommended	Avoid
Dairy products *2–3 cups*	Milk, nondairy milks (soy, almond, cashew, rice), yogurt. Aged hard cheeses.	Malted milk beverages, yogurt with added cookies or granola. Cheese spreads and products containing restricted grains.
Protein foods *2–7 ounce-equivalents*	Fresh meat including beef, pork, poultry, fish; dry beans or legumes; eggs; unflavored nuts and seeds.	Creamed or breaded meat, fish, poultry unless made with allowed flours; commercial products containing restricted grains; some canned meat products and processed lunch or deli meats.
Oils, Solid Fats	Vegetable oils (canola, flaxseed, sesame, olive, peanut, soybean), margarine, butter.	Any salad dressings or mayonnaise containing restricted grains.
Added Sugars/ Desserts	Cakes, cookies, pastries made with gluten-free grains; sorbet and fruit ices; premium ice cream; flavored gelatin; maple syrup, jam, jelly; marshmallows, cocoa powder and chocolate.	Cakes, cookies, pastries made with restricted grains, ice cream cones; some puddings and ice cream with ingredients containing gluten. Licorice, chocolate candy and other candy made with restricted grains.
Fluids/Soup	Water and other fluids, such as coffee, tea, 100% fruit or vegetable juice; gluten-free beer and wine. Broths and soups made with allowed ingredients.	Flavored coffees; beer made with restricted grains. Soups thickened or made with restricted grains.
Snack Foods	Popcorn; plain tortilla chips; some plain potato and corn chips.	Some flavored chips; pretzels.
Condiments	Pure herbs and spices including salt and pepper; most vinegars.	Condiments containing restricted grains such as soy sauce and malt vinegar.

Table 11.10 Sample Menu for Gluten Restricted Diet

Breakfast	Supper
½ c. orange juice	2 oz. tuna on
1 egg	2 slices gluten-free bread with
¾ c. rice or corn cereal	2 tsp. gluten-free dressing
1 slice gluten-free bread or rusk	2 tomato slices
2 tsp. jelly	1 c. leafy greens salad
1 tsp. soft margarine	1 Tbsp. oil and vinegar dressing
1 c. milk	½ c. fruit cocktail
Hot beverage	1 c. milk
Sugar, pepper (optional)	Water

Continued on next page

Table 11.10 Sample Menu for Gluten Restricted Diet Continued from previous page

Lunch	Snack Ideas
2 oz. baked chicken	½ c. melon
½ c. mashed potatoes (made from fresh)	3 cups popcorn
½ c. mixed vegetables	½ c. carrot sticks
1 oz. gluten-free bread or roll	
2 tsp. margarine or butter	
1 c. milk	
Water	

Table 11.11 Gluten-free Snacks from Common Pantry Foods

Fresh apple	Cottage cheese with tomato slices
Canned fruit	Lean lunch meat rolled in lettuce leaves spread with gluten-free salad dressing and mustard
Snack mix (popcorn, raisins, dried cranberries and nuts)	Potato chips with ranch dip
Flavored gelatin cup	Cheese cubes
Pudding cup	Flavored yogurt

REFERENCES

1. Ludvigsson JF, Leffler DA, Bai JC, et al. The Oslo definitions for coeliac disease and related terms. *Gut*. 2013; 62(1):43-52. Doi:10.1136/gutjnl-2011-301346

2. Biesiekierski JR, Iven J. Non-coeliac gluten sensitivity: piecing the puzzle together. *United European Gastroenterol J*. 2015; 3(2):160–165. Doi:10.1177/2050640615578388

3. Academy of Nutrition and Dietetics. Nutrition Care Manual. Celiac Disease Nutrition Therapy. https://www.nutritioncaremanual.org/client_ed.cfm?ncm_client_ed_id=162 Accessed July 17, 2015.

ADDITIONAL RESOURCES

Murray J. *Mayo Clinic Going Gluten Free: Essential Guide to Managing Celiac Disease and Related Conditions*. Birmingham, AL: Oxmoor House; 2014

Cookbooks

Crocker B. *Betty Crocker Gluten-Free Cooking*, Hoboken, NJ: John Wiley and Sons; 2012.

Hasselbeck E. *Deliciously G-Free: Food So Flavorful They'll Never Believe It's Gluten-Free*. New York, NY: Ballantine Books; 2012.

Hunn N. *Gluten-Free on a Shoestring: 125 Easy Recipes for Eating Well on the Cheap*, Cambridge, MA: Da Capo Press; 2012.

Thompson T, Brown M. *Easy Gluten-Free: Expert Nutrition Advice with More than 100 Recipes*. Chicago, IL: Academy of Nutrition and Dietetics; 2011.

Websites

Celiac.com: www.celiac.com

Celiac Support Association: www.csaceliacs.org

Central Iowa Celiac Connection: www.celiacsconnect.com

Gluten Intolerance Group of North America: www.gluten.org

Tri-County Celiac Sprue Support Group: www.tccsg.net

LACTOSE RESTRICTED DIET

Use

The Lactose Restricted Diet is used for patients who cannot digest lactose, the carbohydrate found in milk. Lactose intolerance results from diminished production of lactase enzyme in the small intestine. The degree of sensitivity will vary from person to person; therefore, the diet should be individualized. (1)

Adequacy

The diet will provide the DRIs recommended by the National Academy of Sciences; however, there may be a risk for deficiencies in calcium, riboflavin, and vitamin D depending on food choices and if lactase enzyme is used to aid digestion. Supplementary sources of these nutrients may be advisable.

Diet Principles

1. The diet limits lactose-containing foods according to individual tolerance. Tolerance to lactose varies greatly. For example, one person may have severe symptoms after drinking a small amount of milk, while another person can drink a large amount without having symptoms. Many adolescents and adults may find that they can tolerate up to 12 grams, the amount in 1 cup of milk, when consumed with meals. (1) Individuals may find aged or hard cheeses, such as cheddar or Swiss, and fermented dairy products, such as kefir or yogurt, better tolerated. (2)

2. Read all labels carefully to identify foods containing lactose. Look for the words *lactose, milk, nonfat dry milk, milk solids, skim milk, whey,* or *curds*. Other prepared foods that may contain lactose include commercial breads and baked goods, processed breakfast cereals, instant potatoes, soup and breakfast drink mixes, margarine, lunchmeats (other than kosher), salad dressings, candies and snacks, mixes for pancakes, biscuits, and cookies.

3. Commercially available lactase enzyme may be taken with food, beverages, and some medications as needed.

4. Some medications contain lactose. Individuals with severe lactose intolerance may need to speak with their health care provider to see if other options are needed. (2)

5. Individuals with limited intake of milk and milk products may need additional calcium and vitamin D to meet the Recommended Daily Allowance (RDA) for their age. Dietary intake should be assessed for adequacy to determine if supplementation is needed. (3)

Table 11.12 Lactose Restricted Diet

Food for the Day	Recommended	Contains Lactose - Limit to Tolerance
Vegetables *1-4 cups*	All vegetables and vegetable juices.	Any vegetable prepared with milk or cheese sauce; instant potatoes.
Fruits *1–2.5 cups*	All fruits and fruit juices.	Fruit drinks containing lactose.
Grains *3–10 ounce-equivalents*	Crackers, Italian, French, or Jewish rye bread; cereals, rice, pasta, hominy, oats, barley, wheat, cornmeal, tortillas, rice, and popcorn.	Any bread, cereal, or grain prepared with milk or milk products; instant cereals; dry cereals containing lactose or milk.
Dairy products *2–3 cups*	Lactose-free milk products. Milk treated with lactase enzyme. *Soy, rice, almond, hemp, or oat "milk."	Milk and milk products; buttermilk, yogurt, cocoa mixes. All forms of cheese made with milk.
Protein foods *2–7 ounce-equivalents*	All fresh meat, poultry, fish, shellfish; eggs; peanut butter, dried beans, lentils; nuts, seeds, tofu, kosher prepared meat products.	Meat or meat substitute prepared with milk; cold cuts, wieners, or other meat with added lactose; powdered eggs.
Oils, Solid Fats	Milk-free margarine (kosher margarines do not contain milk); some nondairy cream substitutes; vegetable oils, shortening, lard, bacon, salad dressings made without milk or cheese. Olives, nuts, and seeds. Gravy made without milk.	Butter, margarine, salad dressings, mayonnaise-type salad dressings, sour cream, cream cheese, cream.
Added Sugars	Desserts made without milk; fruit ices, popsicles, gelatin; angel food cake, fruit leather rolls, sugar, corn syrup, maple syrup, honey, jam, jelly, marshmallows, hard candies, gum drops, jelly beans, and fruit pie fillings.	Any dessert, pudding or mix containing lactose; sherbet, ice cream, frozen yogurt, milk chocolate, caramels, cream or chocolate candies.
Fluids/Soup	Broth-based soups; soups made with water, soy milk or other nondairy substitutes. Plain coffee, tea, soft drinks, beer, wine, distilled spirits.	Cream soups, commercial soups containing milk or lactose. Drink mixes containing milk or lactose.
Others	Popcorn, pretzels, plain potato and corn chips; condiments without added milk.	Cheese flavored crackers, cheese curls.

*Other products sold as "milks" but made from plants (e.g., almond, rice, oat, and hemp "milks") may contain calcium and be consumed as a source of calcium, but their overall nutritional content is not similar to dairy milk and fortified soy beverages (soymilk).

Table 11.13 Sample Menu for Lactose Restricted Diet*

Breakfast	Supper
½ c. orange juice	2 oz. tuna on 2 slices whole wheat bread with 2 tsp. mayonnaise
1 egg	
½ c. oatmeal	2 tomato slices
1 slice whole wheat toast	1 c. leafy greens salad
2 tsp. jelly	1 Tbsp. oil and vinegar dressing
1 tsp. soft margarine	½ c. fruit cocktail
1 c. lactose-free milk	1 c. lactose-free milk
Hot beverage	Water
Sugar, pepper (optional)	
Lunch	**Snack Ideas**
2 oz. roasted chicken breast	½ c. cantaloupe
½ c. mashed potatoes with 2 oz. gravy (made without milk)	½ c. carrot sticks
	3 c. popcorn
½ c. mixed vegetables	
1 oz. whole wheat roll	
1 tsp. soft margarine	
1 c. lactose-free milk	
Water	

*Milk substitutes and milk-free foods as suggested above should be used where appropriate.

REFERENCES

1. Suchy FJ, Brannon PM, Carpenter TO, et al. National Institutes of Health consensus development conference: lactose intolerance and health. Ann Intern Med. 2010; 152(12):792-796.

2. National Institute of Diabetes and Digestive and Kidney Diseases: Lactose Intolerance. http://www.niddk.nih.gov/health-information/health-topics/digestive-diseases/lactose-intolerance/Pages/facts.aspx Published May 2014. Updated June 4, 2014. Accessed July 11, 2015.

3. Institute of Medicine, National Academy of Sciences. Dietary Reference Intakes for Calcium and Vitamin D. Washington (DC): National Academies Press (US); 2010.

FRUCTOSE MALABSORPTION AND LOW FODMAP DIET

Fructose malabsorption may require physician prescribed restrictions of fruit, 100% juice, other juices (containing little or no juice), honey, soda pop; commercially made muffins, cakes, pies, and syrups; and anything containing high-fructose corn syrup (HFCS), including ketchup and barbeque sauce. Reading ingredient lists for HFCS is essential. The goal of nutrition therapy is to follow the least restrictive menu while avoiding abdominal discomfort.

Fructose is an important nutrient found naturally occurring in fruit. Fructose is found as free fructose, bound with glucose, and in fructans (present in some vegetables and wheat). During normal digestion, fructose is absorbed in the small intestine. Following absorption, fructose is transported to the liver, where most of the fructose metabolism occurs. When eaten alone or in excess (like a concentrated form of HFCS), it may be poorly absorbed, resulting in symptoms like pain, gas, and diarrhea. (1)

Fructose malabsorption is characterized by the inability to absorb fructose effectively. Malabsorption results in bacterial fermentation, which leads to fatty acid formation, and gases. Gastrointestinal (GI) symptoms associated with fructose malabsorption may include diarrhea, cramping, bloating, and flatulence; which can in turn lead to more severe issues including weight loss, protein energy malnutrition, liver disease, and other nutritional deficiencies. A hydrogen breath test should be the used to determine whether a person has fructose malabsorption. (2, 3)

Fructose consumption has increased recently, due to increased consumption of sweetened beverages and processed foods with added fructose. High Fructose Corn Syrup is a concentrated form of fructose, used to sweeten processed foods such as fruit juices, sodas, and candy, and sports drinks. Excessive fructose intake may lead to liver disease and fructose malabsorption. Also, increased fructose intakes may increase risk of disease by increasing cholesterol levels, obesity, and insulin resistance, along with altered pancreatic enzymes. (2, 3)

Use

The Low FODMAP Diet is used to decrease GI symptoms in persons with fructose malabsorption or Irritable Bowel Syndrome (IBS). FODMAP stands for fermentable oligosaccharides, disaccharides, monosaccharides, and polyols.

Adequacy

The suggested food plan includes foods in amounts that will provide the DRIs recommended by the National Academy of Sciences for adults.

Diet Principles

Excess fructose and fructans can produce acute GI symptoms; therefore, reduction or elimination of the offending carbohydrates may result in improvement. However, every attempt to find a food alternative should be encouraged.

When consuming foods/meals high in FODMAPs, adding glucose may improve tolerance. (6) Glucose tablets may be used instead of food sources, and are available at most pharmacies.

FODMAPs are poorly absorbed carbohydrates that may affect the GI tract and may lead to symptoms of IBS (Irritable Bowel Syndrome).

Some examples of FODMAPs (4):

- Fructose such as fruits, honey, high-fructose corn syrup
- Lactose found in dairy products
- Fructans found in wheat, rye, garlic, onion, chicory
- Galactans found in legumes (e.g., dried beans, lentils, soybeans), cashews, pistachios
- Polyols found in sweeteners containing isomalt, maltitol, mannitol, sorbitol, xylitol, and stone fruits such as avocado, apricots, cherries, nectarines, peaches, and plums as well as some vegetables (e.g., cauliflower, mushrooms).

Table 11.14 Low FODMAP Diet (4, 5, 6)

Food for the Day	Low FODMAP – well tolerated	High FODMAP – limit if not tolerated
Vegetables *1–cups*	Alfalfa, bean sprouts, green beans, bok choy, capsicum (bell pepper), carrot, chives, fresh herbs, choy sum, cucumber, lettuce, tomato, zucchini, eggplant, parsnips, potato, spinach.	Asparagus, artichokes, onions (all), leek bulb, garlic, legumes, sugar snap peas, peas, onion and garlic salts, beetroot, Savoy cabbage, celery, sweet corn, cauliflower, broccoli, Brussels sprouts, mushrooms.
Fruits *1–2.5 cups*	Banana, orange, mandarin oranges, grapes, cantaloupe, blueberries, grapefruit, lemon, lime, passion fruit, raspberries, rhubarb, strawberries.	Apples, pears, mango, nashi pears, watermelon, nectarines, peaches, plums, cherries, persimmons, prunes, apricots, avocado, blackberries, boysenberries.
Grains *3–10 ounce-equivalents*	Gluten-free bread and sourdough spelt bread, crispy rice cereal, oats, gluten-free pasta, rice, quinoa. Gluten-free biscuits, rice cakes, corn thins, popcorn.	Rye, wheat-containing breads, wheat-based cereals with dried fruit, wheat pasta. Rye crackers, wheat-based biscuits. May tolerate wheat and rye products in small amounts.
Dairy Products *2–3 cups*	Lactose-free milk, lactose-free yogurts, hard cheese. (See Chapter 11 for more information on a lactose restricted meal plan).	Cow's milk, yogurt, soft cheeses (e.g., cottage, ricotta), cream, custard, ice cream.
Protein Foods *2–7 ounce equivalents*	Meats, fish, chicken, tofu, tempeh, eggs.	Legumes (e.g., baked beans, kidney beans, lentils, black-eyed peas, garbanzo beans, soybeans).
Oils, Solid Fats	Almonds (<10 nuts), pumpkin seeds, macadamia nuts, peanuts, walnuts, and pine nuts. Margarine, mayonnaise, butter, oil.	Cashews, pistachios.
Added Sugars	Regular sugar (sucrose), maple syrup, glucose.	Honey, sorbitol, mannitol, xylitol, maltitol, isomalt, high-fructose corn syrup, fructose (invert sugar, levulose), agave syrup.
Fluids	Water, coffee, tea.	Soft drinks made with high-fructose corn syrup. Chicory coffee.

Table 11.15 Sample Menu for Low FODMAP Diet

Breakfast	Supper
½ c. orange juice	2 oz. tuna on
1 egg	2 slices gluten-free bread with 2 tsp. mayonnaise
½ c. oatmeal	2 tomato slices
1 slice gluten-free toast	1 c. leafy greens salad
1 tsp. soft margarine	1 Tbsp. oil and vinegar dressing
1 c. lactose-free milk	½ c. mandarin oranges
Hot beverage	1 c. lactose-free milk
Sugar, pepper (optional)	Water
Lunch	**Snack Ideas**
2 oz. roasted chicken breast	½ c. cantaloupe
½ c. mashed potatoes with 2 oz. gravy	½ c. carrot sticks
½ c. green beans	3 c. popcorn
1 oz. gluten-free bread or roll	
1 tsp. soft margarine	
1 c. lactose-free milk	
Water	

FODMAPs are important in bowel health and should not be discouraged unless a person is told to eliminate them by their healthcare professional. A low FODMAP diet should only be followed for 2 to 6 weeks. Then foods may be reintroduced under the care of the health-care team, including a registered dietitian nutritionist. This avoids unnecessary food restrictions and ensures adequate nutrients in the diet. (4)

REFERENCES

1. Laughlin M. Normal roles for dietary fructose in carbohydrate metabolism. *Nutrients.* 2014; 6(8): 3117–3129.

2. Riveros MJ, Parada A, Pettinelli P. Fructose consumption and its health implications; fructose malabsorption and nonalcoholic fatty liver disease. *Nutr Hosp.* 2014; 29(3):491-499.

3. Kolderup A, Svihus B. Fructose metabolism and relation to atherosclerosis, type 2 diabetes, and obesity. *J Nutr Metab.* 2015; 2015: 823081. doi: 10.1155/2015/823081

4. The Monash University low FODMAP diet website. http://www.med.monash.edu/cecs/gastro/fodmap/low-high.html Updated December 18, 2012. Accessed June 30, 2015.

5. Barrett JS. Extending our knowledge of fermentable, short-chain, carbohydrates for managing gastrointestinal symptoms. *Nutr Clin Pract.* 2013; 28(3): 300-306. doi:10.1177/0884533613485790

6. Mansueto P, Seidita A, D'Alcamo A, Carroccio A. Role of FODMAPs in patients with irritable bowel syndrome: a review. *Nutr Clin Pract.* 2015; 30(5):665-682. doi:10.1177/0884533615569886

ADDITIONAL RESOURCES

Scarlata K. Successful Low-FODMAP Living — Experts Discuss Meal-Planning Strategies to Help IBS Clients Better Control GI Distress. *Today's Dietitian. 2012; 14(3):36.* http://www.todaysdietitian.com/newarchives/030612p36.shtml

---

Study Guide Questions

A. Define food allergy and intolerance and explain the differences.

B. What eight foods make up 90% of the diagnosed food allergies?

C. List at least three grains and starches that may be used for the Gluten Restricted Diet.

D. When reading food labels, what ingredients listed would indicate possible gluten content? (Hint: modified food starch)

E. List at least three prepared foods that may contain lactose.

F. What nutrients may be lacking in a lactose-restricted diet?

G. What primary ingredients are avoided on a Low FODMAP diet?

H. Discussion question: Describe communication methods in ensuring staff are aware of critical diet restrictions such as lactose or gluten.

Study Guide Suggested Responses can be found in Appendix 15.

Other Modified Diets

HIGH NUTRIENT DIET

Use

The high nutrient diet is designed to aid the nutritional rehabilitation of malnourished individuals, to provide for persons with elevated needs (e.g., wounds, fractures, drug-nutrient interactions), and to prevent malnutrition in individuals unable to consume a normal volume of food due to low energy needs, lack of appetite, or cognitive impairment.

Adequacy

The High Nutrient Diet is a balanced diet providing all the food groups, macronutrients, and micronutrients, and is more concentrated in micronutrients, protein, and energy than the General Diet. Some individuals may still need commercially prepared oral nutritional supplements and/or multivitamin/mineral supplements if dietary intakes continue to prove inadequate and Dietary Reference Intakes (DRIs) are not met. (1)

Diet Principles

1. **High nutrient foods.** The High Nutrient Diet makes use of enhanced foods, food fortifiers, and nutrient-dense foods to deliver more protein and energy per bite than the General Diet (see Table 12.1).

Table 12.1 Examples of high nutrient foods

Nutrient dense foods (not necessarily high in protein)	Cottage cheese, yogurt and other milk products, whole grains, fruits, vegetables, eggs, peanut butter, legumes, lean meats, poultry, fish, canola and olive oils.
Enhanced foods	**Fortified oatmeal:** 1/2 c. cooked oatmeal, 2 Tbsp. instant nonfat dry milk (NFDM), 1 tsp. canola oil, 2 tsp. sugar or 1 packet non-nutritive sweetener, 1 Tbsp. peanut butter if patient allows, milk to achieve the correct consistency.
	Fortified milk: 8 oz milk, 3 Tbsp. instant NFDM, 2 tsp. sugar or one packet nonnutritive sweetener, vanilla flavor if desired. Blend well.
Food fortifiers	Non-fat dry milk, peanut butter, canola oil, protein powder.

2. **Increasing energy and protein intakes.** Increased energy and protein intakes could be accomplished with the addition of a high nutrient food to one or all meals, larger portions of some high nutrient meal items, or high nutrient between-meal snacks. Excessive increases in portion sizes or total food volume at meals may be ineffective for individuals unable to consume normal amounts of food. Rich pastries, high fat desserts, and candy provide calories but do not significantly contribute to improved nutrition. (2) Table 12.2 lists some strategies for increasing energy and/or protein intakes with nutritious foods. See Appendix 13 "Protein Content of Selected Foods."

Table 12.2 Strategies for increasing dietary protein and/or energy intakes

- Fortified oatmeal at breakfast.
- 2 eggs at breakfast.
- Peanut butter on toast or bread at meals.
- Side dish of cottage cheese.
- Extra ounce of meat or equivalent at lunch or supper.
- Cheese or peanut butter sandwich as a snack.
- Yogurt snack.
- Fortified milk at meals.
- Lactose free commercial oral nutritional supplements may be considered for patients with lactose intolerance.
- Protein powder added to cold beverages or other foods.

3. **Micronutrients.** The micronutrient content of a High Nutrient Diet is higher than the General Diet due to its increased protein and energy content. Nevertheless, the need for vitamin and mineral supplements should be evaluated. Many individuals are unable to consume the DRIs for micronutrients due to low energy needs or lack of appetite with consequent low food intake.

4. **Managing inadequate food consumption.** Interventions for resolving or preventing malnutrition are most effective when they target the cause of the problem. Table 12.3 lists possible causes of malnutrition and possible interventions to consider.

Table 12.3 Managing the causes of inadequate food intake

Possible cause	Possible interventions to consider
Lack of hunger	• Interview patient for food preferences. • Provide higher nutrient beverages (milk based beverages, commercial nutritional supplements). • Use fortified foods. • Offer small portions at meals and nutritious, substantial snacks between meals. • Provide nutritional supplements between meals rather than with meals. • Review medications for drugs causing anorexia or gastrointestinal (GI) discomfort.
Early satiety	• Offer smaller, high nutrient meals and substantial snacks. • Limit beverages at meals; encourage beverages between feedings. • Limit high fat foods; fat can delay gastric emptying.
Loss of taste or smell	• Provide extra condiments and seasonings at the table per patient preference. • Obtain from the patient a list of any disagreeable foods. • Warm foods may be tastier.

Continued on next page

Table 12.3 Managing the causes of inadequate food intake Continued from previous page

Possible cause	Possible interventions to consider
Soreness in the mouth	• Cold foods may be better tolerated. • Straws may help bypass the sore. • Avoid salty, hard or crunchy, spicy, and acidic foods. • Evaluate the mouth for loose teeth, possible infection, and malnutrition related soreness.
Pain	• Review medications for presence of analgesics. • Check patient's positioning to maximize comfort while eating.
Medications causing nausea, abdominal discomfort, drowsiness	• Review medications for drugs that may be contributing to symptoms. • Take meds immediately after a meal, if possible, to buffer the GI effects. • Offer bland foods for patients with nausea. • Cater to food preferences. • Provide meals to patients when they are alert and ready to eat.
Inability to self-feed	• Evaluate for assistive devices (divided plate, large handle utensils, bent utensils, weighted utensils, foods served in separate bowls, spout cups, cut-out cups, mugs, straws). • Provide feeding assistance.
Dementia	• Provide supervision, cueing, or other assistance at meals. • Finger foods may aid self-feeding. • Smaller portions at meals to avoid overwhelming the patient. • Offer nutritious snacks, beverages, and possibly nutritional supplements between meals. • Assistive devices.
Chewing difficulty	• Determine the foods that are difficult to chew. • Provide nutritionally comparable foods that are easier to chew. • Provide a mechanically altered diet. • Determine the health of the mouth; perhaps there is gum disease or infection. • Determine adequacy of the teeth or dentures; a dental appointment may be needed.
Swallowing difficulty	• Refer to the speech therapist for a swallow evaluation. Thickened liquids may be needed.

5. **Nutrition for wound healing.** Nutritional requirements can be higher than normal during wound healing depending on the severity and size of the wound. Table 12.4 summarizes the nutritional recommendations for persons with pressure and surgical wounds.

Table 12.4 Nutritional recommendations for patients with pressure and surgical wounds

Type of wound	Possible interventions to consider
Wounds—pressure.	• **Energy**: Use the Mifflin-St Jeor equation (3, 4) unless indirect calorimetry is available. Clinical judgment should be used when setting energy (calorie) goals to prevent weight gain in normal weight, overweight, and obese patients and to prevent excessive or rapid weight gain in malnourished patients. Hypocaloric, high protein diets are acceptable for obese patients, however, hypocaloric, low protein diets are not. (4)
	• **Protein**: 1.25-1.5 g/kg/day for patients with pressure wounds and malnutrition. (3) Protein recommendations based on ideal body weight (IBW) are suggested for hospitalized obese patients at the level of 1.8-1.9 g/kg IBW (4). Adjust the protein recommendation downward as patient recovers. Assessment of renal function is important to determine tolerance for high protein intakes. Clinical judgment should be used when setting protein goals. (3)
	• **Water**: Water intake should be high enough for adequate hydration and consistent with patient diagnoses. The most commonly used formulas for estimating baseline needs are 1 mL water/1 kcal consumed and 30 mL/kg. The recommendation should be increased for excessive fluid losses with exudate, fever, diarrhea, vomiting, sweating, and when protein and/or solute intakes are high. Care should be taken to avoid overhydration of obese persons, those with congestive heart failure, and renal failure. (3, 5, 6)
	• **Micronutrients**: The historical single nutrient supplementation of high dose vitamin C and zinc have not proven effective for wound healing. Good nutritional status in all micronutrients is ideally achieved through a high quality, balanced diet. Provide vitamin and mineral supplements for those with a poor dietary intake, or those with suspected or confirmed deficiencies. (3)
	• **Oral nutritional supplements**: Provide appropriate oral nutritional supplements if protein or energy needs cannot be met through diet. Efficacy of arginine containing supplements has not been proven; however, arginine supplementation is not contraindicated. (3)
Wounds—surgical. Recommendations apply to major surgical wounds.	• **Energy**: Recommendations depend on the physiological state of the patient and BMI. Obese patients may safely receive hypocaloric nutrition even as low as 22 kcal/kg if protein intakes are at least 2.0 g/kg IBW/day. (7)
	• **Protein**: 1.5-2.5 g/kg IBW/day for critical illness; obese patients receiving hypocaloric nutrition should receive 2.0-2.5 g protein/kg IBW (4, 8). Clinical judgment should be used when setting protein goals. (3)
	• **Micronutrients**: Provide vitamin and mineral supplements for those with a poor dietary intake, or those with suspected or confirmed deficiencies.
	• **Pharmaconutrition**: Arginine, glutamine, n-3 fatty acids, and nucleotides may reduce complications in the healing of surgical wounds. (9, 10, 11, 12) These nutrients are usually provided in combination. Optimal dosages for the individual nutrients have not been established.

6. **Potential for weight changes.** Care must be taken to prevent inappropriate weight changes while attempting to rehabilitate a person's overall nutritional status or heal a wound. Rapid weight gain or weight loss is usually not recommended. Rapid weight gain in individuals who are underweight may result in excessive fat mass; and rapid weight loss in individuals who are overweight or obese increases protein requirements. (13) Weight should be monitored closely and the energy content of meals, snacks, and beverages adjusted accordingly. (14) The energy content of the high nutrient diet should depend on the patient's BMI, rate of recent weight change, and the person's physiological state.

Table 12.5 Sample Menu for High Nutrient Diet

Breakfast	Supper
½ c. orange juice	2 oz. tuna on 2 slices whole wheat bread with
1-2 eggs	1 Tbsp. mayonnaise
½ c. oatmeal (may be fortified)	1 c. leafy green salad with grated parmesan cheese and walnuts
1 slice whole wheat toast	
2 tsp. jelly	1-2 Tbsp. oil and vinegar dressing
1 Tbsp. peanut butter	½ c. fruit cocktail
1 c. whole milk	1 c. whole milk
Hot beverage	Water
Sugar, salt, pepper (optional)	
Lunch	**Snack Ideas**
2-3 oz. roasted chicken	Cheese sandwich (2 slices whole wheat bread, 2 oz. cheese, 1 tsp. mayonnaise)
½ cup mashed "power" potatoes with 2 oz. gravy	
½ c. mixed vegetables	½ c. fortified pudding
1 oz. whole wheat roll	Milkshake or medical nutrition supplement
2 tsp. margarine	3c. popcorn with butter
½ cup strawberry ice cream	
1 c. whole milk	
Water	

REFERENCES

1. National Academy of Sciences, Institute of Medicine, Food and Nutrition Board. Dietary Reference Intakes. United States Department of Agriculture, Food and Nutrition Information Center Web site. http://fnic.nal.usda.gov/dietary-guidance/dietary-reference-intakes/dri-nutrient-reports Accessed August 31, 2015.

2. Bernstein M, Munoz, N. Position of the Academy of Nutrition and Dietetics: Food and nutrition for older adults: promoting health and wellness. *J Acad Nutr Diet.* 2012; 112:1255-1277.

3. Posthauer ME, Banks M, Dorner B, Schols JM. The role of nutrition for pressure ulcer management: national pressure ulcer advisory panel, European pressure ulcer advisory panel, and Pan Pacific pressure injury alliance white paper. *Adv Skin Wound Care.* 2015; 28(4):175-188.

4. Choban P, Dickerson R, Malone A, Worthington P, Compher C, the American Society for Parenteral and Enteral Nutrition. A.S.P.E.N. Clinical Guidelines: Nutrition support of hospitalized adult patients with obesity. *J Parenter Enteral Nutr.* 2013; 37(6):714-744.

5. Dorner B, Posthauer ME, Friedrich EK, Robinson GE. Enteral nutrition for older adults in nursing facilities. *Nutr Clin Pract.* 2011; 26(3):261-272.

6. Dickerson RN, Brown RO. Long-term enteral nutrition support and the risk of dehydration. *Nutr Clin Pract.* 2005; 20(6):646-653.

7. Choban PS, Dickerson RN. Morbid obesity and nutrition support: is bigger different? *Nutr Clin Prac.* 2005; 20(4):480-487.

8. Hoffer LJ, Bistrian BR. Appropriate protein provision in critical illness: a systematic and narrative review. *Am J Clin Nutr.* 2012; 96(3):591-600. doi: 10.3945/ajcn.111.032078

9. Braga M, Wischmeyer PE, Drover J, Heyland DK. Clinical evidence for pharmaconutrition in major elective surgery. *J Parenter Enteral Nutr.* 2013; 37(5 suppl):66S-72S.

10. Evans DC, Martindale RG, Kiraly LN, Jones CM. Nutrition optimization prior to surgery. *Nutr Clin Pract.* 2014; 29(1):10-21.

11. Marik PE, Zaloga GP. Immunonutrition in high-risk surgical patients: a systematic review and analysis of the literature. *J Parenter Enteral Nutr.* 2010; 34(4):378-386.

12. Buijs N, van Bokhorst-de van der Schueren MAE, Langius JAE, et al. Perioperative arginine-supplemented nutrition in malnourished patients with head and neck cancer improves long-term survival. *Am J Clin Nutr.* 2010; 92(5):1151-1156.

13. Soenen S, Martens EAP, Hochstenbach-Waelen A, Lemmens SGT, Westerterp-Pantenga MS. Normal protein intake is required for body weight loss and weight maintenance, and elevated protein intake for additional preservation of resting energy expenditure and fat free mass. *J Nutr.* 2013; 143(5):591-596.

14. Doley J. Nutrition management of pressure ulcers. *Nutr Clin Pract.* 2010; 25(1):50-60.

15. Steiber AL. Chronic kidney disease: considerations for nutrition interventions. *J Parenter Enteral Nutr.* 2014; 38(4): 418-426.

ADDITIONAL RESOURCES

Enhancing Nutritional Value with Fortified Foods: A Resource for Professionals. http://www.dhccdpg.org/local/resources/enhancing_nutritional_value.pdf   Published 2008. Accessed August, 31, 2015.

Leslie WS, Woodward M, Lean ME, Theobald H, Watson L, Hankey CR. Improving the dietary intake of under nourished older people in residential care homes using an energy-enriching food approach: a cluster randomised controlled study. *J Hum Nutr Diet.* 2013; 26(4):387-394. doi: 10.1111/jhn.12020

SMALL PORTIONS DIET

Use

The Small Portions diet follows the principals of the General Diet except portion sizes are reduced for some foods. This diet is appropriate for individuals who would benefit from a reduced portion size for weight maintenance or weight reduction, and for individuals who request a reduced portion (because the portion size offered on the General Diet is too overwhelming).

Small Portion Diet principles may be adjusted to accommodate individual preferences and nutritional needs.

Adequacy

The suggested food plan reduces the calories from the General Diet to prevent undesired weight gain or promote gradual weight loss, depending on the individual's energy needs. It provides adequate protein intake but may not meet all Dietary Reference Intakes (DRIs) of some individuals as recommended by the National Academy of Sciences for adults. The need for vitamin and mineral supplementation should be assessed on an individual basis by the healthcare team. Individuals consuming a small portion diet should be weighed frequently and monitored for poor food intake, resulting in undernutrition.

Diet Principles

1. Meats, meat alternates, or entrée: offer same portion as General Diet.

2. Vegetables: portions range from ¼ to ½ cup for vegetables.

3. Fruits: offer same portion as General Diet.

4. Milk and milk products: offer same portion as General Diet.

5. Grains other than fortified breakfast cereals: portion reduced to half serving; ½ slice of bread, ¼ cup of pasta or rice.

6. Soup: portions range from 4 to 6 ounces.

7. Fluids other than milk: offer same portion as General Diet.

8. Discretionary calories (desserts, alcohol): portion reduced to half serving.

Table 12.6 Sample Menu for Small Portion Diet

Breakfast	Supper
½ c. orange juice	2 oz. tuna on 1 slice whole wheat bread, 2 tsp. mayonnaise
1 egg	
½ c. oatmeal	2 tomato slices
½ slice whole wheat toast	½ c. leafy greens salad
1 tsp. jelly	1 Tbsp. oil and vinegar dressing
1 tsp. soft margarine	½ c. fruit cocktail
1 c. fat-free milk	1 c. fat-free milk
Hot beverage	Water
Sugar, pepper (optional)	
Lunch	**Snack Ideas**
2 oz. roasted chicken breast	½ c. cantaloupe
¼ c. mashed potatoes with 1 oz. gravy	½ c. carrot sticks
⅓ c. mixed vegetables	1 c. popcorn
½ oz. whole wheat roll	
1 tsp. soft margarine	
1 c. fat-free milk	
Water	

ADDITIONAL RESOURCES

Position Paper of the American Dietetic Association: Liberalization of the diet prescription improves quality of life for older adults in long-term care. *J Am Diet Assoc.* 2005; 105(12):1955–1965.

Yager R., Department of Developmental Services, State of California Health and Human Services Agency. Small Diet. In: *Diet Manual.* California; 2010:1.3–1.4. http://www.dds.ca.gov/Publications/docs/DDSDietManual.pdf

Maryland Department of Health and Mental Hygiene, Office of Health Care Quality. Small Diet. In: *Diet Manual for Long-Term Care Residents*. Catonsville, MD; 2014:35-37. http://dhmh.maryland.gov/ohcq/docs/diet_manual_4-3-14.pdf

VEGETARIAN DIETS

Use

Individuals wishing to avoid a diet free of flesh foods (meat, fish, and poultry) and which may or may not exclude egg or dairy products may request a Vegetarian Diet. The following are some of the types of plant-based diets one may choose.

- The Vegan Diet is free from all flesh foods, eggs, and dairy products, and sometimes honey.

- The Lacto-Ovo Vegetarian Diet is free from flesh foods, but includes eggs and dairy products.

- The Ovo Vegetarian Diet is free from flesh foods and dairy foods, but includes eggs.

- The Semi-Vegetarian Diet is a plant-based dietary pattern with occasional beef, pork, poultry or fish; perhaps once or twice a week. Those who follow a Semi-Vegetarian Diet, refer to the General Diet and use meats the individual consumes.

Adequacy

The suggested food plans include foods in amounts that will provide the quantities of nutrients recommended by the National Academy of Sciences for adults. The diet requires additional modifications to meet nutritional needs during illness, pregnancy, lactation, infancy, and childhood.

Diet Principles

1. Obtain an accurate diet history; it is essential in determining limitations and the individual's type of vegetarian diet.

2. Provide adequate nutrients by including mostly foods rich in nutrients and only small amounts of low-nutrient sweets and fats.

3. Limit highly processed grains and other refined carbohydrates to ensure adequate intake of trace nutrients.

4. Careful consideration should be given to the following when planning vegetarian diets:

   a. **Protein.** Plant proteins alone can provide enough amino acids (the building blocks of protein) when a variety of plant proteins are eaten throughout the day and the total caloric intake meets the individual's caloric needs. It is no longer recommended that complementary proteins must be eaten at the same meal. Substitutes for 1 ounce of meat are:

   8 ounces soy milk

   ½ cup cooked dry beans

   2 tablespoons peanut butter or other nut butter

   2 tablespoons nuts or seeds

   4 ounces tofu, ¼ cup tempeh, or 2 ounce meatless burger (soy based)

   1 whole egg or 2 egg whites

   See Appendix 13 for "Protein Content of Selected Foods."

   b. **Calcium.** Calcium intakes in individuals that are lower than that recommended by the National Academy of Sciences may need to increase their intake. See "Calcium

Content of Selected Foods" in Appendix 3 for non-animal sources of calcium. A well-absorbed calcium supplement in divided doses may also be considered.

c.   **Vitamin D.** Individuals who follow most vegetarian diets need to rely on sun exposure, food fortified with vitamin D, and/or vegan supplements to maintain adequate serum levels. Few plant foods are fortified, so those who are following a Vegan Diet may need to rely on vegan supplements.

d.   **Iron.** It is recommended to include sources of iron; such as beans and lentils, raisins, blackstrap molasses, and iron-fortified breads and cereals. Iron in plants is not as readily absorbed as that in meats. To increase iron absorption, include foods rich in vitamin C in the same meal with iron-containing foods. See "Iron Content of Selected Foods" in Appendix 4 and "Vitamin C Content of Selected Foods" in Appendix 10.

e.   **Vitamin B$_{12}$.** Only animal products contain vitamin B$_{12}$. Diets of vegetarians who eat dairy products and eggs may still have risks depending on their intake and vitamin B$_{12}$ status. Good fortified sources include fortified cereals and grain products, fortified soy beverages, and some brands of nutritional (brewer's) yeast. A vitamin B$_{12}$ supplement should be considered based on their physician's guidance. See "Vitamin B$_{12}$ Content of Selected Foods" in Appendix 9.

f.   **Zinc.** Due to the presence of zinc absorption inhibitors in plant foods, the recommendation for those who adhere to vegetarian diet—compared to those who do not—is 50% greater. Foods containing zinc include fortified cereals, legumes, tofu, wheat germ, nuts, nut butters, and seeds.

g.   **n-3 (Omega) Fatty Acids.** Vegetarian diets are generally rich in n-6 fatty acids but they may be marginal in n-3 fatty acids. Vegetarians should include good sources of foods such as flaxseed, walnuts, canola oil, and soy.

5.   Read product labels carefully to avoid hidden ingredients such as meat extracts, animal fats, eggs, and milk.

The following guidelines are for the Lacto-Ovo Vegetarian Diet. You may also refer to the Healthy Vegetarian Eating Pattern in the *2015-2020 Dietary Guidelines for Americans*. (1) Items marked with an asterisk would be omitted from a vegan (no animal products) meal plan.

Table 12.7 Vegetarian Diet

Food for the Day	Recommended	Choose Less Often
Vegetables *1–4 cups*	Any fresh, canned, frozen; tomato juice or vegetable juice cocktail.	Deep-fried or battered and fried vegetables.
Fruits *1–2.5 cups*	Any fresh, canned, frozen, dried; 100% fruit juice, 100% fruit calcium-fortified orange juice.	Fruit canned in heavy syrup.
Grains *3–10 ½ ounce equivalents* *At least half of which are whole grains.*	Whole wheat grain products: pasta, tortillas, waffles, crackers, bread and cereal. Popcorn, oats, millet, quinoa, brown rice.	Enriched grains, or grains with excess sweeteners.

Continued on next page

Table 12.7 Vegetarian Diet Continued from previous page

Food for the Day	Recommended	Choose Less Often
Dairy products *2–3 cups*	Fat-free (skim)*, low-fat (1%)*, or reduced-fat (2%)* milk; low-fat flavored or plain yogurt*, low-fat cheese.*	Whole milk*, chocolate milk*; high-fat cheese.*
Protein foods *1 – 6 ounce-equivalents*	Eggs*, meat analogues, tofu, or tempeh; legumes; soy milk; limited amounts of nuts and nut butters including peanut butter.	Refried beans.
Oils/Fat	Margarine, salad dressings, and vegetable oils.	Butter*, sour cream*, cream cheese*, nondairy creamers containing coconut oil.
Sweets/Desserts	Low-fat, moderately sweetened such as pudding/custard made with fat-free milk*, angel food cake*, graham crackers, vanilla wafers, flavored yogurt*, light ice cream*, frozen yogurt.*	High sugar, high-fat desserts such as pie and pastries, frosted cake, candy, whole-milk puddings* and custards*, ice cream.*
Fluids	Water, bottled and sparkling waters, coffee, herbal tea.	Tea (with meals); carbonated beverages and sweetened flavored, sparkling waters; fruit beverages, drinks and "ades"; beverages containing alcohol.
Other	Vegetable broth, herbs and spices, low sodium seasonings, black strap molasses, brewer's yeast, wheat germ.	Honey*, jelly, and jam; high sodium seasonings.

*These items would be omitted from a vegan (no animal products) meal plan.

Table 12.8 Sample Menu for Lacto-Ovo Vegetarian Diet

Breakfast	Supper
½ c. orange juice	1 oz. low-fat cheese
1 egg or 1 Tbsp. peanut butter	½ c. seasoned pinto beans
½ c. oatmeal	1 c. leafy greens salad
1 slice whole wheat toast	1 Tbsp. oil and vinegar dressing
1 tsp. soft margarine	2 tomato slices
1 c. milk	2 corn tortillas
Hot beverage	1 tsp. soft margarine
Sugar, pepper (optional)	½ c. fruit cocktail
	1 c. milk
	Water

Continued on next page

Table 12.8 Sample Menu for Lacto-Ovo Vegetarian Diet Continued from previous page

Lunch	Snack Ideas
2 oz. meatless burger, soy-based	1 c. cantaloupe
½ c. mashed potatoes (made without chicken stock)	½ c. carrot sticks
½ c. mixed vegetables	3 c. popcorn
1 oz whole wheat roll	6 ounces low-fat yogurt
2 tsp. soft margarine	
1 c. milk	
Water	

Table 12.9 Sample Menu for Vegan Diet

Breakfast	Supper
½ c. orange juice	½ cup seasoned pinto beans
1 Tbsp. peanut butter	1 c. leafy greens salad
½ c. oatmeal made with fortified soy milk	1 Tbsp. oil and vinegar dressing
1 slice whole wheat toast	2 tomato slices
1 tsp. soft margarine	2 corn tortillas
1 c. fortified soy milk	1 tsp. soft margarine
Hot beverage	½ c. fruit cocktail
Sugar, pepper (optional)	1 c. fortified soy milk
	Water

Lunch	Snack Ideas
2-3oz. meatless burger, soy-based	1 c. cantaloupe
½ c. mashed potatoes made with fortified soy milk	½ c. carrot sticks
½ c. mixed vegetables	3 c. popcorn
1 oz. whole wheat roll	6 whole grain crackers with 2 Tbsp. peanut butter
2 tsp. soft margarine	¾ c. cereal with 1 c. fortified soy milk
1 cup strawberries with 3 graham cracker squares	
1 c. fortified soy milk	
Water	

REFERENCES

1. U. S. Department of Health and Human Services and U. S. Department of Agriculture. *2015 – 2020 Dietary Guidelines for Americans*, 8th ed. http://health.gov/dietaryguidelines/2015/guidelines/appendix-5 Published December 2015. Accessed January 13, 2016.

ADDITIONAL RESOURCES

Craig WJ, Mangels AR; American Dietetic Association. Position of the American Dietetic Association: vegetarian diets. J Am Diet Assoc. July 2009; 109(7): 1266-1279.

Messina V, Melina V, Mangels AR. A new food guide for North American vegetarians. J Am Diet Assoc. 2003; 103(6):771-775.

Institute of Medicine, Food and Nutrition Board. Dietary Reference Intakes for Vitamin A, Vitamin K, Arsenic, Boron, Chromium, Copper, Iodine, Iron, Manganese, Molybdenum, Nickel, Silicon, Vanadium, and Zinc. Washington, DC: National Academies Press; 2001. www.nal.usda.gov/fnic/DRI/DRI_Vitamin_A/vitamin_a_full_report.pdf

Websites

Vegetarian Consumer website: www.vegetariannutrition.net

The Vegetarian Resource Group: www.vrg.org

VeganHealth.org: www.veganhealth.org

HALAL DIET

Use

Islam is the world's second largest religion and continues to have rapid growth with more than 23% of the world's population adhering to Islam. (1) Adherents of Islam, known as Muslims, abide by the Qur'an. The Qur'an is a religious text considered to be a revelation from Allah, which is the Arabic word for "God." Included in the Qur'an, along with teachings, revelations, and narratives, are guidelines for how to live life as a Muslim. One set of teachings found in the Qur'an relates to cleanliness; this encompasses dietary laws with respect to permissible foods for consumption and appropriate preparation. Two categories exist regarding what is lawful and unlawful: halal and haram, respectively. Halal is an Arabic term meaning "permissible or lawful," whereas haram means "sinful" or "not permitted." The halal diet, then, refers to foods and beverages that are permissible for Muslims to consume because they satisfy standards of cleanliness, according to the Qur'an. Haram foods and beverages are ones that Muslims must avoid. Also important in the halal diet is the appropriate preparation of certain foods. The practices for food preparation (specifically the slaughtering of animals) exist to ensure sanitary measures are taken. The halal symbol is used as certification to show which food products meet the requirements to comply with the halal dietary laws. There are several organizations that certify halal foods and each has a different symbol.

Adequacy

The suggested food plan includes food in the amounts that will provide the DRIs recommended by the National Academy of Sciences for adults.

Diet Principles

1. The halal diet follows dietary laws according to the Qur'an in order to maintain a person's cleanliness through avoiding certain foods.

2. Foods that have a halal symbol are permissible for consumption because they certifiably do not contain haram ingredients and meet the standards for hygiene and preparation.

3. Meat and poultry must be slaughtered according to Islamic Law for it to be considered halal. (2)

4. All pork and its by-products, carnivorous animals, and birds of prey (i.e., those that hunt with their claws/talons such as a falcon, eagle, kite, hawk) are strictly haram because of hygienic concerns laid out in the Qur'an and should not be consumed by a person following the halal diet. (1)

5. Alcohol and intoxicants are strictly prohibited. (2) This includes any foods made with alcohol such as vanilla extract, sauces, dressings, certain baked goods, candies, or chocolates.

6. Blood and its by-products are considered haram. (2)

7. It is important to read all ingredients on the label to avoid the following: alcohol, animal shortening, broth, gelatin, ham, bacon, lard, l-cysteine, lipase, pepsin, animal rennet, and margarine that contains monoglycerides or diglycerides from an animal source. (1)

8. A registered dietitian nutritionist familiar with the halal diet can assist with further diet planning and provide education to assure nutritional adequacy.

Table 12.10 Halal Diet (3, 4)

Food for the Day	Recommended (Halal)	Avoid (Haram)
Vegetables *1–4 cups*	All vegetables—fresh, frozen, dried, or canned; vegetable juices.	Any vegetables prepared with lard, shortening, bacon, ham, alcohol, or gelatin.
Fruits *1–2.5 cups*	All fruits—fresh, frozen, dried, or canned; fruit juices.	Any fruits prepared with lard, shortening, bacon, alcohol, or gelatin.
Grains *3–10 ounce-equivalents*	Rice, pasta, bread, bread products, crackers, and any grain prepared without Haram ingredients.	Any grains prepared with alcohol, lard, animal shortening, or pure or artificial vanilla extract.
Dairy products *2–3 cups*	Milk and milk products including yogurt, cottage cheese, and cheese (products must be made without animal enzymes).	Any dairy product made with animal rennet, gelatin, lipase, or vanilla extract (pure or artificial).
Protein foods *2–7 ounce-equivalents*	Meat and poultry must be slaughtered according to Islamic law. Seafood, nuts, seeds, eggs, peanut butter, tofu, halal deli meats, dried beans, lentils.	Pork (all types), e.g. bacon, ham, deli meats, sausage. Meats not slaughtered according to Islamic law. Canned beans containing pork.
Oils, Solid Fats	Butter, margarine that does not contain monoglycerides or diglycerides from an animal source, mayonnaise, vegetable oils.	Lard, animal shortening, margarine that contains monoglycerides or diglycerides from an animal source.
Added Sugars, Others	Sugar, honey, syrup, jam, chutney. Beverages: tea, coffee, carbonated beverages, punch.	All alcoholic beverages; foods made with alcohol, artificial or pure vanilla extract; desserts made with gelatin, marshmallows, foods containing blood, broth (made with pork).

Table 12.11 Sample Menu for Halal Diet

Breakfast	Supper
½ c. orange juice	2 oz. tuna on
1 egg	2 slices whole wheat bread with
½ c. oatmeal	2 tsp. mayonnaise
1 slice whole wheat toast	2 tomato slices
1 tsp. soft margarine	1 c. leafy greens salad
2 tsp. jelly	1 Tbsp. oil and vinegar dressing
1 c. milk	½ c. fruit cocktail
Hot beverage	1 c. milk
Sugar, pepper (optional)	Water
Lunch	**Snack Ideas**
2 oz. halal roasted chicken breast	½ c. cantaloupe
½ c. mashed potatoes with fat-free gravy (made without pork)	½ c. carrot sticks
	3 c. popcorn, lower fat, *trans*-fat free, no added salt
½ c. mixed vegetables	
1 oz. wheat roll	
1 tsp. soft margarine	
1 c. milk	
Water	

REFERENCES

1. The Future of World Religions: Population Growth Projections, 2010-2050. Pew Research Center Web site. http://www.pewforum.org/2015/04/02/religious-projections-2010-2050/ Published April 2, 2015. Accessed August 1, 2015.

2. What is Halal? Islamic Food and Nutrition Council of America Web site. http://www.ifanca.org/Pages/staticwebpages.aspx?page=whatisHalal Accessed August 8, 2015.

3. Guide to Understanding Halal Foods. Toronto Public Health Web site. https://www.utsc.utoronto.ca/~facilities/documents/GuidetoHalalFoods.pdf Published 2004. Accessed August 8, 2015.

4. Serving Muslim Patrons Following a Halal Diet: A Quick Halal Guide for Nutrition and Foodservice Professionals. Islamic Food and Nutrition Council of America Web site. http://www.ifanca.org/HFSK/Halal%20Nutrition%20Guide%20for%20Foodservice%20Professionals.pdf Accessed August 1, 2015.

Websites

Certified Halal in the USA: http://photos.state.gov/libraries/amgov/133183/english/P_Certified_Halal_in_the_USA_English.pdf

Halal Research Council: www.halalrc.org

Islamic Food and Nutrition Council of America: www.ifanca.org

KOSHER DIET

Use

Kosher dietary laws followed by some, but not all, adherents to Judaism originated over 2,000 years ago. These dietary laws derived from scholarly interpretations of passages found in the Old Testament of the Bible. The literal meaning of the word kosher is "fit or proper." Kosher does not mean that the food has been "blessed" by the rabbi or other religious authority. It merely connotes that the food has been produced in accordance to relevant dietary laws. At its simplest, the kosher diet mandates a prohibition of the consumption of meat and dairy products at the same meal. It also precludes the cooking together of meat and dairy products. Kosher dietary laws require a complete separation of meat and dairy foods through the use of two separate sets (meat and dairy) of pots and pans, dishes, flatware, as well as cooking and serving utensils. It is also suggested that the individual refrain from eating dairy products for a period of several hours following the consumption of meat. Food products that have been certified as kosher by a local or national religious entity are labeled with a symbol (a variety of such symbols are used in different parts of the United States), which can usually be found on the front of the package label or near the ingredients(s) list. This symbol, called a *hekhsher* indicates that the food ingredients(s), the processes in producing the food, and the food processing plant itself have been inspected to ensure that all kosher dietary laws are being followed.

Adequacy

The suggested food plan includes food in the amounts that will provide the DRIs recommended by the National Academy of Sciences for adults.

Diet Principles

1. This diet follows kosher dietary laws by not combining meat products and dairy products (or its derivatives).

2. Only kosher foods are used in meal preparation. These products are identified by a kosher symbol on the label. If there is no symbol, it is not kosher with the exception of fresh fruits and vegetables. It is important to read the ingredient list on all prepared foods to determine if that product may be used for either a meat or a dairy meal. Care to avoid cross-contamination in food preparation is essential.

3. A kosher animal chews its cud, has split hooves, and includes: cows, goats, sheep, deer, bison, and antelope; all being slaughtered in accordance with religious laws.

4. A kosher fowl includes chickens, domestic geese, turkeys, and doves.

5. A kosher fish must have both fins and scales and includes carp, cod, flounder, haddock, halibut, herring, mackerel, pickerel, pike, salmon, trout, tuna, and whitefish. No "scavenger" species or shellfish are allowed. More information on allowed fish is available at Chabad.org. (1)

6. Any egg from a kosher fowl is considered kosher. Eggs should be checked before use to make sure they are free of blood spots.

7. A kosher dairy product is a milk product from a kosher animal. A dairy food cannot contain any meat or nonkosher products. Dairy foods include milk, butter, yogurt, cheese, cream cheese, and milk derivatives such as sodium caseinate and lactose.

8. Pareve foods are neutral and can be served with either a dairy or meat meal. These foods include raw fruits, vegetables, grains, eggs, pasta, and juice.

9. Fish is considered pareve and may be served with meat or dairy but preferably a dairy meal.

10. In addition to regular kosher laws, there are additional restrictions for Passover. Passover is an eight day festival celebrated in the spring. Wheat, rye, barley, oats, and spelt are avoided during Passover unless the foods are labeled "kosher for Passover." Ashkenazic Jews (most Americans) do not consume the following *kitniyot* foods during Passover: buckwheat, rice, corn, millet, dried beans and peas, peas, green beans, soybeans, edamame, peanuts, fennel, fenugreek, flaxseed, sesame seeds, poppy seeds, sunflower seeds, rapeseed/canola, caraway, cardamom, and mustard. (2)

11. A registered dietitian nutritionist familiar with the kosher diet can assist in diet planning and education to assure nutritional adequacy.

Table 12.12 Kosher Diet

Food for the Day	Recommended	Avoid
Vegetables *1–4 cups*	Fresh vegetables. All canned, frozen, and vegetable juices identified as kosher.	Nonkosher vegetable products or juice. No cream sauces over vegetables are allowed when served with a *meat* meal.
Fruits *1–2.5 cups*	Fresh fruit. All canned, frozen and fruit juices identified as kosher.	Any fruit (except fresh) not identified as kosher.
Grains *3–10 ounce-equivalents*	All baked goods prepared in a kosher kitchen.	Any bakery item not prepared using kosher practices. Any item containing lard.
Dairy products *2–3 cups*	Kosher cheese and other milk products including butter, yogurt, cottage cheese, cream cheese, sour cream and soy milk.	All dairy products when meat is served. Nonkosher cheese.
Protein foods *2–7 ounce-equivalents*	Kosher beef, lamb, mutton, venison, buffalo, or antelope. Kosher chicken, duck, goose, pheasant or turkey. Kosher deli meats, hot dogs. Fish with fins and scales. Eggs from kosher fowl.	Any nonkosher meat or poultry. Pork and rabbit. All shellfish (clams, crab, lobster, oysters, shrimp, and mussels). Eel, frog, shark, octopus, swordfish, catfish. Eggs with blood spots or eggs from nonkosher fowl.
Oils, Solid Fats	Kosher margarines including soy margarine. Nondairy creamers. Kosher mayonnaise, vegetable oil. Olives. Gravy made with kosher meat.	Butter unless served with a *dairy* meal. Nonkosher mayonnaise, salad dressings, and vegetable oils. Milk-containing gravy with *meat* meal.

Continued on next page

Table 12.12 Kosher Diet Continued from previous page

Food for the Day	Recommended	Avoid
Added Sugars, Others	Kosher alcohol, beer and wine.	Dark beer.
	Coffee, tea, powdered drink mixes, carbonated beverages.	Animal fats (bacon, grease, lard).
		Nonkosher desserts.
	Kosher cakes, cookies, candy, chocolate, jam, and jellies.	Nonkosher soups.
	Kosher pudding and ice cream.	Gelatin or products made with gelatin unless identified as kosher.
	Sherbet with dairy meals only.	Marshmallows.
	Any prepared food mixtures prepared under kosher standards.	
	Honey, pepper, salt, sugar, sugar substitutes, and syrup.	

Table 12.13 Sample Menu for Kosher Diet

Breakfast	Supper
½ c. orange juice	2 oz. tuna on
1 egg	2 slices whole wheat bread with
½ c. oatmeal	2 tsp. mayonnaise
1 slice whole wheat toast	2 tomato slices
2 tsp. jelly	1 c. leafy greens salad
1 tsp. soft margarine	1 Tbsp. oil and vinegar dressing
1 c. milk	½ c. fruit cocktail
Hot beverage	1 c. milk
Sugar, pepper (optional)	Water
Lunch	**Snack Ideas**
2 oz. kosher roasted chicken	½ c. cantaloupe
½ c. mashed potatoes (*no milk*—may use nondairy creamer) with 2 oz. gravy (made without milk)	½ c. carrot sticks
	2 kosher cookies
½ c. mixed vegetables	1 c. yogurt
1 oz. whole wheat roll	
1 tsp. soft margarine	
½ c. mandarin oranges	
NO MILK	
Water, Coffee or Tea	

REFERENCES

1. Kosher: A guide to eating Jewishly. Chabad.org website. http://www.chabad.org/library/article_cdo/aid/82675/jewish/Kosher-Fish-List.htm Accessed September 29, 2015.

2. Kitniyot List. OU Kosher website. https://oukosher.org/passover/guidelines/food-items/kitniyot-list/ Accessed September 27, 2015.

Websites

Kosher Handbook: http://www.chabad.org/library/article_cdo/aid/134459/jewish/Handbook.htm

Judaism 101: www.jewfaq.org/kashrut.htm

PHENYLALANINE RESTRICTED DIET

Use

The phenylalanine restricted diet is used for people who lack the enzyme (phenylalanine hydroxylase) necessary to convert phenylalanine to tyrosine, causing a disorder called phenylketonuria (PKU). High amounts of phenylalanine are toxic to the brain and can cause mental retardation. Prior to newborn screening (most states started to screen in the 1960s), individuals with PKU were not identified until the brain damage had occurred. Even though a phenylalanine-restricted diet will not reverse the mental retardation that may have occurred, it may reduce some of the behavior problems these individuals may have. When newborn screening began, infants were placed on the diet at diagnosis and kept on the diet until 5 to 8 years of age when it was thought safe to go off the diet because the most rapid time of brain development was over. As more individuals have been off the diet for longer periods of time, it is apparent that high amounts of phenylalanine continue to be a brain toxin and can cause varying degrees of brain damage. Currently, individuals begin the diet at diagnosis and the recommendation is to continue the diet for life so brain damage does not occur.

Over the past few years, some new treatments for PKU have emerged. Tetrahydrobiopterin or BH4 is a cofactor required for the enzyme phenylalanine hydroxylase to work optimally. A synthetic form of this cofactor marketed under the name of Kuvan® was approved by the FDA in December 2007. Clinical trials indicate that Kuvan® taken orally enhances the efficiency of phenylalanine hydroxylase in some individuals with PKU. This can lead to decreased serum phenylalanine levels or increased natural protein intake.

Another relatively new treatment is the use of large neutral amino acids (LNAA). These are thought to lower the phenylalanine in the brain by competing with phenylalanine to cross the blood-brain barrier. These can be used by individuals who are off diet and find it difficult to return to a phenylalanine-restricted diet, but who wish to see if this improves their mood, memory, or behavior.

Another treatment still in the research phase involves providing the missing enzyme (phenylalanine hydroxylase) in a form that the body can use to break down phenylalanine.

Adequacy

Depending on the type of the special metabolic formula used, the suggested food plan may provide the DRIs recommended by the National Academy of Sciences or may need to be supplemented with a multivitamin and calcium supplement.

Diet Principles

1. The diet eliminates all foods containing natural protein such as meat, fish, poultry, milk, yogurt, cheese, eggs, nuts, seeds, legumes, and peanut butter.

2. Foods containing aspartame are also eliminated because one of the byproducts of aspartame is phenylalanine. Sucralose, acesulfame potassium, and saccharin are allowed.

3. Adequate protein intake is achieved with the use of a metabolic formula that has the phenylalanine removed while the rest of the amino acids remain. Many of the metabolic formulas also provide fat, carbohydrate, vitamins, and minerals.

4. A prescribed amount of phenylalanine is allowed from natural food sources like fruits, vegetables, and grain products.

5. Low protein foods such as pastas, breads, and other baked goods are available to provide calories and variety to the diet without too much phenylalanine. There are also low protein versions for eggs, cheese, meat, and peanut butter.

6. A registered dietitian nutritionist familiar with the phenylalanine restricted diet should assist in diet planning and teaching to assure nutritional adequacy.

Table 12.14 Phenylalanine Restricted Diet

Food for the Day	Recommended	Avoid
Vegetables *1–4 cups*	All fresh, frozen, canned.	Baked beans and other legumes.
Fruits *1–2.5 cups*	Fresh, frozen, canned, dried, fruit juices.	None.
Grains *Amount specified by registered dietitian*	All that will fit within protein allotment. May need to use low protein grains.	None.
Dairy products	Special metabolic formula in the amount prescribed by registered dietitian.	All regular milk, yogurt, cheese.
Protein foods	None.	All meat, poultry, fish, eggs, dried beans or peas, or peanut butter.
Oils, Solid Fats	All are allowed.	None.
Added Sugars	All that will fit into the protein allotment which may include gelatin, sorbets, fruit ices.	Those too high in protein.
Fluids	Water and other fluids, such as coffee, tea, fruit or vegetable juice, lemonade, regular soda.	Beverages containing aspartame, regular milk.

Table 12.15 Sample Menu for Phenylalanine Restricted Diet

Breakfast	Supper
Special metabolic formula	Special metabolic formula
½ c. orange juice	2 tomato slices
½ c. cereal*	1 c. low protein macaroni and cheese
½ cup peaches	1 c. leafy greens salad
1 slice white toast*	1 Tbsp. salad dressing
2 tsp. jelly	½ c. fruit cocktail
1 tsp. soft margarine	Water
Coffee or tea	Coffee or tea
Sugar, salt, pepper (optional)	Sugar, salt, pepper (optional)
Lunch	**Snack Ideas**
Special metabolic formula	½ c. fruit
Low protein cheese pizza	Low protein baked items*
½ c. vegetables	Popsicles®
½ c. mandarin oranges	½ c. carrot or celery sticks
½ c. sorbet	Fruit drinks
Water	Candy with no protein
Coffee or tea	Fruit snacks
Sugar, salt, pepper (optional)	

*Regular or low protein depending on protein allotment

ADDITIONAL RESOURCES

Acosta P, Yannicelli S. *The Ross Metabolic Formula System Nutrition Support Protocols*. Columbus, OH: Ross Products Division, 2001.

Vockley J, Andersson HC, Antshel KM, Braverman NE, et al. Phenylalanine hydroxylase deficiency: diagnosis and management guideline. *Genet Med.* 2014; 16(2):188-200. doi: 10.1038/gim.2013.157

Singh RH, Rohr F, Frazier D, Cunningham A, et al. Recommendations for the nutrition management of phenylalanine hydroxylase deficiency. *Genet Med*. 2014; 16(2): 121-131. doi: 10.1038/gim.2013.179

Schuett V. *Low Protein Food List for PKU*, 3rd ed. CreateSpace; 2010.

Websites

National PKU News: www.pkunews.org

National PKU Alliance: www.npkua.org

Online low protein food list: www.howmuchphe.org

VITAMIN K AND PROTHROMBIN TIME GUIDELINES

The Adequate Intake for Vitamin K is 90 mcg daily for women and 120 mcg daily for men. (1) Too little vitamin K (2) or inconsistent vitamin K intake is a problem for people taking a blood thinning medication called warfarin. Vitamin K helps to clot the blood, therefore a sudden change in vitamin K intake can affect how well warfarin works. The following tests, International Normalized Ratio (INR) and Prothrombin Time (PT), measure the time it takes for the blood to clot. These tests are usually measured at least once a month to make sure they are in the desired range. The amount of vitamin K in the diet should be consistent to keep the INR and PT tests in the recommended range.

Diet Principles

1. Vitamin K intake should be consistent from day to day when taking warfarin.
2. If you take a vitamin supplement containing Vitamin K, be sure to take it every day. Do not take a vitamin supplement that contains more than 100 mcg/day of Vitamin K. (3)

Table 12.16 Foods Very High in Vitamin K (more than 100mcg) (4)

Food	Serving Size	Vitamin K (mcg)
Broccoli, cooked	½ cup	110
Brussel sprouts, frozen, cooked	½ cup	150
Endive, raw	1 cup	116
Greens, beet, cooked	½ cup	349
Greens, collard, frozen, cooked	½ cup	530
Greens, dandelion, raw, chopped	1 cup	428
Greens. mustard, cooked	½ cup	415
Greens, turnip, frozen, cooked	½ cup	425
Kale, frozen, cooked	½ cup	573
Kale, raw	1 cup	113
Onions, green or scallions, raw	½ cup	104
Parsley, raw	10 sprigs	164
Spinach, cooked	½ cup	444
Spinach, raw	1 cup	145
Swiss Chard, cooked	½ cup	287
Swiss Chard, raw	1 cup	299

Table 12.17 Foods High in Vitamin K (45-100mcg) (4)

Food	Serving Size	Vitamin K (mcg)
Asparagus, frozen, cooked	½ cup	72
Broccoli, raw	½ cup	46
Cabbage, green, cooked	½ cup	82
Coleslaw, fast food	½ cup	68
Pomegranate, raw	One 4 inch across	46
Lettuce, green leaf, raw	1 cup	46
Lettuce, romaine, raw	1 cup	48
Noodles, spinach, cooked	½ cup	81
Watercress, raw	1 cup	85

Table 12.18 Foods Moderate in Vitamin K (30-44mcg) (4)

Food	Serving Size	Vitamin K (mcg)
Avocado, raw	1	42
Dried Peas, black-eyed, cooked	½ cup	32
Kiwifruit, raw, sliced	½ cup	36
Okra, frozen, cooked	½ cup	44
Prunes, dried	6 each	34

Additional Information:

- Dietary supplements can alter INR/PT. Use only supplements approved by your health care provider. Dietary supplements to avoid include alfalfa, arnica, bilberry, butchers broom, cat's claw, dong quai, feverfew, forskolin, garlic, ginger, ginkgo, horse chestnut, inositol hexaphosphate, licorice, melilot (sweet clover), pau d'arco, red clover, St. John's wort, sweet woodruff, turmeric, willow bark, and wheat grass. (3, 5)

- Check with your health care provider and/or pharmacist before taking fish oil or vitamin E supplements. (5)

- Alcohol can affect warfarin. Check with your health care provider before including alcohol in your diet. (5)

- Large amounts of cranberry juice (1 quart or more daily) or cranberry juice concentrates in supplements may change the effect of warfarin. (6)

- Take your medications as prescribed and take medications at the same time every day.

- If you are unable to eat for several days, or have ongoing stomach upset, diarrhea or fever, consult your health care provider.

REFERENCES

1. Institute of Medicine. *Dietary reference intakes for vitamin A, vitamin K, arsenic, boron, chromium, copper, iodine, iron, manganese, molybdenum, nickel, silicon, vanadium, and zinc.* Washington, DC: National Academy Press; 2001. http://www.nal.usda.gov/fnic/DRI/DRI_Tables/RDA_AI_vitamins_elements.pdf

2. Sconce EA, Khan TI, Mason J, Noble F, Wynne HA, Kamali F. Patients with unstable control have a poorer dietary intake of vitamin K compared to patients with stable control of anticoagulation. *Thromb Haemost.* 2005; 93(5):872–875.

3. Academy of Nutrition and Dietetics. Nutrition Care Manual. Vitamin K and Medications. https://www.nutritioncaremanual.org/client_ed.cfm?ncm_client_ed_id=120 Accessed August 4, 2015

4. U.S. Department of Agriculture, Agricultural Research Service, Nutrient Data Laboratory. USDA National Nutrient Database for Standard Reference, Release 27 (revised). Version Current: May 2015. Internet: http://www.ars.usda.gov/ba/bhnrc/ndl Accessed September 13, 2015.

5. Important Information to know when you are taking: Warfarin (Coumadin) and Vitamin K. National Institutes of Health Clinical Center website. http://www.cc.nih.gov/ccc/patient_education/drug_nutrient/coumadin1.pdf Published September 5, 2012. Accessed August 4, 2015.

6. Srinivas NR. Cranberry Juice Ingestion and Clinical Drug-Drug Interaction Potentials; Review of Case Studies and Perspectives. *J Pharm Pharm Sci.* 2013; 16(2) 289 – 303. file:///C:/Users/Gateway/Downloads/19126-48332-1-PB%20(2).pdf

GUIDELINES FOR PEPTIC ULCER, GASTRO-ESOPHAGEAL REFLUX DISEASE, AND HIATAL HERNIA

Peptic Ulcer

There is no evidence that a bland diet plays a significant role in the treatment of gastrointestinal disorders. Historically, such a diet was recommended in the treatment of peptic ulcer disease, hiatal hernia, and gastroesophageal reflux disease (GERD). It is now known that most stomach ulcers are caused either by infection with a bacterium called *Helicobacter pylori (H. pylori)* or by use of pain medications such as aspirin, ibuprofen, and other nonsteroidal anti-inflammatory drugs (NSAIDs). (1) Most *H. pylori*-related ulcers can be cured with antibiotics. NSAID-induced ulcers can be cured with time, stomach protective medications, antacids, and avoidance of NSAIDs.

No evidence supports the use of a traditional bland diet nor the consumption of liquid milk to decrease gastric acid secretion or increase the rate of healing. (1) For this reason, the diet should be primarily one that is liberal and individualized because patients differ as to specific food intolerances. There are a few foods that can stimulate gastric secretion and possibly irritate the stomach. It is a limited list and should be based on patient tolerance along with lifestyle changes for the treatment of peptic ulcers. The following recommendations are made:

1. Avoid cigarette smoking, salicylates (aspirin), and other NSAID agents. (1)

2. Avoid or limit alcohol. (1)

3. Individuals currently experiencing ulcers should be encouraged to avoid foods that exacerbate symptoms while also consuming adequate amounts of dietary fiber from fruit and vegetable sources. Previously the following foods were thought to increase symptoms. However, new research shows most people can include them in their diet. You may eat the following foods unless you are actively experiencing peptic ulcers. It is also recommended to avoid/limit these foods if they have been found to cause an individual's symptoms to worsen. (2)

   - black pepper, red pepper and chili powder
   - drinks containing caffeine (e.g., coffee, tea, decaffeinated coffee and tea, cola type soda)

GERD and Hiatal Hernia

Hiatal hernia occurs when a portion of the stomach bulges up into the esophagus. This causes reflux of stomach contents, resulting in heartburn and a bitter or sour taste in the back of the throat. When this happens frequently it is called gastroesophageal reflux disease (GERD). If left untreated, GERD can cause damage to the lining of the esophagus and in severe cases may result in iron-deficiency anemia due to blood loss from the inflamed tissues.

Lifestyle modifications, medications, and diet can manage the symptoms of this disease. The following recommendations are made:

1. Stop smoking to reduce the effect of tobacco on stomach acid production and relaxation of the esophageal muscles. Tobacco also inhibits saliva, which is the body's major buffer. (3)

2. Reduce weight if overweight or obese. (3,4,5,6, 7)

3. Avoid eating 3 hours before sleep. (3)

4. Raise the head of the bed by 6-9 inches. (7)

5. Avoid wearing tight fitting clothing. (8)

6. Sit upright when eating and eat in a relaxed environment. (8)

7. Consume small, frequent meals rather than 3 large meals per day. (9)

8. Previously the following foods were thought to increase symptoms. New research shows most people can include them in their diet. You may eat the following foods unless they cause symptoms to worsen. (3,6,7,10,11)

   - chocolate
   - coffee and other highly caffeinated beverages
   - peppermint and spearmint
   - high fat foods
   - tomato products and onions
   - black and red pepper
   - alcoholic beverages
   - citrus fruits

REFERENCES

1. Peptic Ulcer Disease. National Institute of Diabetes and Digestive and Kidney Diseases. http://www.niddk.nih.gov/health-information/health-topics/digestive-diseases/peptic-ulcer/Pages/eating-diet-nutrition.aspx Published November 13, 2014. Accessed August 27, 2015.

2. Krenitsky, JS, Decher, N. Medial nutrition therapy for upper gastrointestinal tract disorders. In: Mahan, LK, Escott-Stump, S, Raymond, JL, eds. *Krause's Food and the Nutrition Care Process*, 13th ed. St. Louis, MO: Elsevier/Saunders; 2012: 592-609.

3. Kang JH, Kang JY. Lifestyle measures in the management of gastro-oesophageal reflux disease: clinical and pathophysiological considerations. *Ther Adv Chronic Dis.* 2015; 6(2):51-64. doi: 10.1177/2040622315569501

4. Hampel H, Abraham NS, El-Serag HB. Meta-Analysis: Obesity and the Risk for Gastroesophageal Reflux Disease and Its Complications. *Ann Intern Med.* 2005; 143:199-211. doi:10.7326/0003-4819-143-3-200508020-00006

5. Ruhl CE, Everhart JE. Overweight, but not high dietary fat intake, increases risk of gastroesophageal reflux disease hospitalization: the NHANES I Epidemiologic Followup Study. First National Health and Nutrition Examination Survey. *Ann Epidemiol.* 1999; 9(7):424-435.

6. Dore MP, Maragkoudakis E, Fraley K, et al. Diet, Lifestyle and Gender in Gastro-Esophageal Reflux Disease. *Dig Dis Sci.* 2008; 53(8):2027-2032.

7. Kaltenbach, T, Crockett, S, Gerson, LB. Are lifestyle measures effective in patients with gastroesophageal reflux disease? An evidence-based approach. *Arch Intern Med.* 2006; 166:965-971.

8. Treatment for Gastroesophageal Reflux (GER) and Gastroesophageal Reflux Disease (GERD). National Institute of Diabetes and Digestive and Kidney Diseases. http://www.niddk.nih.gov/health-information/health-topics/digestive-diseases/ger-and-gerd-in-adults/Pages/treatment.aspx Published November 13, 2014. Accessed August 25, 2015.

9. Jarosz M, Taraszewska A. Risk factors for gastroesophageal reflux disease: the role of diet. *Prz Gastroenterol.* 2014; 9(5):297-301. doi: 10.5114/pg.2014.46166.

10. Bujanda L. The effects of alcohol consumption upon the gastrointestinal tract. *Am J Gastroenterol.* 2000; 95(12):3374-3382. doi:10.1111/j.1572-0241.2000.03347

11. Dent J, El-Serag HB, Wallander MA, Johansson S. Epidemiology of gastro-oesophageal reflux disease: a systematic review. *Gut* 2005;54:710-717 doi:10.1136/gut.2004.051821

ADDITIONAL RESOURCES

Moskovitz DN, Saltzman J, Kim YI, et al. The aging gut. In: Chernoff R, ed. *Geriatric Nutrition the Health Professional's Handbook*, 3rd ed. Sudberry, MA: James and Bartlett; 2006:241-242.

Websites

Cleveland Clinic Digestive Disease Institute: www.clevelandclinic.org/digestivedisease

Mayo Clinic: www.mayoclinic.com/health/pepticulcer/DS00242

National Digestive Diseases Information Clearinghouse a service of the NIDDK: www.niddk.nih.gov/health-information/health-topics/digestive-diseases

NUTRITION GUIDELINES FOR GOUT

Gout is a form of arthritis with a strong association to dietary intake. Historically gout was known as the "rich man's disease" as it tended to be linked with the frequent consumption of rich foods and alcohol. Gout is most predominant in men but does occur in women after menopause. The age of an individual may increase the likelihood of developing gout. Other factors that are linked to gout include: genetics, gender, age, medical condition, medications, and lifestyle factors. (1)

While the onset of gout may be affected by lifestyle factors such as stress and age, dietary patterns have also been shown to play a role. Foods high in purine content, specifically those foods of animal origin, may increase symptoms of gout. Therefore, the purine found in meats should be limited to Dietary Guidelines for Americans recommendations (Chapter 1). Alternatively, the protein found in non-meat sources is preferred (low-fat or nonfat dairy products, eggs, nut butters, and tofu). Vegetable sources of protein have not been shown to increase symptoms of gout. (2) Recently, studies have found the intake of cherries and cherry extract to decrease the risk of gout attacks. (3) This research has only been conducted in small sample sizes and warrants further research before recommendations can safely be made.

Lifestyle modifications, the use of medications, and diet can aid in managing this disease. During a gout flare up, adoption of the following diet principles are recommended (1):

1. Avoid alcohol during a flare up. Limit alcohol during remission. (4) Beer has been found to have the greatest effect on uric acid levels. Foods high in purines increase uric acid levels, which can lead to uric acid crystals being deposited in joints.

2. Limit meat, fish and poultry to 4-6 ounces per day. During this time, protein from non-meat sources is recommended, such noted above. Avoid organ meats such as liver, and limit sardines and shellfish as they are high in purines. (4)

3. Consume more than 8 cups of fluids daily. (5) This is recommended both during an attack and during remission.

4. Maintain a healthy weight and avoid high protein diets. (5)

REFERENCES

1. Academy of Nutrition and Dietetics. Nutrition Care Manual. Gout. https://www.nutritioncaremanual.org/topic.cfm?ncm_toc_id=29929 Accessed July 7, 2015.

2. Choi HK, Atkinson K, Karlson EW, Willett W, Curhan, G. Purine-rich foods, dairy and protein intake, and the risk of gout in men. N Engl J Med.2004; 350:1093-1103. doi: 10.1056/NEJMoa035700

3. Zhang Y, Neogi T, Chen C, Chaisson C, Hunter D, Choi HK. Cherry Consumption and the Risk of Recurrent Gout Attacks. Arthritis and rheumatism. 2012; 64(12):4004-4011. doi:10.1002/art.34677

4. Khanna D, Fitzgerald JD, Khanna PP, et al. 2012 American College of Rheumatology Guidelines for Management of Gout. Part 1: Systematic nonpharmacologic and pharmacologic therapeutic approaches to hyperuricemia. *Arthritis Care* Res. 2012; 64(10):1431-1446.

5. Jordan KM, Cameron JS, Snaith M, et al. British Society for Rheumatology and British Health Professionals in Rheumatology guideline for the management of gout. *Rheumatology.* 2007; 46(8):1372-1374.

Study Guide Questions

A. List at least three uses for the High Nutrient Diet.

B. List at least three common food fortifiers on a High Nutrient Diet.

C. What are five causes of inadequate food intake?

D. In what situation should a Small Portions Diet be ordered?

E. When planning a Vegan Diet, which excludes all animal products, what nutrients should be given special consideration?

F. What individuals may follow a Halal diet?

G. Describe three diet principles in treating a person with phenylketonuria (PKU).

H. List at least three lifestyle changes that may be helpful for persons with gastroesophageal reflux disease (GERD).

I. Discussion Question: How and where can you purchase the appropriate foods on specialized diets if food and beverage items are not available from your primary vendor?

Study Guide Suggested Responses can be found in Appendix 15.

Dining Assistance/ Special Needs

FINGER FOOD DIET

Use

The Finger Food Diet is appropriate for persons who exhibit the need to eat with their fingers even after training to improve hand movements to maintain utilization of utensils. The Finger Food Diet is often used in those with Alzheimer's disease, other dementia or cognitive impairment, especially those who are unable to sit still to eat; those with arthritic hands; or those with certain neuromuscular disorders including those with severe tremors.

Adequacy

The diet, if carefully chosen from suggested foods, meets the Dietary Reference Intakes (DRIs) recommended by the National Academy of Sciences for adults. The General Diet should form the basis of this diet but it can be adapted for those on therapeutic diets, with only such modifications as to prompt self-feeding and promote independence. This diet modification can also be applied to those on a chopped texture and those receiving various portion sizes.

Diet Principles

1. All foods offered on this diet are given in a form that can be easily handled with the person's fingers; without risk of spilling significant amounts.

2. Food should be cut in bite-sized pieces, slices, wedges, or made into sandwiches.

3. People who resist being fed, are combative, or have difficulty manipulating utensils may increase their caloric intake and stabilize their weight if presented with most of their food in finger food form, bite size pieces.

4. Individuals may benefit from this eating approach to decrease frustration, enhance dignity and self-esteem, and increase morale and motivation. Improvement in appetite may also occur.

5. A person served finger foods should be in complete control over what they eat, when they eat, and how much they eat. Using this in place of traditional meals may prolong a person's independence and stimulate them to eat more frequently.

6. The person's acceptance of finger foods may determine the appropriateness in relation to dignity. The person's diet can be adjusted to promote the highest degree of independence for feeding themselves.

7. The encouragement to self-feed may lead to greater mobility in otherwise inactive individuals, resulting in enhanced strength and coordination and expanded range of motion.

8. Individuals may benefit from a feeding assistant providing verbal cues or demonstrating eating behavior with fingers.

9. Foods offered should be nutrient dense and should be good sources of fiber.

10. Pacing and restlessness in some individuals may elevate energy expenditure beyond that estimated by conventional calculation. Finger foods that can be consumed on the go will help some people increase their energy intake.

11. Adequate fluid intake should be encouraged. Ample opportunities to drink liquids should be provided.

12. Persons on consistency altered diets will need further modifications to some of the suggested foods listed in the Tables 13.1 and 13.2.

Table 13.1 Finger Food Diet

Food for the Day	Recommended
Vegetables *1–4 cups*	Bite-size cooked vegetables such as baby carrots, sweet potato, broccoli, cauliflower, whole mushrooms, baked or steamed baby potatoes, French fries, potato wedges, tater tots, waffle fries; fresh vegetables such as tomato quarters, cherry tomatoes cut in half; vegetable juice served in a mug.
Fruits *1–2.5 cups*	Cut-up fresh fruits, grapes cut in half, drained chunk canned fruits, dried fruit, fruit molded in firm gelatin; whole, fresh fruit may be served if the individual can bite off pieces; fruit juice served in a mug.
Grains *3–10 ounce-equivalents*	Breads, buns, muffins, biscuits, crackers, pita bread, tortillas, pancakes, French toast, waffles, cereal bars, granola bars, bite-size dry cereal without milk, cooked cereal with milk served in a mug.
Dairy products *2–3 cups*	Any fluid milk (may be served in mugs), cheese sticks, cubes, or slices.
Protein foods *2–7 ounce-equivalents*	Tender cut-up meats; roasts, meatballs, patties, cutlets, nuggets, chicken fingers/tenders, fish cakes, fish sticks, cocktail sausage, luncheon meats, omelets, deviled eggs, hard cooked eggs, firmly cooked scrambled/fried eggs, mini quiches, fried tofu cubes, pizza slices, burritos, foods that can easily be made into sandwiches or put on tortilla or pita bread.
Oils, Solid Fats	Nuts, peanut butter, table spreads, salad dressings, mayonnaise, sweet or sour cream, creamers and toppings, applied as appropriate before serving. Gravies and sauces can be served in a side dish for dipping.
Added Sugars	Cookies, cake, donuts, turnovers, bar cookies, custard pie, ice cream bars, ice cream sandwiches, finger gelatin; ice cream, sorbet, yogurt or pudding served in ice cream cone.
Soups	Strained or blended soups served in a mug.
Fluids	Any (may be served in mugs).

Table 13.2 Sample Menu for Finger Food Diet

Breakfast	Supper
1 orange, divided into sections	Blended vegetable soup served in mug
1 hard-boiled egg, firm	Tuna salad sandwich, quartered
½ c. bite-size shredded wheat	4 tomato quarters
1 slice whole wheat toast, quartered	1 Tbsp. oil and vinegar dressing
2 tsp. jelly	½ c. chunk fruit cocktail, drained
1 tsp. soft margarine	1 c. milk
1 c. milk	Water
Hot beverage	
Sugar, pepper (optional)	
Lunch	**Snack Ideas**
2 oz. chicken tenders	½ c. melon slices/cubes
½ c. boiled potato, cut up	3 c. popcorn
½ c. mixed vegetables, drained	1 oz. cheese cubes
1 oz. whole wheat roll	
2 tsp. soft margarine	
1 c. milk	
Water	

Foods to avoid

1. Any small foods that may be hard to pick up due to dexterity problems (e.g., corn, peas, rice).
2. Any slippery foods that may be difficult to pick up due to agility problems (e.g., fruits in heavy syrup, macaroni in cheese sauce, noodles in sauce).
3. Crumbly foods such as some cakes and cookies.

Tips

Serving food in large bowls instead of on plates, and offering spoons instead of forks may be helpful. The use of adaptive equipment such as plate stabilizers, plate guards, weighted utensils, rocking knives, nosey cups, covered or spouted cups, and cups or mugs with large or double handles may be useful in certain instances.

Cutting foods such as meats, cheese, fruits, and vegetables into strips or wedges provides an easy way to grasp the foods that allows easy self-feeding. Foods cut into bite-size cubes are easy to pick up with the fingers.

Pasta such as gnocchi, rotini, tortellini, ravioli, or novelty shapes are recommended because they are thicker and easier to pick up.

Sandwiches, pancakes, waffles, toast, bread, quick breads or cake should be cut into quarters or sliced into sticks.

Serving liquids, including soups (most often pureed for safety) and thin cooked cereal, in mugs or with a straw will often facilitate intake.

An occupational therapist consultation may prove beneficial. Individuals should be assessed for the need for and ability to use adaptive equipment.

ADDITIONAL RESOURCES

Pouyet V, Giboreau A, Benattar L, Cuvelier G. Attractiveness and consumption of finger foods in elderly Alzheimer's disease patients. *Food Quality and Preference*. 2014; 34: 62-69.

Website

Alzheimer's Association. Eating. 2012. www.alz.org

GUIDELINES FOR INDIVIDUALS WITH DEMENTIA

Individuals with dementia are at risk for weight loss and poor nutritional intake. (1) Successful interventions for treatment and prevention of inadequate nutrition focus on the causes of the problem. Energy and nutrient intakes can be increased in individuals with the appropriate interventions. (2, 3, 4, 5) Individuals at each stage of dementia should be allowed to do as much for themselves as possible, and also provided with adequate assistance and support to assure good nutritional status. Flexibility is required of caregivers so that feeding assistance is tailored to each person and adjusted as the person changes. Families can provide important information about food preferences and feeding strategies. Pain can lead to insufficient food intake and must be controlled. Medications should be reviewed for side effects such as drowsiness that impact food intake or cause altered nutrient metabolism.

The following is a list of feeding guidelines to consider at mealtimes to promote safe, oral intake and a positive dining environment. (6, 7, 8)

1. **Positioning.** The individual should maintain an upright, vertical position in a chair or wheelchair with feet supported on the floor, on foot rests, or on a foot stool. The person should ideally be sitting at a 90-degree angle with the floor or may be slightly leaned forward. If the individual must be fed in bed or a recliner chair, adjust the chair or bed to achieve as close to the desired vertical position as possible. Pillows can be helpful for proper alignment and positioning. An upright position should be maintained for at least 30 minutes after meals to prevent reflux. Avoid tilting the head back as this increases the risk for aspiration. Caregivers should sit at eye level to promote a chin tuck swallow.

2. **Encouraging adequate food intake**. Provide foods that stimulate the appetite by their appearance, smell, and taste. Regularly provide the person's favorite foods. Identify the food to the person as you give it. Make positive remarks, such as "Doesn't this look good?!" or "It all smells so good!" Enhance the flavor of food with condiments and seasonings according to personal preference. If the individual must be fed, try alternating warm and cold foods to maintain interest. Fortified, nutrient-dense foods and supplements may be provided as appropriate.

3. **Encouraging independence.** Foster independence by providing finger foods, cueing, appropriate assistive devices (divided plate, large handle utensils, bent utensils, weighted utensils, foods served in separate bowls, spout cups, cut-out cups, mugs, straws), or practicing the hand-over-hand technique. Feeding a person the first few bites of food may set the self-feeding behavior in motion, after which the spoon can be handed to the person.

4. **Preventing distractions.** The dining environment must be pleasant and friendly. Limit distractions and control noise through efficient meal service. Serving only one or two foods at a time may help reduce the person's decision making. Use the simplest of table settings. Serve meals on plain (no patterns) dishes of bright colors to help the individual distinguish between the food and the dish. Focus on the person to keep him or her on task. Staff should avoid inappropriate conversation, loud laughter, or shouting across the room. Disagreeing or reality orientation may be counterproductive with advanced dementia. It is better to acknowledge the resident's current mentation with acceptance

and patience. Play only soft, familiar music or no music at all. Serving smaller groups of people at a time may help achieve a calmer dining room atmosphere. A consistent seating arrangement can provide familiarity and lessen anxiety.

5. **Providing the correct diet texture.** Observe and report signs of chewing and swallowing difficulties (i.e., coughing, throat clearing, gurgling, abnormal rate of eating, excessive chewing or no chewing at all, pocketing food, spilling food or liquids from the mouth, and recurring pneumonia). These may require changes in food texture or thickened liquids. Foods with combination textures, such as chunky soups or casseroles with rice, and foods that are crumbly and fall apart easily, such as corn, peas, rice, bacon, and chips, are difficult to form into a bolus and swallow safely. Offer small bites (1 teaspoon) and sips, alternate liquids and solids to promote a safe swallow. Be sure food has been completely swallowed before offering a beverage. For some individuals, the use of a straw forcefully propels the liquid to the back of the throat before the normal swallow reflex is triggered. Therefore, straws are generally not used for patients with swallowing difficulty unless approved by the speech therapist. See Chapter 3, Consistency Altered Diets, for more information.

    Never feed with a syringe. Syringe feeding rapidly forces liquefied food to the back of the throat and increases the risk of aspiration. In addition, syringe feeding is viewed as force feeding and is considered unacceptable in a person with dementia.

6. **Allowing plenty of time to eat**. People with dementia may eat slowly and require longer mealtimes, however, excessive time at the table may tire the person leading to inadequate intakes. If a meal cannot be consumed in 30 to 45 minutes, consider serving smaller meals and offering nutritious snacks at times the individual is alert and rested. Perhaps the individual needs a mechanically altered diet to reduce excessive chewing. If the person gets up at night for a couple hours, take the opportunity to offer a nutritious food and/or beverage. Nontraditional times and places may be necessary to maintain good nutrition and hydration.

7. **Nutrition directives and care planning**. Many people with advanced dementia are unable to express likes and dislikes adequately. Monitor resident for cueing signs of fullness, unacceptance or refusal of food and fluids such as turning the head away from items offered, clamping mouth shut, letting food and fluids run out of mouth, or physically pushing utensil away from mouth. Be familiar with the resident's care plan for nutrition interventions desired by the resident and/or family. Family may wish for comfort cares with the understanding that nutrition parameters may decline. At that time, it is appropriate to honor refusal of food and fluids and not force any type of feeding. (9)

REFERENCES

1. Thomas DR, Kamel HK, Morley JE. Nutritional deficiencies in long-term care. Part II: management of protein energy malnutrition and dehydration. *Supplement to Annals of Long Term Care*. February 2004:8–14. http://www.annalsoflongtermcare.com/attachments/1079364363-NutritionLTC.pdf

2. Bernstein M, Munoz N. Position of the Academy of Nutrition and Dietetics: food and nutrition for older adults: promoting health and wellness. *J Acad Nutr Diet*. 2012; 112(8):1255-1277.

3. Germain I, Dufresne T, Gray-Donald K. A novel dysphagia diet improves the nutrient intake of institutionalized elders. *J Am Diet Assoc*. 2006; 106(10):1614–1623.

4. Salas-Salvado J, Torres M, Planas M, et al. Effect of oral administration of a whole formula diet on nutritional and cognitive status in patients with Alzheimer's disease. *Clin Nutr*. 2005; 24(3):390–397.

5. Ryan M, Salle A, Favreau AM, et al. Oral supplements differing in fat and carbohydrate content: effect on the appetite and food intake of undernourished elderly patients. *Clin Nutr.* 2004; 23(4):683–689.

6. Food, Eating and Alzheimer's. Alzheimer's Association Website. http://www.alz.org/living_with_alzheimers_eating.asp Published 2015. Accessed August 13, 2015.

7. Hellen CR. *Alzheimer's Disease Activity-Focused Care,* 2nd ed. Woburn, MA: Butterworth-Heinemann; 1998.

8. Finley B. Nutritional needs of the person with Alzheimer's disease: practical approaches to quality care. *J Amer Diet Assoc.* 1997; 97(Suppl 2):S177–S180.

9. Academy of Nutrition and Dietetics. Practice Paper of the Academy of Nutrition and Dietetics: Ethical and legal issues in feeding and hydration. http://www.eatrightpro.org/resource/practice/position-and-practice-papers/practice-papers/practice-paper-ethical-and-legal-issues-in-feeding-and-hydration Published June 2013. Accessed January 13, 2016.

NUTRITION FOR INDIVIDUALS WITH DEVELOPMENTAL DISABILITIES

The term "Developmental Disabilities" covers a large group of chronic conditions that can be cognitive, physical, or a combination of the two. Those that are cognitive in nature are referred to as intellectual disabilities (formerly mental retardation). (1) Developmental disabilities appear before the 22nd birthday and typically impact day-to-day functioning throughout one's lifetime due to physical, learning, language, or behavioral impairments. (2, 3)

Nutrition-Related Issues

Adults with developmental disabilities experience higher rates of nutrition-related risks and risk factors including overweight and underweight, gastrointestinal dysfunction, asthma, cardiovascular disease, diabetes, osteoporosis, and oral-hygiene issues. (4, 5, 6, 7) These nutrition risk factors are often not inherent to the developmental disability itself, but are instead related to secondary conditions which may be preventable. (5, 8)

Table 13.3 highlights common nutrition concerns among select developmental disabilities. It is important to note nutrition concerns vary from condition to condition, and because of large variability in the disease process often from person to person. (9) Therefore, the provision of routine nutrition screening and individualized nutrition assessment and intervention when needed is of paramount importance. (10)

Feeding Concerns

Problems with oral-motor control and swallowing can lead to discomfort, poor nutritional status, dehydration, aspiration, and asphyxiation; and if left unaddressed can be life-threatening. (11, 12) Signs of impaired swallowing function (coughing, choking, wet breathing, changes in respiration or face color) or other eating difficulties should trigger further evaluation and intervention for dysphagia. (12-14) For more on this topic, see Chapter 3.

1. **Gastrointestinal Concerns.** Gastrointestinal (GI) disease which includes reflux, delayed gastric emptying, constipation, and diarrhea is frequent in those with a developmental disability. (15, 16) Gastroesophageal reflux (GERD) affects 75% of those with neurological impairment, and may result in a loss of nutrients when presenting with frequent episodes of vomiting. (9, 17) Upwards of 70% of individuals with developmental disabilities residing in a long term care setting develop constipation. (18) This constipation may be caused or worsened by prolonged inactivity, low muscle tone, and/or inadequate fluid and fiber intake. (19) Though autism spectrum disorders are not typically seen as

Table 13.3 Nutrition Side-Effects of Common Developmental Disabilities

Condition	Cerebral Palsy	Spina Bifida	Autism Spectrum Disorders	Down Syndrome	Prader Willi
Description	Nonprogressive condition of muscle control or coordination resulting from brain injuries during fetal development; can variably affect different parts of the body, communication and cognition	Incomplete closure of the neural tube during fetal development resulting in a lesion along the spinal cord. Level of muscle weakness and paralysis depends on the level of the lesion (high or low along the spinal cord) (23)	Characterized by impairments in communication and social interaction in addition to restricted and/or repetitive behaviors(23)	Chromosomal condition resulting in cognitive delay that often occurs with other developmental and health conditions (28)	Chromosomal condition associated with cognitive delay and abnormal food-related behaviors
Feeding Concerns	Aspiration related to dysphagia; impaired motor skills can limit self-feeding	Aspiration related to dysphagia; impaired motor skills can limit self-feeding; abnormal gag reflux(23)	Sensorimotor issues may lead to selective eating, elimination of entire food groups and frequent meal-time behaviors	Low muscle tone can lead to difficulties closing mouth chewing, and swallowing; may eat very slowly (limiting nutrient intake) or rapidly (increasing risk for aspiration)(29)	Distorted sense of hunger/satiety leading to excessive intake and consumption of non-food items
Gastrointestinal Concerns	GERD Gut dysmotility with constipation	Constipation Gut dysmotility	Possible increase in incidence of GI symptoms including constipation and GERD (20)	Constipation related to hypotonia, low activity and/or low fiber diet Increased incidence of celiac disease (28)	Constipation (30)

Continued on next page

Table 13.3 Nutrition Side-Effects of Common Developmental Disabilities Continued from previous page

Condition	Cerebral Palsy	Spina Bifida	Autism Spectrum Disorders	Down Syndrome	Prader Willi
Nutrient Requirements	Possible increased energy needs with athetoid CP and hypertonia Decreased energy needs with hypotonia and decreased physical activity (23)	Decreased energy needs may be due to factors related to short stature, hypotonia, and decreased physical activity; presence of pressure ulcers may temporarily increase energy, protein, fluid, and micronutrient needs	Though nutrition needs not affected by an autism diagnosis, selective eating can lead to micronutrient deficiencies	Energy needs are often decreased due to low muscle tone and short stature	Short stature contributing to decreased energy needs (may be addressed through growth hormones); hypotonia and problems with muscle coordination, leading to decreased physical activity levels and decreased energy needs
Growth & Weight Status	Adults at risk for both under and overweight based on their ability to eat, muscle tone and activity level	Adults at risk for being overweight	May be at risk for overweight / obesity	Adults at risk for overweight and obesity due to short stature, hypotonia and decreased opportunities for physical activity	Obesity common in later childhood and adulthood due to low energy needs paired with lack of satiety
Other	Contractures can make weight and length assessment difficult		Many families of those with autism explore alternative therapies which may exclude significant sources of nutrition and/or increase risk for drug-nutrient interactions	Higher risk for hypothyroidism which may affect weight gain (27)	

*Modified from Journal of the Academy of Nutrition and Dietetics, 115(4), Ptomey LT, Wittenbrook W, Position of the Academy of Nutrition and Dietetics: nutrition services for individuals with intellectual and developmental disabilities and special health care needs, pp. 593-608. 2015 (10) with permission from Elsevier.

physical conditions, constipation and diarrhea are also far more common in this group of individuals compared to the general public. (20)

GI disturbances often lead to pain and anxiety. Because many individuals with developmental disabilities are unable to articulate and communicate such discomfort, GI issues may remain unaddressed for long periods of time as they are instead seen as behavioral manifestations. Behaviors that may indicate GI discomfort include increased irritability, stereotypy, and hyperactivity, social withdrawal, and sudden food avoidance or aversion. (19, 20) Such sudden behavior problems particularly with the introduction of food should prompt evaluation for GI disorders. (20)

2. **Enteral Feedings**. Enteral feedings (or tube feedings) may be required to meet nutrition and hydration needs in those who are not able to maintain weight/proper growth or are at risk for aspiration pneumonia and/or dysphagia. (21, 22) Enteral feedings may be used in combination with oral feeding or as the sole source of nutrition. Those who require the use of low-calorie formulas may also need additional micronutrient and protein to supplement the formula. Some individuals with feeding tubes may also require additional fluid, protein and micronutrients, particularly with the use of high energy density formulas. (9) Any oral feeding that is safe should be encouraged for socialization and preservation of oral motor skills. (22) Ongoing nutrition evaluation/intervention can help balance oral feedings and tube feedings with the need for growth, weight maintenance, or weight loss.

Nutrient Requirements

Certain developmental disabilities alter an individual's nutrient needs, while other conditions interfere with adequate nutrient intakes. (23) Nutrition requirements vary greatly based on the specific diagnosis, the severity of the condition including muscle atrophy and spasticity, extent of mobility, age, medications, and feeding problems. (10, 21)

1. **Calorie Requirements.** Conventional methods used to estimate calorie requirements are not always accurate for those with developmental disabilities. (24) In order to determine an appropriate calorie prescription, more than one method/equation may be required along with assessment of weight/growth history, review of laboratory data and food intake records, observation of meal times, consideration of age and need for growth, and interview with the individual when possible. (21) Calorie needs may be greater in those with muscle spasticity, cystic fibrosis, and need for wound healing. (24-26) Conditions that cause short stature, low muscle tone and limited activity or mobility may also decrease energy needs compared to the general population. (12) Because of the large variability in calorie needs amongst individuals with developmental disabilities along with the possible need for continued growth, ongoing weight-gain and BMI evaluation are important to ensure the assessed nutrition needs indeed match the individual's needs for consistent growth or weight maintenance. (9)

2. **Macronutrient Composition.** In most cases carbohydrate, protein, and fat distribution does not differ from recommendations made for the general population and the DRIs should be utilized. (22) There are some instances in which macronutrient intake must be controlled as with metabolic conditions or maximized (increased protein for cystic fibrosis and wound healing). (23)

3. **Vitamins and Minerals.** Few medical conditions have a primary effect on an individual's micronutrient needs. Exceptions include Wilson's disease, William's Syndrome (limit supplemental vitamin D and calcium), and other metabolic disorders. (23) Largely, nutrient requirements are the same for physically healthy people with or without developmental disabilities. (5) In general the primary concerns around altered micronutrient needs are associated with medication-nutrient interactions. (23)

4. **Drug Nutrient Interaction/Alternative Nutrition**. It is common for individuals with developmental disabilities to take numerous prescription and nonprescription

medications in addition to using various complementary and alternative therapies. (12, 27) Multiple medications and long-term use of certain medications or treatments and their potential side effects are often factors impacting nutrition status and gastrointestinal function. (12) Table 13.4 highlights common medications used by those with developmental disabilities along with possible nutrition side-effects.

Table 13.4 Common Drug-Nutrient Interactions with Developmental Disabilities

Drug	Nutrition-Related Side-Effects
Antibiotics	Diarrhea, nausea, vomiting; destroys "good" intestinal bacteria; altered absorption of minerals, fats, and proteins
Anticonvulsants	Decrease absorption or stores of vitamins D, K, B6 and B12; folate, calcium
Antipsychotics	Decreased absorption of sodium and potassium; increased appetite with weight gain
Antireflux Medications	Long-term loss of iron, vitamin B12 and calcium, nausea, diarrhea
Antispasmodics	Nausea, abdominal pain leading to decreased appetite; constipation; altered taste; difficulty swallowing (23)
Corticosteroids	Bone loss due to depletion of calcium and phosphorous; altered glucose levels; increased appetite with weight gain; altered absorption/stores of vitamin D, protein, zinc, vitamin C and potassium; fluid retention with need to limit sodium; reflux, vomiting, and diarrhea
Diuretics	Loss of potassium, magnesium, calcium and folate stores; nausea, diarrhea and vomiting leading to poor appetite
Laxatives	Depletion of fat-soluble vitamins with long-term use
Stimulants	Decreased appetite leading to weight loss

Modified from: © Academy of Nutrition and Dietetics. Behavioral Health Nutrition Dietetic Practice Group and Pediatric Nutrition Practice Group. Pocket Guide to Children with Special Health Care and Nutritional Needs. Chicago, IL; 2012 (22). Reprinted with permission.

Weight Status

Obesity rates for adults with disabilities are 58% higher than for adults without disabilities. (12) Factors contributing to a higher incidence of overweight and obesity include poor eating habits, medications that contribute to weight gain, physical limitations and inactivity, lack of social opportunities, inadequate financial support, and depression. (12) Body composition is another factor that may contribute to unhealthy levels of weight gain. As highlighted in Table 13.3, low muscle tone is common among several developmental disabilities. (23) Because fat is not as dense/heavy as muscle, adults with low muscle tone may benefit from a BMI at the lower end of the "acceptable" range to maintain a healthy percentage of body fat. (23)

Though the incidence of being underweight in adults with developmental disabilities is not as common as being overweight or obese, the issue remains disproportionately high compared to adults without developmental disabilities. (5) This can be linked with difficulties self-feeding, chewing/swallowing deficits, and food aversions amongst other issues addressed earlier in this chapter. (5)

Height and weight measurements in individuals with developmental disabilities can be difficult to obtain when scoliosis, contractures, neuromuscular, sensory, or compliance issues are present. (22) To calculate desired body weight, it may be necessary to use multiple methods such as arm span measurement, triceps skinfold, and sitting height. (23) Measurement techniques should be used consistently and follow a facility's protocol to ensure weight assessments are accurate and nutrient needs estimates are based on relevant data. (26)

REFERENCES

1. Frequently asked questions on intellectual disability. American Association on Intellectual and Developmental Disabilities website. http://aaidd.org/intellectual-disability/definition/faqs-on-intellectual-disability#.VbJut3iztO8 Updated 2013. Accessed July 24, 2015.

2. Rubin L, Crocker A. *Developmental Disabilities: Delivery of Medical Care for Children and Adults*. Philadelphia, PA: Lea & Febiger; 1989.

3. Still in the Shadows with Their Future Uncertain: A Report on Family and Individual Needs for Disability Supports (FINDS), 2011. The Arc website. http://www.thearc.org/document.doc?id=3672 Update June, 2011. Accessed July 24, 2015.

4. Facts about Developmental Disabilities. Centers for Disease Control and Prevention website. http://www.cdc.gov/ncbddd/developmentaldisabilities/facts.html Updated July 9, 2015. Accessed July 24, 2015.

5. Humphries K, Traci M, Seekins T. Nutrition and adults with intellectual or developmental disabilities: systematic literature review results. Intellect Dev Disabil. 2009; 47(3): 163-185. doi: 10.1352/1934-9556-47.3.163

6. Rimmer JH, Yamaki K, Lowry BM, Wang E, Vogel LC. Obesity and obesity-related secondary conditions in adolescents with intellectual/developmental disabilities. *J Intellect Disabil Res*. 2010; 54(9): 787-794. doi: 10.1111/j.1365-2788.2010.01305.x

7. Morgan JP, Minihan PM, Stark PC, et al. The oral health status of 4,732 adults with intellectual and developmental disabilities. *J Am Dent Assoc*. 2012; 143(8): 838-846. http://www.ncbi.nlm.nih.gov/pmc/articles/PMC4527687/

8. Disability and Health. Healthy People 2020 website. http://www.healthypeople.gov/2020/topics-objectives/topic/disability-and-health Updated August 11, 2015. Accessed August 25, 2015.

9. Marchand V, Motil KJ; NASPGHAN Committee on Nutrition. Nutrition support for neurologically impaired children: a clinical report of the North American Society for Pediatric Gastroenterology, Hepatology, and Nutrition. *J Pediatr Gastroenterol Nutr*. 2006; 43(1): 123-135.

10. Ptomey L, Wittenbrook W. Position of the Academy of Nutrition and Dietetics: nutrition services for individuals with intellectual and developmental disabilities and special health care needs. *J Acad Nutr Diet*. 2015; 115(4): 593-608. doi: 10.1016/j.jand.2015.02.002

11. Sullivan PB, Lambert B, Rose M, Ford-Adams M, Johnson A, Griffiths P. Prevalence and severity of feeding and nutritional problems in children with neurological impairment: Oxford Feeding Study. *Dev Med Child Neurol*. 2000; 42(10): 674–680. doi: 10.1111/j.1469-8749.2000.tb00678.x

12. Cushing P, Spear D, Novak P, et al. Academy of Nutrition and Dietetics: standards of practice and standards of professional performance for registered dietitians (competent, proficient, and expert) in intellectual and developmental disabilities. *J Acad Nutr Diet*. 2012; 112(9): 1454-1464. doi: 10.1016/j.jand.2012.06.365

13. Arvedson JC. Assessment of pediatric dysphagia and feeding disorders: clinical and instrumental approaches. *Dev Disabil Res Rev*. 2008; 14(2): 118-127. doi: 10.1002/ddrr.17

14. Chadwick DD, Jolliffe J. A descriptive investigation of dysphagia in adults with intellectual disabilities. *J Intellect Disabil Res*. 2009; 53(1): 29-43. doi: 10.1111/j.1365-2788.2008.01115.x

15. Chong SK. Gastrointestinal problems in the handicapped child. *Curr Opin Pediatr*. 2001; 13(5): 441-446.

16. Somerville H, Tzannes G, Wood J, et al. Gastrointestinal and nutritional problems in severe developmental disability. *Dev Med Child Neurol.* 2008; 50(9): 712-716. doi: 10.1111/j.1469-8749.2008.03057.x

17. Ravelli AM, Milla PJ. Vomiting and gastroesophageal motor activity in children with disorders of the central nervous system. *J Pediatr Gastroenterol Nutr.* 1998; 26(1): 56-63

18. Böhmer C, Taminiau J, Klinkenberg-Knol E, Meuwissen S. The prevalence of constipation in institutionalized people with intellectual disability. *J Intellect Disabil Res.* 2001; 45: 212-218. doi: 10.1046/j.1365-2788.2001.00300.x

19. Sullivan P. Gastrointestinal disorders in children with neurodevelopmental disabilities. *Dev Disabil Res Rev.* 2008; 14: 128-136. doi: 10.1002/ddrr.18

20. Chaidez V, Hansen R, Hertz-Picciotto I. Gastrointestinal problems in children with autism, developmental delays or typical development. J Autism Dev Disord. 2014; 44: 1117-27. doi: 10.1007/s10803-013-1973-x

21. Van Riper C, Wallace L; American Dietetic Association. Position of the American Dietetic Association: Providing nutrition services for people with developmental disabilities and special health care needs. J Am Diet Assoc. 2010; 110(2): 296-307. doi: http://dx.doi.org/10.1016/j.jada.2009.12.003

22. Behavioral Health Nutrition Dietetic Practice Group and Pediatric Nutrition Practice Group. Academy of Nutrition and Dietetics Pocket Guide to Children with Special Health Care and Nutritional Needs. Chicago, IL: Academy of Nutrition and Dietetics; 2012.

23. Washington State Department of Health. *Nutrition Interventions for Children with Special Health Care Needs*, 3rd ed. Olympia, WA: Washington State Department of Printing; 2010. http://here.doh.wa.gov/materials/nutrition-interventions/15_CSHCN-NI_E10L.pdf Accessed from Pacific West MCH Distance Learning Network Self-Study: Nutrition for children with special needs: http://depts.washington.edu/pwdlearn/web/intro.php on July 31, 2015.

24. American Dietetic Association Behavioral Health Nutrition Dietetic Practice Group. *The Adult with Intellectual and Developmental Disabilities: A Resource Tool for Nutritional Professionals*. Chicago, IL: Academy of Nutrition and Dietetics; 2008.

25. Williams J, Barbul A. Nutrition and wound healing. *Crit Care Nurs Clin North Am.* 2012; 24(2): 179-200. doi.org/10.1016/j.ccell.2012.03.001

26. Wittenbrook, W. Nutritional Assessment and Intervention in Cerebral Palsy. *Pract Gastroenterol.* 2011; 16, 21-32. http://www.medicine.virginia.edu/clinical/departments/medicine/divisions/digestive-health/nutrition-support-team/nutrition-articles/WittenbrookArticle.pdf

27. Kiefer D, Pitluk J, Klunk K. An overview of CAM: components and clinical uses. *Nutr Clin Pract.* 2009; 24(5): 549-559. doi: 10.1177/0884533609342437

28. Bull M; Committee on Genetics. Clinical Report - Health supervision for children with Down syndrome. *Pediatrics.* 2011; 128: 393-406. doi: 10.1542/peds.2011-1605

29. Smith C, Teo Y, Simpson S. An observational study of adults with Down syndrome eating independently. *Dysphagia.* 2014; 29(1):52-60. doi: 10.1007/s00455-013-9479-4

30. Kuhlmann L, Joensson I, Froekjaer J, Krogh K, Farholt S. A descriptive study of colorectal function in adults with Prader-Willi Syndrome: high prevalence of constipation. *BMC Gastroenterol.* 2014; 14:63. doi: 10.1186/1471-230X-14-63

Study Guide Questions

A. List two foods in each food group that would be appropriate for a Finger Food Diet.

B. Describe in detail six guidelines for feeding individuals with dementia.

C. List five types of adaptive equipment that may be utilized to maintain an individual's independence in dining.

D. What are unique health concerns associated in individuals with developmental disabilities?

E. Discussion question: In observing dining assistance for residents with dementia, how can the dining atmosphere be enhanced to encourage independence in dining and promotion of oral intake?

Study Guide Suggested Responses can be found in Appendix 15.

Appendices

Appendix

Body Mass Index Table (kg/m²)

Simplified Diet Manual, Twelfth Edition. Edited by Paula Watkins.
© 2016 Iowa Academy of Nutrition and Dietetics.

Body Mass Index Table (kg/m^2) or (lb/in^2 × 703)

	Normal						Overweight					Mild Obesity				
BMI	19	20	21	22	23	24	25	26	27	28	29	30	31	32	33	34
Height (inches)	Body Weight (pounds)															
58	91	96	100	105	110	115	119	124	129	134	138	143	148	153	158	162
59	94	99	104	109	114	119	124	128	133	138	143	148	153	158	163	168
60	97	102	107	112	118	123	128	133	138	143	148	153	158	163	168	174
61	100	106	111	116	122	127	132	137	143	148	153	158	164	169	174	180
62	104	109	115	120	126	131	136	142	147	153	158	164	169	175	180	186
63	107	113	118	124	130	135	141	146	152	158	163	169	175	180	186	191
64	110	116	122	128	134	140	145	151	157	163	169	174	180	186	192	197
65	114	120	126	132	138	144	150	156	162	168	174	180	186	192	198	204
66	118	124	130	136	142	148	155	161	167	173	179	186	192	198	204	210
67	121	127	134	140	146	153	159	166	172	178	185	191	198	204	211	217
68	125	131	138	144	151	158	164	171	177	184	190	197	203	210	216	223
69	128	135	142	149	155	162	169	176	182	189	196	203	209	216	223	230
70	132	139	146	153	160	167	174	181	188	195	202	209	216	222	229	236
71	136	143	150	157	165	172	179	186	193	200	208	215	222	229	236	243
72	140	147	154	162	169	177	184	191	199	206	213	221	228	235	242	250
73	144	151	159	166	174	182	189	197	204	212	219	227	235	242	250	257
74	148	155	163	171	179	186	194	202	210	218	225	233	241	249	256	264
75	152	160	168	176	184	192	200	208	216	224	232	240	248	256	264	272
76	156	164	172	180	189	197	205	213	221	230	238	246	254	263	271	279

Source: Adapted from Clinical Guidelines on the Identification, Evaluation, and Treatment of Overweight and Obesity in Adults: The Evidence Report. National Heart, Blood and Lung Institute, part of the National Institutes of Health and U.S. Department of Health & Human Service. http://www.nhlbi.nih.gov/files/docs/guidelines/ob_gdlns.pdf Published September 1998. Accessed June 24, 2015.

BMI Calculator: http://www.nhlbi.nih.gov/health/educational/lose_wt/BMI/bmicalc.htm

Body Mass Index Table (kg/m²) or (lb/in² × 703) Continued from previous page

	Moderate Obesity				Extreme Obesity										Super Obese				
35	36	37	38	39	40	41	42	43	44	45	46	47	48	49	50	51	52	53	54

Body Weight (pounds)

35	36	37	38	39	40	41	42	43	44	45	46	47	48	49	50	51	52	53	54
167	172	177	181	186	191	196	201	205	210	215	220	224	229	234	239	244	248	253	258
173	178	183	188	193	198	203	208	212	217	222	227	232	237	242	247	252	257	262	267
179	184	189	194	199	204	209	215	220	225	230	235	240	245	250	255	261	266	271	276
185	190	195	201	206	211	217	222	227	232	238	243	248	254	259	264	269	275	280	285
191	196	202	207	213	218	224	229	235	240	246	251	256	262	267	273	278	284	289	295
197	203	208	214	220	225	231	237	242	248	254	259	265	270	278	282	287	293	299	304
204	209	215	221	227	232	238	244	250	256	262	267	273	279	285	291	296	302	308	314
210	216	222	228	234	240	246	252	258	264	270	276	282	288	294	300	306	312	318	324
216	223	229	235	241	247	253	260	266	272	278	284	291	297	303	309	315	322	328	334
223	230	236	242	249	255	261	268	274	280	287	293	299	306	312	319	325	331	338	344
230	236	243	249	256	262	269	276	282	289	295	302	308	315	322	328	335	341	348	354
236	243	250	257	263	270	277	284	291	297	304	311	318	324	331	338	345	351	358	365
243	250	257	264	271	278	285	292	299	306	313	320	327	334	341	348	355	362	369	376
250	257	265	272	279	286	293	301	308	315	322	329	338	343	351	358	365	372	379	386
258	265	272	279	287	294	302	309	316	324	331	338	346	353	361	368	375	383	390	397
265	272	280	288	295	302	310	318	325	333	340	348	355	363	371	378	386	393	401	408
272	280	287	295	303	311	319	326	334	342	350	358	365	373	381	389	396	404	412	420
279	287	295	303	311	319	327	335	343	351	359	367	375	383	391	399	407	415	423	431
287	295	304	312	320	328	336	344	353	361	369	377	385	394	402	410	418	426	435	443

Fiber Content of Selected Foods

Food Description	Measure	Total Dietary Fiber (g)
Bran, ready-to-eat cereals	½ cup	14.2–19.2
Avocado, raw	1	13.5
Raisin bran, ready-to-eat cereals	1 cup	6.7-8.1
Beans (navy, pinto, black, kidney, lima, white), cooked	½ cup	6.3–9.6
Peas, split, cooked	½ cup	8.2
Potato, baked, flesh and skin	1 large	6.9
Pomegranate, raw	half 4 inch across	5.65
Pears, raw	1 medium	5.5
Beans, baked, canned, plain	½ cup	5.2
Soybeans, mature cooked	½ cup	5.2
Vegetables, mixed, canned, cooked	½ cup	4.7
Peas, green, cooked	½ cup	4.4
Raspberries, raw	½ cup	4.0
Pumpkin, canned	½ cup	3.6
Spinach, frozen, cooked	½ cup	3.5
Almonds	1 ounce	3.5
Sweet potato, cooked, flesh	½ cup	3.3
Spaghetti, whole-wheat, cooked	½ cup	3.1
Sunflower seed kernels	1 ounce	3.1
Squash, winter, cooked	½ cup	2.9
Banana	1small	2.6
Quinoa, cooked	½ cup	2.6
Raisins, seeded	¼ cup	2.5
Peanuts, dry-roasted	1 ounce	2.4
Prunes	3	2.0
Whole wheat bread	1ounce slice	1.7

Source: U.S. Department of Agriculture, Agricultural Research Service, Nutrient Data Laboratory. USDA National Nutrient Database for Standard Reference, Release 27 (revised). Version Current: May 2015. For a comprehensive list of selected foods containing fiber, refer to Nutrient Data Laboratory Home Page, http://www.ars.usda.gov/ba/bhnrc/ndl

Dietary Reference Intakes (DRIs) for fiber can be found at http://fnic.nal.usda.gov/dietary-guidance/dietary-reference-intakes/dri-tables-and-application-reports

Appendix

Calcium Content of Selected Foods

Food Description	Measure	Calcium (mg)
Fortified ready-to-eat cereals, Total®	¾ cup	1,000
Cheese, ricotta, part skim milk	½ cup	337
Yogurt, fruit, low-fat	8-oz container	313
Yogurt, plain, low-fat	8-oz container	311
Cheese, mozzarella, part skim milk	1 ½ ounces	305
Cream of wheat cereal, cooked	1 cup	303
Soymilk, unsweetened, with added calcium	1 cup	301
Milk, nonfat	1 cup	299
Cheese, cheddar	1 ½ ounces	284
Milk, whole	1 cup	276
Milk, chocolate, reduced fat	1 cup	272
Tofu, firm, prepared with calcium sulfate and magnesium chloride	½ cup	253
Cheese, cottage, low-fat, 2% milkfat, 1 cup	1 cup	251
Yogurt, Greek, nonfat vanilla	8 ounces	202-240
Fish, salmon, pink, canned, solids with bone and liquid	3 ounces	181
Collards, frozen, cooked	½ cup	179
Orange juice, calcium fortified	½ cup	175
Macaroni and cheese, box mix, prepared	1 cup	161
Spinach, frozen, cooked	½ cup	145
Pudding, vanilla, prepared with milk	½ cup	138-143
Almonds, roasted	¼ cup	114
Sardines, canned with bone	2 small	92
Ice cream, vanilla	½ cup	84
Fortified ready-to-eat cereal, puffed rice	1 cup	1

Source: U.S. Department of Agriculture, Agricultural Research Service, Nutrient Data Laboratory. USDA National Nutrient Database for Standard Reference, Release 27 (revised). Version Current: May 2015. For a comprehensive list of selected foods containing calcium, refer to Nutrient Data Laboratory Home Page, http://www.ars.usda.gov/ba/bhnrc/ndl

Dietary Reference Intakes (DRIs) for Calcium can be found at http://fnic.nal.usda.gov/dietary-guidance/dietary-reference-intakes/dri-tables-and-application-reports

Appendix

Iron Content of Selected Foods

Food Description	Measure	Iron (mg)
Fortified ready-to-eat cereals (various)	1 cup	4.4–28.4
Cream of wheat cereal, cooked	1 cup	10.0
Beans, baked, canned, with pork and tomato sauce	½ cup	3.98
Liver, beef, cooked	2 ounces	3.93
Lentils, cooked	½ cup	3.29
Spinach, cooked	½ cup	3.2
Beans (white, kidney, lima, black, pinto), cooked	½ cup	1.79–3.31
Clams, cooked	3 ounces	2.39
Baby food, cereal, rice, dry	2 Tbsp	2.38
Sunflower seed kernels, toasted	¼ cup	1.4–2.3
Edamame, cooked	½ cup	1.76
Cashew nuts, roasted	1 ounce	1.72
Beef, ground, 85% lean meat, cooked	2 ounces	1.66
Oysters, canned	1 ounce	1.54
Sesame seed butter, tahini	1 Tbsp	1.34
Almonds, dry roasted	1 ounce (22 nuts)	1.06
Molasses	1 Tbsp	0.94
Macaroni, enriched, cooked	½ cup	0.90
Pork, shoulder, whole, lean only, cooked	2 ounces	0.85
Egg, whole, cooked, scrambled	1 large	0.80
Hummus	2 Tbsp	0.73
Chicken, canned, no broth	2 ounces	0.72
Whole wheat bread	1 ounce slice	0.70
Peanut butter, chunk style	2 Tbsp	0.61
Fish, tuna, white, canned in water, drained	2 ounces	0.55

Source: U.S. Department of Agriculture, Agricultural Research Service, Nutrient Data Laboratory. USDA National Nutrient Database for Standard Reference, Release 27 (revised). Version Current: May 2015. For a comprehensive list of selected foods containing iron, refer to Nutrient Data Laboratory Home Page, http://www.ars.usda.gov/ba/bhnrc/ndl

Dietary Reference Intakes (DRIs) for Iron can be found at http://fnic.nal.usda.gov/dietary-guidance/dietary-reference-intakes/dri-tables-and-application-reports

Appendix

Folate Content of Selected Foods

Food Description	Measure	Folate, DFE (mcg)
Fortified ready-to-eat cereals (various)	1 cup	3–1362
Kellogg's All-Bran® Original cereal	1 cup	1362
Chicken liver, cooked	1	254
Edamame, frozen, cooked	½ cup	241
Lentils, cooked	½ cup	179
Beans (pinto, black, kidney)	½ cup	115–147
Spinach, frozen, cooked	½ cup	115
Noodles, egg, cooked, enriched	½ cup	110
Pretzels, hard, plain, salted	10 pretzel twists	100
Broccoli, cooked	½ cup	84
Macaroni, cooked, enriched	½ cup	83
Rice, white, long-grain, prepared, enriched	½ cup	77
Sunflower seeds, toasted	1 ounce	67
Romaine lettuce, shredded	1 cup	64
Pomegranate, raw	half 4 inch across	53
Bread, raisin, enriched	1 ounce slice	44
Quinoa, cooked	½ cup	39
English walnuts	1 ounce	28
Salmon, Atlantic wild, cooked	3 ounces	25
Orange juice, unsweetened, diluted	½ cup	24
Egg, whole, cooked, scrambled	1 large	22
Cashew nuts, roasted	1 ounce	20
Yogurt, vanilla	6 ounces	19
Almonds, dry roasted	1 ounce	16
Bread, whole wheat	1 ounce slice	12
Beef, ground, 80/20 patty, cooked	3 ounces	8
Cheese, cheddar	1 ounce	7
Rice, brown, long-grain, cooked	½ cup	4
Macaroni, whole wheat, cooked	½ cup	4
Puffed rice cereal, fortified	1 cup	3

Continued on next page

Simplified Diet Manual, Twelfth Edition. Edited by Paula Watkins.
© 2016 Iowa Academy of Nutrition and Dietetics.

Folate Content of Selected Foods Continued from previous page

Source: U.S. Department of Agriculture, Agricultural Research Service, Nutrient Data Laboratory. USDA National Nutrient Database for Standard Reference, Release 27 (revised). Version Current: May 2015. For a comprehensive list of selected foods containing folate, refer to Nutrient Data Laboratory Home Page, http://www.ars.usda.gov/ba/bhnrc/ndl

Dietary Reference Intakes (DRIs) for folate can be found at http://fnic.nal.usda.gov/dietary-guidance/dietary-reference-intakes/dri-tables-and-application-reports

Appendix

Magnesium Content of Selected Foods

Food Description	Measure	Magnesium (mg)
Sesame seed kernels, toasted	¼ cup	111
Muffin, oat bran, 2 ounce muffin	1	90
Spinach, frozen, cooked	½ cup	78
Almonds	1 ounce (22 nuts)	78
Cashews	1 ounce	74
Beans, white, black, lima, navy, pinto, cooked	½ cup	43–63
Soymilk, original, unfortified	1 cup	61
Quinoa, cooked	½ cup	59
Peanuts, roasted	1 ounce	50
Edamame, frozen, cooked	½ cup	50
Potato, baked, flesh and skin	1 medium	48
Molasses	1 Tbsp	48
Yogurt, plain, skim milk	8-oz container	43
Rice, brown, long-grain, cooked	½ cup	42
Sunflower seed kernels, dry roasted	1 ounce	37
Oatmeal, cooked	½ cup	32
Peanut butter, smooth style	1 Tbsp	27
Milk, fluid, nonfat	1 cup	27
Hazelnut spread, chocolate flavored	2 Tbsp	24
Macaroni, whole wheat, cooked	½ cup	21
Corn muffin, 2 ounce muffin	1	18
Pomegranate, raw	Half 4 inch across	17
Sesame seed butter, tahini	1 Tbsp	14

Source: U.S. Department of Agriculture, Agricultural Research Service, Nutrient Data Laboratory. USDA National Nutrient Database for Standard Reference, Release 27 (revised). Version Current: May 2015. For a comprehensive list of selected foods containing magnesium, refer to Nutrient Data Laboratory Home Page, http://www.ars.usda.gov/ba/bhnrc/ndl

Dietary Reference Intakes (DRIs) for magnesium can be found at http://fnic.nal.usda.gov/dietary-guidance/dietary-reference-intakes/dri-tables-and-application-reports

Appendix

Potassium Content of Selected Foods

Food Description	Measure	Potassium (mg)
Potato, baked, flesh and skin	1 medium	952
Avocado, California, raw without skin or seed	1	690
Tomato products, canned, paste	¼ cup	669
Beet greens, boiled, drained	½ cup	654
Yogurt, plain, skim milk	8-oz container	579
Beans (lima, kidney, navy, white, black)	½ cup	305–552
Tomato products, canned, puree	½ cup	549
Cantaloupe, cubes	1 cup	427
Banana, raw	1 medium	422
Sweet potato, canned, vacuum pack	½ cup	398
Milk, skim	1 cup	382
Prune juice	½ cup	353
Pomegranate, raw	half 4 inch across	333
Pork, roasted, lean only	3 ounces	317
Potatoes, mashed, home-prepared, whole milk added	½ cup	311
Tuna, yellowfin, cooked	2 ounces	299
Beans, baked, canned, with pork and sweet sauce	½ cup	288
Spinach, frozen, boiled, drained	½ cup	287
Beef, ground, 85% lean patty, cooked	3 ounces	270
Tomato juice, canned	½ cup	264
Beets, boiled, drained	½ cup	259
Raisins, seedless	1 ounce	212
Pear, raw	1 medium	206
Almonds, roasted	1 ounce	198
Orange juice, frozen concentrate, unsweetened, diluted	½ cup	197
Watermelon, diced	1 cup	170
Potatoes, mashed, made from granules with milk and water added	½ cup	163

Continued on next page

Simplified Diet Manual, Twelfth Edition. Edited by Paula Watkins.
© 2016 Iowa Academy of Nutrition and Dietetics.

Potassium Content of Selected Foods Continued from previous page

Source: U.S. Department of Agriculture, Agricultural Research Service, Nutrient Data Laboratory. USDA National Nutrient Database for Standard Reference, Release 27 (revised). Version Current: May 2015. For a comprehensive list of selected foods containing potassium, refer to Nutrient Data Laboratory Home Page, http://www.ars.usda.gov/ba/bhnrc/ndl

Dietary Reference Intakes (DRIs) for potassium can be found at http://fnic.nal.usda.gov/dietary-guidance/dietary-reference-intakes/dri-tables-and-application-reports

Appendix

Vitamin A Content of Selected Foods

Food Description	Measure	Vitamin A, RAE (mcg)
Liver- Lamb, Beef, Turkey, Pork	1 oz	1116-2205
Sweet potato, cooked, without skin	½ cup mashed	1290
Braunschweiger (liver sausage), pork	1 oz	1196
Carrots, raw	1 cup, chopped	1069
Sweet potato, cooked, baked in skin	½ cup	961
Pumpkin, canned	½ cup	953
Carrots, canned	½ cup	815
Carrots, frozen, cooked	½ cup	617
Squash, winter, butternut, cooked, baked	½ cup cubes	572
Spinach, canned, drained	½ cup	524
Collards, frozen, cooked	½ cup	489
Kale, frozen, cooked	½ cup	478
Mixed vegetables, canned, drained	½ cup	475
Spinach, cooked, drained	½ cup	471
Sweet potato, canned, syrup pack	½ cup	449
Turnip greens, frozen, cooked	½ cup	441
Cereals, ready-to-eat, assorted brands	¾ cup	0-434
Squash, winter, butternut, frozen, cooked	½ cup mashed	200
Apricots, canned, heavy syrup, drained	½ cup	160
Lettuce, romaine, raw	1 cup shredded	205
Mixed vegetables, frozen, cooked	½ cup	195
Milk, with added vitamin A	1 cup	150
Cantaloupe, raw	½ cup, balls	149
Spinach, raw	1 cup	141
Peppers, sweet, red, raw	½ cup, chopped	117
Mandarin oranges, canned, drained	½ cup	53
Asparagus, canned	½ cup	49
Broccoli, frozen, cooked	½ cup	47
Peaches, canned, heavy syrup, drained	½ cup	34

Continued on next page

Simplified Diet Manual, Twelfth Edition. Edited by Paula Watkins.
© 2016 Iowa Academy of Nutrition and Dietetics.

Vitamin A Content of Selected Foods Continued from previous page

Source: US Department of Agriculture, Agricultural Research Service, Nutrient Data Laboratory. USDA National Nutrient Database for Standard Reference, Release 27 (revised). Version Current: May 2015. For a comprehensive list of selected foods containing Vitamin A, refer to Nutrient Data Laboratory Home Page, http://www.ars.usda.gov/ba/bhnrc/ndl

Dietary Reference Intakes (DRIs) for Vitamin A can be found at http://fnic.nal.usda.gov/dietary-guidance/dietary-reference-intakes/dri-tables-and-application-reports

Vitamin B$_{12}$ Content of Selected Foods

Food Description	Measure	Vitamin B$_{12}$ (mcg)
Mollusks, clam, cooked	1 oz	28
Liver- Turkey, Pork, Beef, Lamb	1 oz	5-24
Soup, clam chowder, New England	1 cup	11.5
Soup, clam chowder, Manhattan style	1 cup	7.92
Cereals, ready-to-eat	0.67 cup	0-6
Mollusks, oyster, farmed/wild, cooked	1 oz	4.5-5
Fish, mackerel, king, raw	1 oz	4.4
Almond milk	8 oz	3.0
Crustaceans, crab, cooked	1 oz	2.9
Fish, herring, Pacific, raw	1 oz	2.8
Fish, tuna, fresh, bluefin, raw	1 oz	2.7
Beef, plate steak, boneless, cooked	1 oz	2.1
Soymilk	8 oz	2.0
Fish, salmon, sockeye, cooked	1 oz	1.6
Milk, nonfat	1 cup	1.2
Fish, tuna, canned in water, drained	1 oz	0.8
Beef, ground , cooked	1 oz	0.8
Cottage cheese, low-fat	4 oz	0.7
Egg, whole, cooked	1 large	0.5
Pork, roast, cooked	1 oz	0.3
Turkey, cooked	1 oz	0.3
Chicken, breast, skinless, cooked	1 oz	0.1
Bacon	1 slice	0.1

Source: US Department of Agriculture, Agricultural Research Service, Nutrient Data Laboratory. USDA National Nutrient Database for Standard Reference, Release 27 (revised). Version Current: May 2015. For a comprehensive list of selected foods containing Vitamin B$_{12}$, refer to Nutrient Data Laboratory Home Page, http://www.ars.usda.gov/ba/bhnrc/ndl

Dietary Reference Intakes (DRIs) for Vitamin B$_{12}$ can be found at http://fnic.nal.usda.gov/dietary-guidance/dietary-reference-intakes/dri-tables-and-application-reports

Appendix

Vitamin C Content of Selected Foods

Food Description	Measure	Vitamin C, total ascorbic acid (mg)
Guava, raw	½ cup	188
Peppers, sweet, yellow, raw	½ large pepper	170
Pomegranate, raw	half 4 inch across	144
Tomato juice, canned	½ cup	85
Kiwifruit, green, raw	½ cup	83
Orange juice, fresh	½ cup	62
Peppers, sweet, green, raw	½ cup chopped	60
Oranges, raw	½ cup sections	47.9
Apple juice, with added ascorbic acid	½ cup	47.8
Pineapple, raw	½ cup chunks	46.5
Orange juice, frozen concentrate, diluted	½ cup	45
Strawberries, raw	½ cup halves	44.7
Mandarin oranges	½ cup	42.6
Broccoli, raw	½ cup	40.6
Peas, edible-podded, cooked	½ cup	38.3
Broccoli, frozen, chopped, cooked	½ cup	36.9
Grapefruit, raw	½ cup with juice	35.9
Brussels sprouts, frozen, cooked	½ cup	35.4
Melons, cantaloupe, raw	½ cup balls	32.5
Mandarin oranges, canned, drained	½ cup	32
Grape juice, with added ascorbic acid	½ cup	31.6
Mangos, raw	½ cup pieces	30
Cauliflower, frozen, cooked	½ cup pieces	28.2
Tomatoes, red, ripe, cooked	½ cup	27.3
Kale, cooked	½ cup chopped	26.7
Tomato products, canned, sauce	½ cup	26.2
Cabbage, red, raw	½ cup chopped	25.3
Asparagus, canned, drained	½ cup	22.3
Sweet potato, cooked	½ cup mashed	21
Raspberries, frozen, red, sweetened	½ cup thawed	20.6

Continued on next page

Simplified Diet Manual, Twelfth Edition. Edited by Paula Watkins.
© 2016 Iowa Academy of Nutrition and Dietetics.

Vitamin C Content of Selected Foods Continued from previous page

Source: US Department of Agriculture, Agricultural Research Service, Nutrient Data Laboratory. USDA National Nutrient Database for Standard Reference, Release 27 (revised). Version Current: May 2015. For a comprehensive list of selected foods containing Vitamin C, refer to Nutrient Data Laboratory Home Page, http://www.ars.usda.gov/ba/bhnrc/ndl

Dietary Reference Intakes (DRIs) for Vitamin C can be found at http://fnic.nal.usda.gov/dietary-guidance/dietary-reference-intakes/dri-tables-and-application-reports

Appendix

Vitamin D Content of Selected Foods

Food Description	Measure	Vitamin D2 + D3 (mcg*)
Fish oil, cod liver	1 tsp	11.2
Mushrooms, portabella, UV light exposed, grilled	½ cup sliced	8.0
Fish, swordfish, cooked, dry heat	1 oz	4.7
Fish, farmed rainbow trout, cooked, dry heat	1 oz	4.5
Fish, salmon, pink, canned, drained	1 oz	4.1
Milk, nonfat, with added Vitamin D	1 cup	2.9
Soymilk with added calcium and Vitamin D	1 cup	2.9
Cereals, ready-to-eat, assorted brands	1 cup	0-2.5
Yogurt, fruit variety, nonfat, fortified Vitamin D	6 oz	2.2
Mushrooms, Chanterelle, raw	½ cup	1.5
American cheese, Vitamin D fortified	1 slice (2/3 oz)	1.3
Orange juice, from concentrate, added Vitamin D	½ cup	1.25
Egg, whole, cooked	1 large	1.0

Source: US Department of Agriculture, Agricultural Research Service, Nutrient Data Laboratory. USDA National Nutrient Database for Standard Reference, Release 27 (revised). Version Current: May 2015. For a comprehensive list of selected foods containing Vitamin D, refer to Nutrient Data Laboratory Home Page, http://www.ars.usda.gov/ba/bhnrc/ndl

*1 mcg = 40 IU

Dietary Reference Intakes (DRIs) for Vitamin D can be found at http://fnic.nal.usda.gov/dietary-guidance/dietary-reference-intakes/dri-tables-and-application-reports

Appendix

Vitamin E Content of Selected Foods

Food Description	Measure	Vitamin E (alpha-tocopherol) (mg)
Cereals, ready-to-eat, assorted brands	1 cup	0-13.6
Seeds, sunflower seed kernels, dry roasted	1 oz	7.4
Nuts, almonds, dry roasted	1 oz	6.78
Oil, wheat germ	1 tsp	6.72
Soymilk, enhanced	1 cup	6.12
Nuts, hazelnuts, blanched	1 oz	4.92
Nuts, almond paste	1 oz	3.84
Nuts, mixed, dry roasted, with peanuts	1 oz	3.1
Peanut butter, smooth	2 Tbsp	2.91
Oil, hazelnut	1 tsp	2.14
Spinach, canned, drained	½ cup	2.08
Oil, sunflower	1 tsp	1.86
Oil, almond	1 tsp	1.78
Margarine-like spread, BENECOL® light	1 tsp	1.74
Sweet potato, cooked	½ cup mashed	1.54
Oil, vegetable	1 tsp	1.0
Margarine-like, vegetable oil spread	1 tsp	0.99
Oil, canola	1 tsp	0.81
Avocado, raw	2 Tbsp pureed	0.77
Oil, olive, salad or cooking	1 tsp	0.65
Oil, soybean, salad or cooking	1 tsp	0.55

Source: US Department of Agriculture, Agricultural Research Service, Nutrient Data Laboratory. USDA National Nutrient Database for Standard Reference, Release 27 (revised). Version Current: May 2015. For a comprehensive list of selected foods containing Vitamin E, refer to Nutrient Data Laboratory Home Page, http://www.ars.usda.gov/ba/bhnrc/ndl

Dietary Reference Intakes (DRIs) for Vitamin E can be found at http://fnic.nal.usda.gov/dietary-guidance/dietary-reference-intakes/dri-tables-and-application-reports

Appendix

Protein Content of Selected Foods

Food Description	Measure	Protein (g)
Yogurt, Greek, nonfat, plain	6 ounces	17.3
Soybeans, cooked	½ cup	15.7
Tofu, firm ,raw, prepared with calcium sulfate	¼ cup	9.9
Evaporated milk, nonfat	½ cup	9.7
Dried beans and peas (black, kidney, lima, navy, pinto and white beans; lentils; split peas), cooked	½ cup	7.3-8.7
Beef, fish, poultry, pork, cooked, lean only	1 ounce	5.7-8.6
Edamame, cooked	½ cup	8.4
Milk, nonfat	1 cup	8.3
Cheese (cheddar, mozzarella, Swiss)	1 ounce	6.8-7.6
Yogurt, fruit variety, nonfat	6 ounces	7.5
Peanut butter, smooth style	2 Tbsp	7.1
Soymilk, unsweetened	1 cup	6.9
Peanuts, dry-roasted	1 ounce	6.9
Egg, large, scrambled	1	6.0
Milk, dry, instant, nonfat	¼ cup	6.0
Cottage cheese, 2% milkfat	¼ cup	5.9
Almonds	1 ounce (22 nuts)	5.9
Peanut butter, powdered*	2 Tbsp	5
Quinoa, cooked	½ cup	4.0
Pudding, instant, prepared with 2% milk, vanilla	½ cup	3.7
Ice cream, vanilla	½ cup	2.3
Hazelnut spread, chocolate flavored	2 Tbsp	2.0
Almond milk, vanilla	1 cup	1.0

Source: U.S. Department of Agriculture, Agricultural Research Service, Nutrient Data Laboratory. USDA National Nutrient Database for Standard Reference, Release 27 (revised). Version Current: May 2015. For a comprehensive list of selected foods containing protein, refer to Nutrient Data Laboratory Home Page, http:// www.ars.usda.gov/ba/bhnrc/ndl

*information from manufacturer

Dietary Reference Intakes (DRIs) for protein can be found at http://fnic.nal.usda.gov/dietary-guidance/dietary-reference-intakes/dri-tables-and-application-reports

14

Appendix

Choose Your Foods: Food Lists for Diabetes*
THE FOOD LISTS

The following chart shows the amount of nutrients in 1 choice from each list.

Food List	Carbohydrate (grams)	Protein (grams)	Fat (grams)	Calories
Carbohydrates				
Starch: breads; cereals; grains and pasta; starchy vegetables; crackers and snacks; and beans, peas, and lentils	15	3	1	80
Fruits	15	—	—	60
Milk and Milk Substitutes				
Fat-free, low-fat (1%)	12	8	0–3	100
Reduced-fat (2%)	12	8	5	120
Whole	12	8	8	160
Nonstarchy Vegetables	5	2	—	25
Sweets, Desserts, and Other Carbohydrates	15	varies	varies	varies
Proteins				
Lean	—	7	2	45
Medium-fat	—	7	5	75
High-fat	—	7	8	100
Plant-based	varies	7	varies	varies
Fats	—	—	5	45
Alcohol (1 alcohol equivalent)	varies	—	—	100

* © Academy of Nutrition and Dietetics. *Choose Your Foods: Food Lists for Diabetes.* 2014. Reprinted with permission.

Simplified Diet Manual, Twelfth Edition. Edited by Paula Watkins.
© 2016 Iowa Academy of Nutrition and Dietetics.

STARCH

Breads, cereals, grains (including pasta and rice), starchy vegetables, crackers and snacks, and beans, peas, and lentils are starches. In general, **1 starch choice** is:

- ½ cup of cooked cereal, grain, or starchy vegetable
- ⅓ cup of cooked rice or pasta
- 1 oz of a bread product, such as one slice of bread
- ¾ oz to 1 oz of most snack foods (some snack foods may also have extra fat)

Nutrition Tips

- A choice on the **Starch** list has 15 grams of carbohydrate, 3 grams of protein, 1 gram of fat, and 80 calories.
- For health benefits, at least half of your servings of grains each day should be whole grains.

Selection Tips

- Choose starches that are low in fat as often as possible.
- Starchy vegetables, baked goods, and grains that are prepared with fat count as 1 starch choice and 1 fat choice.
- For many starchy foods (bagels, muffins, dinner rolls, buns), a general rule of thumb is 1 oz equals 1 choice. Because of their large size, some foods have more carbohydrate and calories than you might think. For example, a large bagel may weight 4 oz and equal 4 starch choices.
- For specific information about a specific food, read the Nutrition Facts panel on its food label.

Bread

Food	Serving Size
Bagel	¼ large bagel (1 oz)
Biscuit	1 biscuit (2 ½ inches across)
Breads, loaf-type	
white, whole-grain, French, Italian, pumpernickel, rye, sourdough, unfrosted raisin or cinnamon	1 slice (1 oz)
reduced-calorie, light	2 slices (1 ½ oz)
Breads, flat-type (flatbreads)	
chapatti	1 oz
ciabatta	1 oz
naan	3¼-inch square (1oz)
pita (6 inches across)	½ pita
roti	1 oz
sandwich flat buns, whole-wheat	1 bun, including top and bottom (1 ½ oz)
taco shell	2 taco shells (each 5 inches across)
tortilla, corn	1 small tortilla (6 inches across)
tortilla, flour	1 small tortilla (6 inches across) or ⅓ large tortilla (10 inches across)

Continued on next page

Food	Serving Size
Cornbread	1 ¾-inch cube (1 ½ oz)
English muffin	½ muffin
Hot dog bun or hamburger bun	½ bun (¾ oz)
Pancake	1 pancake (4 inches across, ¼ inch thick)
Roll, plain	1 small roll (1 oz)
Stuffing, bread	⅓ cup
Waffle	1 waffle (4-inch square or 4 inches across)

Cereals

Food	Serving Size
Bran cereal (twigs, buds or flakes)	½ cup
Cooked cereals (oats, oatmeal)	½ cup
Granola cereal	¼ cup
Grits, cooked	½ cup
Muesli	¼ cup
Puffed cereal	1 ½ cups
Shredded wheat, plain	½ cup
Sugar-coated cereal	½ cup
Unsweetened, ready-to-eat cereal	¾ cup

Grains (Including Pasta and Rice)

Unless otherwise indicated, serving sizes are for cooked grains.

Food	Serving Size
Barley	⅓ cup
Bran, dry	
oat	¼ cup
wheat	½ cup
Bulgur	½ cup
Couscous	⅓ cup
Kasha	½ cup
Millet	⅓ cup
Pasta, white or whole-wheat (all shapes and sizes)	⅓ cup
Polenta	⅓ cup
Quinoa, all colors	⅓ cup
Rice, white, brown, and other colors and types	⅓ cup
Tabbouleh (tabouli), prepared	½ cup
Wheat germ, dry	3 Tbsp
Wild rice	½ cup

Starchy Vegetables

All of the serving sizes for starchy vegetables on this list are for cooked vegetables.

Food	Serving Size
Breadfruit	¼ cup
Cassava or dasheen	⅓ cup
Corn	½ cup
on cob	4- to 4½-inch piece (½ large cob)
Hominy	¾ cup
Mixed vegetables with corn or peas	1 cup
Marinara, pasta, or spaghetti sauce	½ cup
Parsnips	½ cup
Peas, green	½ cup
Plantain	⅓ cup
Potato	
baked with skin	¼ large potato (3 oz)
boiled, all kinds	½ cup or ½ medium potato (3 oz)
mashed, with milk and fat	½ cup
French fried (oven-baked)*	1 cup (2 oz)
Pumpkin puree, canned, no sugar added	¾ cup
Squash, winter (acorn, butternut)	1 cup
Succotash	½ cup
Yam or sweet potato, plain	½ cup (3½ oz)

*Note: Restaurant-style French Fries are on the **Fast Foods** list

Crackers and Snacks

Note: Some snacks are high in fat. Always check food labels.

Food	Serving Size
Crackers	
animal	8 crackers
crispbread	2 to 5 pieces (¾ oz)
graham, 2 ½-inch square	3 squares
nut and rice	10 crackers
oyster	20 crackers
round, butter-type*	6 crackers
saltine-type	6 crackers
sandwich-style, cheese or peanut butter filling*	3 crackers
whole-wheat, baked	5 regular 1½-inch squares or 10 thins (¾ oz)

Continued on next page

Food	Serving Size
Granola or snack bar	1 bar (¾ oz)
Matzoh, all shapes and sizes	¾ oz
Melba toast	4 pieces (each about 2 by 4 inches)
Popcorn	
no fat added	3 cups
with butter added**	3 cups
Pretzels	¾ oz
Rice cakes	2 cakes (4 inches across)
Snack chips	
baked (potato, pita)	about 8 chips (¾ oz)
regular (tortilla, potato)**	about 13 chips (1 oz)

*Count as 1 starch choice + 1 fat choice (l starch choice plus 5 grams of fat)

**Count as 1 starch choice + 2 fat choices (1 starch choice plus 10 grams of fat)

Note: For other snacks, see the **Sweets, Desserts, and Other Carbohydrates** list.

Beans, Peas, and Lentils

The choices on this list count as 1 starch choice + 1 lean protein choice.

Food	Serving Size
Baked beans, canned	⅓ cup
Beans (black, garbanzo, kidney, lima, navy, pinto, white), cooked or canned, drained and rinsed	½ cup
Lentils (any color), cooked	½ cup
Peas (black-eyed and split), cooked or canned, drained and rinsed	½ cup
Refried beans, canned	½ cup

Note: Beans, lentils and peas are also found on the **Protein** list.

FRUITS

Fresh, frozen, canned, and dried fruits and fruit juices are on this list. In general, **1 fruit choice** is:

- ½ cup of canned or frozen fruit
- 1 small fresh fruit (¾ to 1 cup)
- ½ cup of unsweetened fruit juice
- 2 tablespoons of dried fruit

Nutrition Tips

- A choice on the **Fruits** list has 15 grams of carbohydrate, 0 grams of protein, 0 grams of fat, and 60 calories.
- Fresh, frozen, and dried fruits are good sources of fiber. Fruit juices contain very little fiber. Choose fruits instead of juices whenever possible.
- Citrus fruits, berries, and melons are good sources of vitamin C.

Selection Tips

- Some fruits on the list are measured by weight. The weights include skin, core, seeds and rind. Use a food scale to weigh fresh fruits and figure out how many choices you are eating.

- Read the Nutrition Facts panel on food labels of packaged fruits and juices. If 1 serving has more than 15 grams of carbohydrate, you may need to adjust the size of the serving to fit with the choices in your Eating Plan.

- Serving sizes for canned fruits on the **Fruits** list are for the fruit and a small amount of juice (1 to 2 tablespoons).

- Food labels for fruits and fruit juices may contain the words "no sugar added" or "unsweetened." This means that no sugar, other than the sugar from the fruit itself, has been added. It does not mean the food contains no sugar.

- Fruit canned in extra-light syrup has the same amount of carbohydrate per serving as canned fruit labeled "no sugar added" or "juice pack." All canned fruits on the **Fruits** list are based on one of these three types of pack. Avoid fruit canned in heavy syrup.

Fruits

The weights listed include skin, core, seeds, and rind.

Food	Serving Size
Apple, unpeeled	1 small apple (4 oz)
Apples, dried	4 rings
Applesauce, unsweetened	½ cup
Apricots	
canned	½ cup
dried	8 apricot halves
fresh	4 apricots (5½ oz total)
Banana	1 extra-small banana, about 4 inches long (4 oz)
Blackberries	1 cup
Blueberries	¾ cup
Cantaloupe	1 cup diced
Cherries	
sweet, canned	½ cup
sweet, fresh	12 cherries (3½ oz)
Dates	3 small (deglet noor) dates or 1 large (medjool) date
Dried fruits (blueberries, cherries, cranberries, mixed fruit, raisins)	2 Tbsp
Figs	
dried	3 small figs
fresh	1 ½ large or 2 medium figs (3½ oz total)

Continued on next page

Food	Serving Size
Fruit cocktail	½ cup
Grapefruit	
fresh	½ large grapefruit (5½ oz)
sections, canned	¾ cup
Grapes	17 small grapes (3 oz total)
Guava	2 small guava (2½ oz total)
Honeydew melon	1 cup diced
Kiwi	½ cup sliced
Loquat	¾ cup cubed
Mandarin oranges, canned	¾ cup
Mango	½ small mango (5½ oz) or ½ cup
Nectarine	1 medium nectarine (5½ oz)
Orange	1 medium orange (6½ oz)
Papaya	½ papaya (8 oz) or 1 cup cubed
Peaches	
canned	½ cup
fresh	1 medium peach (6 oz)
Pears	
canned	½ cup
fresh	½ large pear (4 oz)
Pineapple	
canned	½ cup
fresh	¾ cup
Plantain, extra-ripe (black), raw	¼ plantain (2 ¼ oz)
Plums	
canned	½ cup
dried (prunes)	3 prunes
small	2 small plums (5 oz total)
Pomegranate seeds (arils)	½ cup
Raspberries	1 cup
Strawberries	1 ¼ cup whole berries
Tangerine	1 large tangerine (6 oz)
Watermelon	1 ¼ cups diced

Fruit Juice

Food	Serving Size
Apple juice/cider	½ cup
Fruit juice blends, 100% juice	⅓ cup
Grape juice	⅓ cup
Grapefruit juice	½ cup
Orange juice	½ cup
Pineapple juice	½ cup
Pomegranate juice	½ cup
Prune juice	⅓ cup

MILK AND MILK SUBSTITUTES

Different types of milk, milk products, and milk substitutes are included on this list. However, certain types of milk and milk-like products are found in other lists:

- Cheeses are on the **Protein** list (because they are rich in protein and have very little carbohydrate).
- Butter, cream, coffee creamers, and unsweetened nut milks are on the **Fats** list.
- Ice cream and frozen yogurt are on the **Sweets, Desserts, and Other Carbohydrates** list.

Nutrition Tips

- Milk and yogurt are good sources of calcium and protein.
- Greek yogurt contains more protein and less carbohydrate than most other yogurts.
- Types of milk and yogurt that are high in fat (2% or whole milk) have more saturated fat, cholesterol, and calories than low-fat or fat-free milk and yogurt.
- Children older than 2 years and adults should choose lower-fat varieties of milk and milk products, such as fat-free (skim) or low-fat (1%) milk or low-fat or nonfat yogurt.

Selection Tips

- 1 cup equals 8 fluid oz or ½ pint.

One milk choice has 12 grams of carbohydrate and 8 grams of protein and:

- One fat-free (skim) or low-fat (1%) milk choice has 0-3 grams of fat and 100 calories per serving.
- One reduced-fat (2%) milk choice has 5 grams of fat and 120 calories per serving.
- One whole milk choice has 8 grams of fat and 160 calories per serving.

Milk and Yogurts

Food	Serving Size	Choices per Serving
Fat-free (skim) or low-fat (1%)		
milk, buttermilk, acidophilus milk, lactose-free milk	1 cup	1 fat-free milk
evaporated milk	½ cup	1 fat-free milk
yogurt, plain or Greek; may be sweetened with an artificial sweetener	⅔ cup (6 oz)	1 fat-free milk
chocolate milk	1 cup	1 fat-free milk + 1 carbohydrate
Reduced-fat (2%)		
milk, acidophilus milk, kefir, lactose-free milk	1 cup	1 reduced-fat milk
yogurt, plain	⅔ cup (6 oz)	1 reduced-fat milk
Whole		
milk, buttermilk, goat's milk	1 cup	1 whole milk
evaporated milk	½ cup	1 whole milk
yogurt, plain	1 cup (8 oz)	1 whole milk
chocolate milk	1 cup	1 whole milk + 1 carbohydrate

Other Milk Foods and Milk Substitutes

Food	Serving Size	Choices per Serving
Eggnog		
fat-free	⅓ cup	1 carbohydrate
low-fat	⅓ cup	1 carbohydrate + ½ fat
whole milk	⅓ cup	1 carbohydrate + 1 fat
Rice drink		
plain, fat-fee	1 cup	1 carbohydrate
flavored, low-fat	1 cup	2 carbohydrates
Soy milk		
light or low-fat, plain	1 cup	½ carbohydrate + ½ fat
regular, plain	1 cup	½ carbohydrate + 1 fat
Yogurt with fruit, low-fat	⅔ cup (6 oz)	1 fat-free milk + 1 carbohydrate

Note: Unsweetened nut milks (such as almond milk and coconut milk) are on the **Fats** list.

NONSTARCHY VEGETABLES

Vegetables that contain a small amount of carbohydrate and few calories are on this list. (Vegetables that contain higher amounts of carbohydrate and calories can be found on the **Starch** list.) In general, **1 nonstarchy vegetable choice** is:

- ½ cup of cooked vegetables or vegetable juice
- 1 cup of raw vegetables

If you eat 3 cups or more of raw vegetables or 1 ½ cups or more of cooked nonstarchy vegetables in a meal, count them as 1 carbohydrate choice.

Nutrition Tips

- A choice on the **Nonstarchy Vegetables** list has 5 grams of carbohydrate, 2 grams of protein, 0 grams of fat, and 25 calories.
- Nonstarchy and starchy vegetables both contain important nutrients. Try to choose a variety of vegetables and **eat at least 2 to 3 nonstarchy vegetable choices daily.**
- Fresh, plain vegetables have no added salt. When choosing canned or frozen vegetables, read food labels and look for low-sodium or no-salt-added varieties. If these are not available, you can drain and rinse canned vegetables to reduce their sodium content.
- Read the Nutrition Facts panel on labels for canned and frozen vegetables. In addition to sodium, some products have added fats and sauces, which increase the calories and carbohydrate.
- Read labels on canned vegetable juices, too, and choose no-salt-added or low-sodium products.
- Vegetables that are deep in color, such as dark green or dark yellow vegetables, offer many nutritional benefits. Good daily choices include spinach, kale, broccoli, romaine, carrots, and peppers.
- Good sources of vitamin C include broccoli, brussels sprouts, cauliflower, greens, peppers, spinach, and tomatoes.
- Vegetables from the cruciferous family are rich in nutrients and offer health benefits. Eat them several times each week. Choices include bok choy, broccoli, brussels sprouts, cabbage, cauliflower, collards, kale, kohlrabi, radishes, rutabaga, and turnips.
- Many vegetables are a good source of dietary fiber.
- Raw sprouts, such as alfalfa or bean sprouts, may cause foodborne illness. For this reason, you should not eat raw sprouts.

Selection Tips

- One cup of raw vegetables is a portion about the size of a baseball or your fist.
- The tomato sauce referred to in this list is different from spaghetti/pasta sauce, which usually contains added sugar and is on the **Starchy Vegetables** list.

Nonstarchy Vegetables

Amaranth leaves (Chinese spinach)	Hearts of palm
Artichoke	Jicama
Artichoke hearts (no oil)	Kale
Asparagus	Kohlrabi

Continued on next page

Baby corn	Leeks
Bamboo shoots	Mixed vegetables (without starchy vegetables, legumes, or pasta)
Bean sprouts (alfalfa, mung, soybean)	Mushrooms, all kinds, fresh
Beans (green, wax, Italian, yard-long beans)	Okra
Beets	Onions
Broccoli	Pea pods
Broccoli slaw, packaged, no dressing	Peppers (all varieties)
Brussels sprouts	Radishes
Cabbage (green, red, bok choy, Chinese)	Rutabaga
Carrots	Sauerkraut, drained and rinsed
Cauliflower	Spinach
Celery	Squash, summer varieties (yellow, pattypan, crookneck, zucchini)
Chayote	Sugar pea snaps
Coleslaw, packaged, no dressing	Swiss chard
Cucumber	Tomato
Daikon	Tomatoes, canned
Eggplant	Tomato sauce (unsweetened)
Fennel	Tomato/vegetable juice
Gourds (bitter, bottle, luffa, bitter melon)	Turnips
Green onions or scallions	Water chestnuts
Greens (collard, dandelion, mustard, purslane, turnip)	

Note: Salad greens (like arugula, chicory, endive, lettuce, radicchio, romaine, and watercress) are on the **Free Foods** list.

SWEETS, DESSERTS, AND OTHER CARBOHYDRATES

Foods from this list have added sugars or fat. However, you can substitute food choices from this list for other carbohydrate-containing foods.

Nutrition Tips

- A carbohydrate choice on this list has 15 grams of carbohydrate and about 70 calories.

- Choose foods from this list less often. They do not have as many vitamins or minerals or as much fiber as the choices on the **Starch**, **Fruits**, and **Milk and Milk Substitutes** lists. Balance your meal by eating foods from other food lists to get the nutrients your body needs.

- Many of the foods on the **Sweets, Desserts, and Other Carbohydrates** list contain more than a single choice of carbohydrate. Some will also count as one or more fat choices.

- The serving sizes for foods on this list are small because these foods are high in calories.

Selection Tips

- Read the Nutrition Facts panel on the food label to find the serving size and nutrient information. Remember: The label serving size may be different from the serving size used in this food list.

- Many sugar-free, fat-free, or reduced-fat products are made with ingredients that contain carbohydrate. These types of food often have the same amount of carbohydrate as the regular foods they are replacing. Talk with your registered dietitian nutritionist (RDN) to find out how to fit these foods into your Eating Plan.

Common Measurements

Dry	Liquid
3 tsp = 1 Tbsp	4 Tbsp = ¼ cup
4 oz = ½ cup	8 oz = 1 cup or ½ pint
8 oz = 1 cup	

Beverages, Soda, and Sports Drinks

Food	Serving Size	Choices per Serving
Cranberry juice cocktail	½ cup	1 carbohydrate
Fruit drink or lemonade	1 cup (8 oz)	2 carbohydrates
Hot chocolate, regular	1 envelope (2 Tbsp or ¾ oz) added to 8 oz water	1 carbohydrate
Soft drink (soda), regular	1 can (12 oz)	2 ½ carbohydrates
Sports drink (fluid replacement type)	1 cup (8 oz)	1 carbohydrate

Brownies, Cake, Cookies, Gelatin, Pie, and Pudding

Food	Serving Size	Choices per Serving
Biscotti	1 oz	1 carbohydrate + 1 fat
Brownie, small, unfrosted	1 ¼-inch square, ⅞ inch high (about 1 oz)	1 carbohydrate + 1 fat
Cake		
angel food, unfrosted	$\frac{1}{12}$ of cake (about 2 oz)	2 carbohydrates
frosted	2-inch square (about 2 oz)	2 carbohydrates + 1 fat
unfrosted	2-inch square (about 1 oz)	1 carbohydrate + 1 fat
Cookies		
100-calorie pack	1 oz	1 carbohydrate + ½ fat
chocolate chip cookies	2 cookies (2 ¼ inches across)	1 carbohydrate + 2 fats
gingersnaps	3 small cookies, 1 ½ inches across	1 carbohydrate

Continued on next page

Brownies, Cake, Cookies, Gelatin, Pie, and Pudding Continued from previous page

Food	Serving Size	Choices per Serving
large cookie	1 cookie, 6 inches across (about 3 oz)	4 carbohydrates + 3 fats
sandwich cookies with crème filling	2 small (about ⅔ oz)	1 carbohydrate + 1 fat
sugar-free cookies	1 large or 3 small cookies (¾–1 oz)	1 carbohydrate + 1 to 2 fats
vanilla wafer	5 cookies	1 carbohydrate + 1 fat
Cupcake, frosted	1 small (about 1 ¾ oz)	2 carbohydrates + 1 to 1 ½ fats
Flan	½ cup	2 ½ carbohydrates + 1 fat
Fruit cobbler	½ cup (3 ½ oz)	3 carbohydrates + 1 fat
Gelatin, regular	½ cup	1 carbohydrate
Pie		
commercially prepared fruit, 2 crusts	⅙ of 8-inch pie	3 carbohydrates + 2 fats
pumpkin or custard	⅛ of 8-inch pie	1 ½ carbohydrates + 1 ½ fats
Pudding		
regular (made with reduced-fat milk)	½ cup	2 carbohydrates
sugar-free or sugar- and fat-free (made with fat-free milk)	½ cup	1 carbohydrate

Candy, Spreads, Sweets, Sweeteners, Syrups, and Toppings

Food	Serving Size	Choices per Serving
Blended sweeteners (mixtures of artificial sweeteners and sugar)	1½ Tbsp	1 carbohydrate
Candy		
chocolate, dark or milk type	1 oz	1 carbohydrate + 2 fats
chocolate "kisses"	5 pieces	1 carbohydrate + 1 fat
hard	3 pieces	1 carbohydrate
Coffee creamer, nondairy type		
powdered, flavored	4 tsp	½ carbohydrate + ½ fat
liquid, flavored	2 Tbsp	1 carbohydrate
Fruit snacks, chewy (pureed fruit concentrate)	1 roll (¾ oz)	1 carbohydrate
Fruit spreads, 100% fruit	1 ½ Tbsp	1 carbohydrate
Honey	1 Tbsp	1 carbohydrate
Jam or jelly, regular	1 Tbsp	1 carbohydrate
Sugar	1 Tbsp	1 carbohydrate

Continued on next page

Candy, Spreads, Sweets, Sweeteners, Syrups, and Toppings Continued from previous page

Food	Serving Size	Choices per Serving
Syrup		
chocolate	2 Tbsp	2 carbohydrates
light (pancake-type)	2 Tbsp	1 carbohydrate
regular (pancake-type)	1 Tbsp	1 carbohydrate

Condiments and Sauces

Food	Serving Size	Choices per Serving
Barbeque sauce	3 Tbsp	1 carbohydrate
Cranberry sauce, jellied	¼ cup	1 ½ carbohydrates
Curry sauce	1 oz	1 carbohydrate + 1 fat
Gravy, canned or bottled	½ cup	½ carbohydrate + ½ fat
Hoisin sauce	1 Tbsp	½ carbohydrate
Marinade	1 Tbsp	½ carbohydrate
Plum sauce	1 Tbsp	½ carbohydrate
Salad dressing, fat-free, cream-based	3 Tbsp	1 carbohydrate
Sweet-and-sour sauce	3 Tbsp	1 carbohydrate

Note: You can also check the **Fats** and **Free Foods** list for other condiments.

Doughnuts, Muffins, Pastries, and Sweet Breads

Food	Serving Size	Choices per Serving
Banana nut bread	1-inch slice (2 oz)	2 carbohydrates + 1 fat
Doughnut		
cake, plain	1 medium doughnut (1 ½ oz)	1 ½ carbohydrates + 2 fats
hole	2 holes (1 oz)	1 carbohydrate + 1 fat
yeast-type, glazed	1 doughnut, 3 ¾ inches across (2 oz)	2 carbohydrates + 2 fats
Muffin		
regular	1 muffin (4 oz)	4 carbohydrates + 2½ fats
lower-fat	1 muffin (4 oz)	4 carbohydrates + ½ fat
Scone	1 scone (4 oz)	4 carbohydrates + 3 fats
Sweet roll or Danish	1 pastry (2 ½ oz)	2 ½ carbohydrates + 2 fats

Frozen Bars, Frozen Desserts, Frozen Yogurt, and Ice Cream

Food	Serving Size	Choices per Serving
Frozen pops	1	½ carbohydrate
Fruit juice bars, frozen, 100% juice	1 bar (3 oz)	1 carbohydrate
Ice cream		
fat-free	½ cup	1 ½ carbohydrates
light	½ cup	1 carbohydrate + 1 fat
no-sugar-added	½ cup	1 carbohydrate + 1 fat
regular	½ cup	1 carbohydrate + 2 fats
Sherbet, sorbet	½ cup	2 carbohydrates
Yogurt, frozen		
fat-free	⅓ cup	1 carbohydrate
regular	½ cup	1 carbohydrate + 0 to 1 fat
Greek, lower-fat or fat-free	½ cup	1 ½ carbohydrates

PROTEIN

Meat, fish, poultry, cheese, eggs, and plant-based foods are all sources of protein and have varying amounts of fat. Foods from this list are divided into four groups based on the amount of fat they contain. These groups are lean protein, medium-fat protein, high-fat protein, and plant-based protein. The following chart shows you what one protein choice includes.

	Carbohydrate (grams)	Protein (grams)	Fat (grams)	Calories
Lean protein	—	7	2	45
Medium-fat protein	—	7	5	75
High-fat protein	—	7	8	100
Plant-based protein	varies	7	varies	varies

Some meals may have more than 1 protein choice. For example, a breakfast sandwich may be made with 1 ounce cheese and 1 egg. Since 1 ounce of cheese counts as 1 protein choice and 1 egg counts as 1 protein choice, this meal would contain 2 protein choices. As another example, if you eat 3 ounces of cooked chicken at dinner, this portion would equal 3 protein choices because each ounce counts as 1 protein choice. Some snacks may also contain protein. Talk to your RDN to find out how many protein choices to eat each day.

Nutrition Tips

- Many types of fish (halibut, herring, mackerel, salmon, sardines, trout, and tuna) are rich in omega-3 fats, which may help reduce risk for heart disease. Choose fish (not commercially fried fish fillets) two or more times each week.
- Whenever possible, choose lean meats because they have less saturated fat and cholesterol than medium-fat and high-fat meats.
  - Select grades of meat that are the leanest.

- Choice grades have a moderate amount of fat.
- Prime cuts of meat have the highest amount of fat.

Selection Tips

- Read labels to find foods low in fat and cholesterol. Try for 5 grams of fat or less per protein choice (serving size, usually 1 oz)
- Read labels to find "hidden" carbohydrate. For example, meatless or vegetable burgers may contain quite a bit of carbohydrate. Check the Nutrition Facts panel on the label to see if the total carbohydrate in 1 serving is close to 15 grams. If it is close to 15 grams, count it as 1 carbohydrate choice and 1 protein choice.
- Processed meats, such as hot dogs and sausages, are often high in fat and sodium. Look for lower-fat and lower-sodium versions.

Portion Sizes

Portion size is an important part of meal planning. The **Protein** list is based on cooked weight (for example, 4 oz of raw meat is equal to 3 oz of cooked meat) after the bone and fat have been removed. Try using the following comparisons to help estimate portion sizes:

- 1 oz cooked meat, poultry, or fish is about the size of a small matchbox.
- 3 oz cooked meat, poultry, or fish is about the size of a deck of playing cards.
- 2 tablespoons peanut butter is about the size of a golf ball.
- The palm of a woman's hand is about the size of 3 to 4 oz of cooked, boneless meat. The palm of a man's hand is about the size of 4 to 6 oz of cooked, boneless meat.
- 1 oz of cheese is about the size of 4 dice.

Cooking Tips

- Bake, poach, steam or boil instead of frying.
- Roast, broil, or grill meat on a rack to drain off fat during cooking.
- Trim off visible fat or skin.
- Use a nonstick spray or a nonstick pan to brown or fry foods.
- Meat or fish that is breaded with cornmeal, flour, or dried bread crumbs contains carbohydrate. Count 3 tablespoons of one of these dry starches as 15 grams of carbohydrate.

Ground Beef Labeling

Some ground beef is labeled by cut, and others are labeled by lean-to-fat percentages. Ground beef is highest in fat, about 30% fat, followed by ground chuck, about 20% fat. Ground round and ground sirloin each have about 11% fat. However, the grade of the meat stated on the label does not always indicate how lean the meat is. All packaged ground beef has some fat. Look for lean ground beef choices such as 90% lean/10% fat.

Lean Protein

Note: 1 oz is usually the serving size for meat, fish, poultry, or hard cheeses.

Food	Serving Size
Beef: ground (90% or higher lean/10% or lower fat); select or choice grades trimmed of fat: roast (chuck, round, rump, sirloin), steak (cubed, flank, porterhouse, T-bone), tenderloin	1 oz
Beef jerky	½ oz

Continued on next page

Food	Serving Size
Cheeses with 3 grams of fat or less per oz	1 oz
Curd-style cheeses: cottage-type (all kinds); ricotta (fat-free or light)	¼ cup (2 oz)
Egg substitutes, plain	¼ cup
Egg whites	2
Fish	
fresh or frozen, such as catfish, cod, flounder, haddock, halibut, orange roughy, tilapia, trout	1 oz
salmon, fresh or canned	1 oz
sardines, canned	2 small sardines
tuna, fresh or canned in water or oil and drained	1 oz
smoked: herring or salmon (lox)	1 oz
Game: buffalo, ostrich, rabbit, venison	1 oz
Hot dog with 3 grams of fat or less per oz Note: may contain carbohydrate	1 hot dog (1¾ oz)
Lamb: chop, leg, or roast	1 oz
Organ meats: heart, kidney, liver Note: May be high in cholesterol.	1 oz
Oysters, fresh or frozen	6 medium oysters
Pork, lean	
Canadian bacon	1 oz
ham	1 oz
rib or loin chop/roast, tenderloin	1 oz
Poultry, without skin: chicken; Cornish hen; domestic duck or goose (well-drained of fat); turkey; lean ground turkey or chicken	1 oz
Processed sandwich meats with 3 grams of fat or less per oz: chipped beef, thin-sliced deli meats, turkey ham, turkey pastrami	1 oz
Sausage with 3 grams of fat or less per oz	1 oz
Shellfish: clams, crab, imitation shellfish, lobster, scallops, shrimp	1 oz
Veal: cutlet (no breading), loin chop, roast	1 oz

Medium-Fat Protein

Food	Serving Size
Beef trimmed of visible fat: ground beef (85% or lower lean/15% or higher fat), corned beef, meatloaf, prime cuts of beef (rib roast), short ribs, tongue	1 oz
Cheeses with 4 to 7 grams of fat per oz: feta, mozzarella, pasteurized processed cheese spread, reduced-fat cheeses	1 oz
Cheese, ricotta (regular or part-skim)	¼ cup (2 oz)
Egg	1 egg

Continued on next page

Food	Serving Size
Fish; any fried	1 oz
Lamb: ground, rib roast	1 oz
Pork: cutlet, ground, shoulder roast	1 oz
Poultry with skin: chicken, dove, pheasant, turkey, wild duck, or goose; fried chicken	1 oz
Sausage with 4–7 grams of fat per oz	1 oz

High-Fat Protein

These foods are high in saturated fat, cholesterol, and calories and may raise blood cholesterol levels if eaten on a regular basis. Try to eat 3 or fewer choices from this group per week.

Food	Serving Size
Bacon, pork	2 slices (1 oz each, before cooking)
Bacon, turkey	3 slices (½ oz each before cooking)
Cheese, regular: American, blue-veined, brie, cheddar, hard goat, Monterey jack, Parmesan, queso, and Swiss	1 oz
Hot dog: beef, pork, or combination	1 hot dog (10 hot dogs per 1 lb-sized package)
Hot dog: turkey or chicken	1 hot dog (10 hot dogs per 1 lb-sized package)
Pork: sausage, spareribs	1 oz
Processed sandwich meats with 8 grams of fat or more per oz: bologna, hard salami, pastrami	1 oz
Sausage with 8 grams fat or more per oz: bratwurst, chorizo, Italian, knockwurst, Polish, smoked, summer	1 oz

Note:

- Beans, peas, and lentils are also found on the **Starch** list.
- Nut butters in smaller amounts are found in the **Fats** list.
- Canned beans, lentils, and peas can be high in sodium unless they're labeled *no-salt-added* or *low-sodium*. Draining and rinsing canned beans, peas, and lentils reduces sodium content by at least 40%.

Plant-Based Proteins

Because carbohydrate content varies among plant-based proteins, read food labels.

Food	Serving Size	Choices per Serving
"Bacon" strips, soy-based	2 strips (½ oz)	1 lean protein
Baked beans, canned	⅓ cup	1 starch + 1 lean protein
Beans (black, garbanzo, kidney, lima, navy, pinto, white), cooked or canned, drained and rinsed	½ cup	1 starch + 1 lean protein

Continued on next page

Food	Serving Size	Choices per Serving
"Beef" or "sausage" crumbles, meatless	1 oz	1 lean protein
"Chicken" nuggets, soy-based	2 nuggets (1 ½ oz)	½ carbohydrate + 1 medium-fat protein
Edamame, shelled	½ cup	½ carbohydrate + 1 lean protein
Falafel (spiced chickpea and wheat patties)	3 patties (about 2 inches across)	1 carbohydrate + 1 high-fat protein
Hot dog, meatless, soy-based	1 hot dog (1 ½ oz)	1 lean protein
Hummus	⅓ cup	1 carbohydrate + 1 medium-fat protein
Lentils, any color, cooked or canned, drained and rinsed	½ cup	1 starch + 1 lean protein
Meatless burger, soy-based	3 oz	½ carbohydrate + 2 lean proteins
Meatless burger, vegetable-and starch-based	1 patty (about 2 ½ oz)	½ carbohydrate + 1 lean protein
Meatless deli slices	1 oz	1 lean protein
Mycoprotein ("chicken" tenders or crumbles), meatless	2 oz	½ carbohydrate + 1 lean protein
Nut spreads: almond butter, cashew butter, peanut butter, soy nut butter	1 Tbsp	1 high-fat protein
Peas: (black-eyed and split peas), cooked or canned, drained and rinsed	½ cup	1 starch + 1 lean protein
Refried beans, canned	½ cup	1 starch + 1 lean protein
"Sausage" breakfast-type patties, meatless	1 (1 ½ oz)	1 medium-fat protein
Soy nuts, unsalted	¾ oz	½ carbohydrate + 1 medium-fat protein
Tempeh, plain, unflavored	¼ cup (1 ½ oz)	1 medium-fat protein
Tofu	½ cup (4 oz)	1 medium-fat protein
Tofu, light	½ cup (4 oz)	1 lean protein

FATS

The fats on this list are divided into three groups, based on the main type of fat they contain:

- **Unsaturated fats** primarily come from vegetable sources and are considered healthy fats.
  - **Monounsaturated fats**
  - **Polyunsaturated fats** (including omega-3 fats)
- **Saturated fats** primarily come from animal sources and are considered unhealthy fats.

Trans **fat,** a product of food processing, is an unhealthy fat and should be avoided (see below).

Nutrition Tips

- A choice on the **Fats** list contains 5 grams of fat and 45 calories. In general, **1 fat choice** equals:
  - 1 teaspoon of oil or solid fat
  - 1 tablespoon of salad dressing
- All fats are high in calories. Limit serving sizes for good nutrition and health.
- Limit the amount of fried foods you eat.
- Choose unsaturated fats instead of saturated and *trans* fats whenever possible.
- Nuts and seeds are good sources of unsaturated fats and have small amounts of fiber and protein. Eat them in moderation to control calories.
- Good sources of omega-3 fatty acids include:
  - Fish such as albacore tuna, halibut, herring, mackerel, salmon, sardines, and trout.
  - Flaxseeds and English walnuts.
  - Oils such as canola, soybean, flaxseed, and walnut.

Selection Tips

- Check the Nutrition Facts panel on food labels for serving sizes. One fat choice is based on a serving size that has 5 grams of total fat. Remember: The label serving size may be different than the serving size used in this food list.
- The food label lists total fat grams, saturated fat grams, and *trans* fat grams per serving. When most of the total fat come from saturated fat, the food is listed on the Saturated Fats list.
- When selecting fats, consider replacing saturated fats with monounsaturated fats and polyunsaturated fats that are good sources of omega-3 fats. Talk with your RDN about the best choices for you.
- Choose liquid oils instead of solid fats, such as butter, lard, shortening, or margarine, for cooking or baking.
- Read ingredient lists. Replace fats or spreads that include partially hydrogenated oils (*trans* fats) in the ingredient list with products containing oils that do NOT include the words "partially hydrogenated" or "hydrogenated."
- When selecting margarine, choose a type that either lists liquid vegetable oil (*trans* fat-free) as the first ingredient or lists water as the first ingredient and liquid vegetable oil as the second ingredient.
- Soft or tub margarines have less saturated fat than stick margarines and are a healthier choice. Select *trans* fat-free soft margarines.

Trans Fat

Avoid *trans* fat. Most *trans* fats found in foods are made in a process that changes vegetable oils into semi-solid fats. Partially hydrogenated and hydrogenated fats are types of processed *trans* fats and should be avoided. *Trans* fats can often be found in the following types of foods:

- Solid shortening, stick margarines, and some tub margarines
- Crackers, candies, cookies, snack foods, fried foods, baked goods, coffee creamers, and other food items made with partially hydrogenated vegetable oils.

Keep in mind that some foods claiming to be *trans* fat-free may still contain *trans* fat. Foods only need to have less than ½ gram of *trans* fat per serving to be labeled *trans* fat-free.

Unsaturated Fats—Monounsaturated Fats

Food	Serving Size
Almond milk (unsweetened)	1 cup
Avocado, medium	2 Tbsp (1 oz)
Nut butters (*trans* fat-free): almond butter, cashew butter, peanut butter (smooth or crunchy)	1 ½ tsp
Nuts	
almonds	6 nuts
Brazil	2 nuts
cashews	6 nuts
filberts (hazelnuts)	5 nuts
macadamia	3 nuts
mixed (50% peanuts)	6 nuts
peanuts	10 nuts
pecans	4 halves
pistachios	16 nuts
Oil: canola, olive, peanut	1 tsp
Olives	
black (ripe)	8 large
green, stuffed	10 large
Spread, plant stanol ester-type	
light	1 Tbsp
regular	2 tsp

Unsaturated Fats - Polyunsaturated Fats

Food	Serving Size
Margarine	
lower-fat spread (30–50% vegetable oil, *trans* fat-free)	1 Tbsp
stick, tub (*trans* fat-free), or squeeze (*trans* fat-free)	1 tsp
Mayonnaise	
reduced-fat	1 Tbsp
regular	1 tsp
Mayonnaise-style salad dressing	
reduced-fat	1 Tbsp
regular	2 tsp

Continued on next page

Food	Serving Size
Nuts	
pignolia (pine nuts)	1 Tbsp
walnuts, English	4 halves
Oil: corn, cottonseed, flaxseed, grapeseed, safflower, soybean, sunflower	1 tsp
Salad dressing	
reduced-fat (Note: May contain carbohydrate.)	2 Tbsp
regular	1 Tbsp
Seeds	
flaxseed, ground	1 ½ Tbsp
pumpkin, sesame, sunflower	1 Tbsp
Tahini or sesame paste	2 tsp

Saturated Fats

Food	Serving Size
Bacon, cooked, regular or turkey	1 slice
Butter	
reduced-fat	1 Tbsp
stick	1 tsp
whipped	2 tsp
Butter blends made with oil	
reduced-fat or light	1 Tbsp
regular	1 ½ tsp
Chitterlings, boiled	2 Tbsp (½ oz)
Coconut, sweetened, shredded	2 Tbsp
Coconut milk, canned, thick	
light	⅓ cup
regular	1 ½ Tbsp
Cream	
half-and-half	2 Tbsp
heavy	1 Tbsp
light	1 ½ Tbsp
whipped	2 Tbsp
Cream cheese	
reduced-fat	1 ½ Tbsp (¾ oz)
regular	1 Tbsp (½ oz)
Lard	1 tsp

Continued on next page

Food	Serving Size
Oil: coconut, palm, palm kernel	1 tsp
Salt pork	¼ oz
Shortening, solid	1 tsp
Sour cream	
reduced-fat or light	3 Tbsp
regular	2 Tbsp

Similar Foods in Other Lists

- Bacon and peanut butter, when used in smaller amounts, are counted as fat choices. When used in larger amounts, they are counted as high-fat protein choices (see the **Protein** list).
- Fat-free salad dressings are on the **Sweets, Desserts, and Other Carbohydrates** list.
- Look for whipped topping and fat-free products, such as margarines, salad dressings, mayonnaise, sour cream, and cream cheese, on the **Free Foods** list.

FREE FOODS

A "free" food is any food or drink choice that has less than 20 calories and 5 grams or less of carbohydrate per serving.

Nutrition Tip

- Some free foods contain sodium (salt). Examples of high-sodium seasonings or condiments include soy sauce, flavored salts (such as garlic salt and celery salt), and lemon pepper. Use these seasonings less often and in small amounts.

Selection Tips

- If a "free" is listed with a serving size, that means the calories and/or carbohydrate are near the limits defined for "free." Limit yourself to 3 servings or fewer of that food per day, and spread the servings throughout the day. If you eat all 3 servings at once, the carbohydrate in the food may raise your blood glucose level like 1 carbohydrate choice would.
- Food and drink choices listed here without a serving size can be used whenever you like.

Low Carbohydrate Foods

Food	Serving Size
Candy, hard (regular or sugar-free)	1 piece
Fruits	
Cranberries or rhubarb, sweetened with sugar substitute	½ cup
Gelatin dessert, sugar-free, any flavor	
Gum, sugar-free	
Jam or jelly, light or no-sugar-added	2 tsp
Salad greens (such as arugula, chicory, endive, escarole, leaf or iceberg lettuce, purslane, romaine, radicchio, spinach, watercress)	
Sugar substitutes (artificial sweeteners)	

Continued on next page

Food	Serving Size
Syrup, sugar-free	2 Tbsp
Vegetables: any **raw** nonstarchy vegetables (such as broccoli, cabbage, carrots, cucumber, tomato)	½ cup
Vegetables: any **cooked** nonstarchy vegetables (such as carrots, cauliflower, green beans)	¼ cup

Reduced-Fat or Fat-Free Foods

Food	Serving Size
Cream cheese, fat-free	1 Tbsp (½ oz)
Coffee creamers, nondairy	
liquid, flavored	1 ½ tsp
liquid, sugar-free, flavored	4 tsp
powdered, flavored	1 tsp
powdered, sugar-free, flavored	2 tsp
Margarine spread	
fat-free	1 Tbsp
reduced-fat	1 tsp
Mayonnaise	
fat-free	1 Tbsp
reduced-fat	1 tsp
Mayonnaise-style salad dressing	
fat-free	1 Tbsp
reduced-fat	2 tsp
Salad dressing	
fat-free	1 Tbsp
fat-free, Italian	2 Tbsp
Sour cream, fat-free or reduced-fat	1 Tbsp
Whipped topping	
light or fat-free	2 Tbsp
regular	1 Tbsp

Artificial Sweeteners

Sugar substitutes, alternatives, or replacements that are approved by the Food and Drug Administration (FDA) are safe to use. Each sweetener is tested for safety before it can be marketed and sold. Common types include:

- Aspartame, neotame (blue packet)
- Monk fruit (orange packet)
- Saccharin (pink packet)

- Stevia (green packet) (Note: The whole leaf or crude form of stevia is not FDA-approved.)
- Sucralose (yellow packet)

Note: Blended sweeteners (mixtures of a sweetener and sugar (sucrose) are found in the **Sweets** list.

Condiments

Food	Serving Size
Barbecue sauce	2 tsp
Catsup (ketchup)	1 Tbsp
Chili sauce, sweet, tomato-type	2 tsp
Horseradish	
Hot pepper sauce	
Lemon juice	
Miso	1 ½ tsp
Mustard	
honey	1 Tbsp
brown, Dijon, horseradish-flavored, wasabi-flavored, or yellow	
Parmesan cheese, grated	1 Tbsp
Pickle relish (dill or sweet)	1 Tbsp
Pickles	
dill	1 ½ medium pickles
sweet, bread and butter	2 slices
sweet, gherkin	¾ oz
Salsa	¼ cup
Soy sauce, light or regular	1 Tbsp
Sweet-and-sour sauce	2 tsp
Taco sauce	1 Tbsp
Vinegar	
Worcestershire sauce	
Yogurt, any type	2 Tbsp

Free Snack Suggestions

When you are hungry between meals, try to choose whole foods as snacks instead of highly processed options. The foods listed below are examples of healthy free-food snacks:

- ½ choice from the **Nonstarchy Vegetables** list; for example, ½ cup raw broccoli, carrots, celery, cucumber, or tomato
- ½ choice from the nuts and seeds portion of the **Fats** list; for example, 8 pistachios, 3 almonds, 4 black olives, or 1 ½ tsp sunflower seeds
- ⅓ choice from the **Fruits** list; for example, ¼ cup blueberries or blackberries, ⅓ cup melon, 6 grapes, or 2 tsp dried fruits

- ½ choice from the **Lean Protein** list; for example, ½ slice of fat-free cheese or ½ oz lean cooked meat
- ¼ choice from the Starch list; for example, 2 animal crackers, 1½ saltine-type crackers, ¾ cup no-fat-added popcorn, ½ regular-sized rice or popcorn cake

Drinks/Mixes

• Bouillon broth, consommé	• Diet soft drinks, sugar-free
• Bouillon or broth, low-sodium	• Drink mixes (powder or liquid drops), sugar-free
• Carbonated or mineral water	• Tea, unsweetened or with sugar substitute
• Club soda	• Tonic water, sugar-free
• Cocoa powder, unsweetened (1 Tbsp)	• Water
• Coffee, unsweetened or with sugar substitute	• Water, flavored, sugar-free

Seasonings

• Flavoring extracts (for example, vanilla, almond, or peppermint)	• Kelp
	• Nonstick cooking spray
• Garlic, fresh or powder	• Spices
• Herbs, fresh or dried	• Wine, used in cooking

COMBINATION FOODS

Many of the foods you eat, such as casseroles and frozen entrees, are mixed together in various combinations. These "combination" foods do not fit into any one choice list. This list of some typical "combination" food choices will help you fit these foods into your Eating Plan. Ask your RDN about the nutrient information for other combination foods you would like to eat, including your own recipes. One carbohydrate choice in this list has 15 grams of carbohydrate and about 70 calories.

Entrees

Food	Serving Size	Choices per Serving
Casserole-type entrees (tuna noodle, lasagna, spaghetti with meatballs, chili with beans, macaroni and cheese)	1 cup (8 oz)	2 carbohydrates + 2 medium-fat proteins
Stews (beef/other meats and vegetables)	1 cup (8 oz)	1 carbohydrate + 1 medium-fat protein + 0 to 3 fats

236

Frozen Meals/Entrees

Food	Serving Size	Choices per Serving
Burrito (beef and bean)	1 burrito (5 oz)	3 carbohydrates + 1 lean protein + 2 fats
Dinner-type healthy meal (includes dessert and is usually less than 400 calories)	About 9-12 oz	2 to 3 carbohydrates + 1 to 2 lean proteins + 1 fat
"Healthy"-type entree (usually less than 300 calories)	About 7–10oz	2 carbohydrates + 2 lean proteins
Pizza		
Cheese/vegetarian, thin crust	¼ of a 12 inch pizza (4 ½-5 oz)	2 carbohydrates + 2 medium-fat proteins
Meat topping, thin crust	¼ of a 12 inch pizza (5 oz)	2 carbohydrates + 2 medium-fat proteins + 1 ½ fats
Cheese/vegetarian or meat topping, rising crust	1/6 of 12-inch pizza (4 oz)	2 ½ carbohydrates + 2 medium-fat proteins
Pocket sandwich	1 sandwich (4 ½ oz)	3 carbohydrates + 1 lean protein + 1 to 2 fats
Pot pie	1 pot pie (7 oz)	3 carbohydrates + 1 medium-fat protein + 3 fats

Salads (Deli-Style)

Food	Serving Size	Choices per Serving
Coleslaw	½ cup	1 carbohydrate + 1 ½ fats
Macaroni/pasta salad	½ cup	2 carbohydrates + 3 fats
Potato salad	½ cup	1 ½ to 2 carbohydrates + 1 to 2 fats
Tuna salad or chicken salad	½ cup (3 ½ oz)	½ carbohydrate + 2 lean proteins + 1 fat

Soups

Food	Serving Size	Choices per Serving
Bean, lentil, or split pea soup	1 cup (8 oz)	1½ carbohydrates + 1 lean protein
Chowder (made with milk)	1 cup (8 oz)	1 carbohydrate + 1 lean protein + 1 ½ fats
Cream (made with water)	1 cup (8 oz)	1 carbohydrate + 1 fat
Miso soup	1 cup (8 oz)	½ carbohydrate + 1 lean protein
Ramen noodle soup	1 cup (8 oz)	2 carbohydrates + 2 fats

Continued on next page

Food	Serving Size	Choices per Serving
Rice soup/porridge (congee)	1 cup (8oz)	1 carbohydrate
Tomato soup (made with water), borscht	1 cup (8 oz)	1 carbohydrate
Vegetable beef, chicken noodle, or other broth-type soup (including "healthy"-type soups, such as those lower in sodium and/or fat	1 cup (8 oz)	1 carbohydrate + 1 lean protein

FAST FOODS

The choices in the **Fast Foods** list are not specific fast food meals or items, but are estimates based on popular foods. You can get specific nutrition information for almost every fast food or restaurant chain. Ask the restaurant or check its website for nutrition information about your favorite fast foods. One carbohydrate choice has 15 grams of carbohydrate and about 70 calories.

Main Dishes/Entrees

Food	Serving Size	Choices per Serving
Chicken		
Breast, breaded and fried*	1 (about 7 oz)	1 carbohydrate + 6 medium-fat proteins
Breast, meat only**	1	4 lean proteins
Drumstick, breaded and fried*	1 (about 2 ½ oz)	½ carbohydrate + 2 medium-fat proteins
Drumstick, meat only**	1	1 lean protein + ½ fat
Nuggets or tenders	6 (about 3 ½ oz)	1 carbohydrate + 2 medium-fat proteins + 1 fat
Thigh, breaded and fried*	1 (about 5 oz)	½ carbohydrate + 3 medium-fat proteins + 2 fats
Thigh, meat only**	1	2 lean proteins + ½ fat
Wing, breaded and fried*	1 wing (about 2 oz)	½ carbohydrate + 2 medium-fat proteins
Wing, meat only**	1 wing	1 lean protein
Main dish salad (grilled chicken-type, no dressing or croutons)	1 salad (about 11 ½ oz)	1 carbohydrate + 4 lean proteins
Pizza		
Cheese, pepperoni or sausage, regular or thick crust	1/8 of a 14 inch pizza (about 4 oz)	2 ½ carbohydrates + 1 high-fat protein + 1 fat
Cheese, pepperoni or sausage, thin crust	1/8 of a 14 inch pizza (about 2 ¾ oz)	1 ½ carbohydrates + 1 high-fat protein + 1 fat
Cheese, meat, vegetable, regular crust	1/8 of a 14 inch pizza (about 5 oz)	2 ½ carbohydrates + 2 high-fat proteins

*Definition and weight refer to food **with** bone, skin, and breading.

Definition refers to above food **without bone, skin, and breading.

Asian

Food	Serving Size	Choices per Serving
Beef/chicken/shrimp with vegetables in sauce	1 cup (about 6 oz)	1 carbohydrate + 2 lean proteins + 1 fat
Egg roll, meat	1 egg roll (about 3 oz)	1 ½ carbohydrates + 1 lean protein + 1½ fats
Fried rice, meatless	1 cup	2 ½ carbohydrates + 2 fats
Hot-and-sour soup	1 cup	½ carbohydrate + ½ fat
Meat with sweet sauce	1 cup (about 6 oz)	3 ½ carbohydrates + 3 medium-fat proteins + 3 fats
Noodles and vegetables in sauce (chow mein, lo mein)	1 cup	2 carbohydrates + 2 fats

Mexican

Food	Serving Size	Choices per Serving
Burrito with beans and cheese	1 small burrito (about 6 oz)	3½ carbohydrates + 1 medium-fat protein + 1 fat
Nachos with cheese	1 small order (about 8 nachos)	2 ½ carbohydrates + 1 high-fat protein + 2 fats
Quesadilla, cheese only	1 small order (about 5 oz)	2 ½ carbohydrates + 3 high-fat proteins
Taco, crisp, with meat and cheese	1 small taco (about 3 oz)	1 carbohydrate + 1 medium-fat protein + ½ fat
Taco salad with chicken and tortilla bowl	1 salad (1 lb, including tortilla bowl)	3½ carbohydrates + 4 medium-fat proteins + 3 fats
Tostada with beans and cheese	1 small tostada (about 5 oz)	2 carbohydrates + 1 high-fat protein

Sandwiches

Food	Serving Size	Choices per Serving
Breakfast Sandwiches		
Breakfast burrito with sausage, egg, cheese	1 burrito (about 4 oz)	1 ½ carbohydrates + 2 high-fat proteins
Egg, cheese, meat on an English muffin	1 sandwich	2 carbohydrates + 3 medium-fat proteins + ½ fat
Egg, cheese, meat on a biscuit	1 sandwich	2 carbohydrates + 3 medium-fat proteins + 2 fats

Continued on next page

Food	Serving Size	Choices per Serving
Sausage biscuit sandwich	1 sandwich	2 carbohydrates + 1 high-fat protein + 4 fats
Chicken Sandwiches		
grilled with bun, lettuce, tomatoes, spread	1 sandwich (about 7 ½ oz)	3 carbohydrates + 4 lean proteins
crispy, with bun, lettuce, tomatoes, spread	1 sandwich (about 6 oz)	3 carbohydrates + 2 lean proteins + 3 ½ fats
Fish sandwich with tartar sauce and cheese	1 sandwich (5 oz)	2 ½ carbohydrates + 2 medium-fat proteins + 1 ½ fats
Hamburger		
regular with bun and condiments (catsup, mustard, onion, pickle)	1 burger (about 3 ½ oz)	2 carbohydrates + 1 medium-fat protein + 1 fat
4 oz meat with cheese, bun, and condiments (catsup, mustard, onion, pickle)	1 burger (about 8 ½ oz)	3 carbohydrates + 4 medium-fat protein + 2 ½ fats
Hot dog with bun, plain	1 hot dog (about 3 ½ oz)	1 ½ carbohydrates + 1 high-fat protein + 2 fats
Submarine sandwich (no cheese or sauce)		
less than 6 grams fat	One 6-inch sub	3 carbohydrates + 2 lean proteins
regular	One 6-inch sub	3 carbohydrates + 2 lean proteins + 1 fat
Wrap, grilled chicken, vegetables, cheese, and spread	1 small wrap (about 4 to 5 oz)	2 carbohydrates + 2 lean proteins + 1 ½ fats

Sides/Appetizers

Food	Serving Size	Choices per Serving
French fries	1 small order (about 3 ½ oz)	2 ½ carbohydrates + 2 fats
	1 medium order (about 5 oz)	3 ½ carbohydrates + 3 fats
	1 large order (about 6 oz)	4 ½ carbohydrates + 4 fats
Hashbrowns	1 cup/medium order (about 5 oz)	3 carbohydrates + 6 fats
Onion rings	1 serving (8 to 9 rings, about 4 oz)	3 ½ carbohydrates + 4 fats
Salad, side (no dressing, croutons or cheese)	1 small salad	1 nonstarchy vegetable

Food	Serving Size	Choices per Serving
Coffee, latte (fat-free milk)	1 small order (about 12 oz)	1 fat-free milk
Coffee, mocha (fat-free milk, no whipped cream)	1 small order (about 12 oz)	1 fat-free milk + 1 carbohydrate
Milkshake, any flavor	1 small shake (about 12 oz)	5 ½ carbohydrates + 3 fats
	1 medium shake (about 16 oz)	7 carbohydrates + 4 fats
	1 large shake (about 22 oz)	10 carbohydrates + 5 fats
Soft-serve ice cream cone	1 small	2 carbohydrates + ½ fat

ALCOHOL

Nutrition Tips

- In general, 1 alcohol equivalent (½ oz absolute alcohol, also known as ethanol or ethyl alcohol) has about 100 calories.

Selection Tips

- Women who choose to drink alcohol should limit alcohol to 1 serving or less per day. Men who choose to drink alcohol should limit alcohol to 2 servings or less per day.
- To reduce your risk of low blood glucose (hypoglycemia), especially if you take insulin or a diabetes pill that increases insulin, never drink alcohol on an empty stomach. Always eat a carbohydrate food when you are having an alcoholic beverage.
- While alcohol does not directly affect blood glucose levels, be aware of the carbohydrate in alcoholic beverages, such as mixed drinks, beer, and wine. The carbohydrate may raise your blood glucose levels.
- Check with your RDN if you would like to fit alcohol into your Eating Plan.

One alcohol equivalent or choice (½ oz absolute alcohol) has about 100 calories.

One carbohydrate choice has 15 grams of carbohydrate and about 70 calories.

Alcoholic Beverage	Serving Size	Choices per Serving
Beer		
light (less than 4.5% abv)	12 fl oz	1 alcohol equivalent + ½ carbohydrate
regular (about 5% abv)	12 fl oz	1 alcohol equivalent + 1 carbohydrate
dark (more than 5.7% abv)	12 fl oz	1 alcohol equivalent + 1 to 1 ½ carbohydrates
Distilled spirits (80 or 86 proof): vodka, rum, gin, whiskey, tequila	1 ½ fl oz	1 alcohol equivalent

Continued on next page

Alcoholic Beverages Continued from previous page

Alcoholic Beverage	Serving Size	Choices per Serving
Liqueur, coffee (53 proof)	1 fl oz	½ alcohol equivalent + 1 carbohydrate
Sake	1 fl oz	½ alcohol equivalent
Wine		
champagne/sparkling	5 fl oz	1 alcohol equivalent
dessert (sherry)	3 ½ fl oz	1 alcohol equivalent + 1 carbohydrate
dry, red or white (10%abv)	5 fl oz	1 alcohol equivalent

Note: The abbreviation "%abv" refers to the percentage of alcohol by volume.

15

Appendix

Study Guide Suggested Responses

The following are suggested responses to Study Guide Questions in this book. Many questions have several acceptable answers. Responses comparable to those given here should be considered correct.

CHAPTER 1

A. www.ChooseMyPlate.gov

B. Fruits, Vegetables, Grains, Protein Foods, and Dairy

C. Dark-green vegetables: 1 ½ cups per week
Red and orange vegetables: 5 ½ cups per week
Legumes (beans and peas): 1 ½ cups per week
Starchy vegetables: 5 cups per week
Other vegetables: 4 cups per week

D. 8 oz seafood per week for Healthy U.S.-Style Eating Pattern compared to 15 oz seafood per week for the Healthy Mediterranean-Style Eating Pattern.

E. Dark-green and Red & Orange vegetable subgroups. List any four vegetables from the dark-green and red & orange vegetable subgroups in Table 1.3.

CHAPTER 2

A. Iron, folate, choline, iodine, calcium, and vitamin D.

B. See Appendix 5.

C. Benefits to infant nutrition: gastrointestinal function, immune system, and the potential beneficial influence on neurodevelopment and chronic diseases of childhood.

D. Honey should be avoided; avoid water contaminated from lead pipes, nitrates, or bacteria; avoid foods that children could choke on.

E. Make mealtime enjoyable; children make food choices and determine how much is consumed; include snacks of high nutrient content, meat should be tender and moist encourage finger foods, fat and cholesterol should not be limited until 2 years of age

F. See Table 2.7

G. Changes in economic, functional, physiological, and psychosocial conditions.

H. Implement a general diet if at all possible; keep the diet as liberal as possible even for diabetes, high cholesterol, and weight management; use vitamin supplementation if nutrition assessment confirms these are necessary; obesity may be managed with simple diet modifications; consider previous food habits and patterns; meet individual daily caloric needs; offer adequate protein to meet the DRIs or higher; individualize diet to promote glycemic control; ensure adequate calcium and vitamin D intake; include key micronutrients as recommended; promote fluid intake; adjust diet textures to meet chewing and swallowing needs; promote cooking techniques that maintain nutrient density; utilize finger foods as needed; serve foods at regular meal times; encourage social contact; consider factors such as depression and alcohol use in promoting adequate nutrition.

I. Menu based on MyPlate for Older Adults should include: bright colored vegetables, deep-colored fruits, whole, enriched or fortified grains, low or non-fat dairy, high quality proteins listed, liquid vegetable oils, fluids such as water, tea, coffee, fat-free milk and soup.

J. Since total and resting energy requirements decrease progressively with age, it can be challenging to maintain nutritional status since vitamin and mineral needs often remain constant, or may even increase for many nutrients. Consider how foods might be fortified to increase nutrient density in the daily diet as compared to the use of liquid supplements. Tailor the diet based on the preferences of the patient.

CHAPTER 3

A. Stroke, head or neck injury, cancer, cerebral palsy, dementia, or other illness as a result of aging.

B. A physician, a swallowing therapist (speech language pathologist or occupational therapist), a dietitian, and a nurse all play a part in assessing a patient's needs for dietary interventions that keep the patient safe and adequately nourished. Assessment includes swallowing abilities, fatigue, nutrient intake, need for adaptive equipment, and tolerance to food and fluid texture modifications.

C. See Principles of Consistency Alteration.

D. Thin, Nectar-like, Honey-like, and Spoon-thick.

E. Modify the diet plan written for Chapter 2 using guidelines for the Mechanical Soft diet and Nectar-like liquids in Chapter 3.

F. Measure out the total number of portions of required pureed servings based on the planned therapeutic diet. Add the appropriate liquid or thickeners to obtain the appropriate consistency, flavor, and nutrient density. Divide the total volume by the number of original servings pureed, utilizing a standard portioning utensil to serve. Portion sizes of foods often change in volume after they have been pureed.

G. Consider adding ingredients that enhance the original flavor, including condiments that would be served for patients on a general diet. In addition, consider how the appearance of the texture-modified foods might be enhanced by the appropriate shapes, molding, and garnishing.

CHAPTER 4

A. Clear liquid diets may be prescribed for patients with an acute gastrointestinal illness to prevent dehydration; or in conditions when it is necessary to minimize fecal residue, such as bowel preparation for surgery or a gastrointestinal procedure. It also has been used to reintroduce foods following a period with no oral intake when poor tolerance or aspiration is anticipated.

B. Juices, gelatin, broth, popsicles, tea, and coffee.

C. See tables 4.3 and 4.4 in Chapter 4 for the Full Liquid Diet

D. Enteral nutrition may be ordered for patients who are physically or psychologically unable to take food by mouth in amounts that will meet nutrient requirements.

E. Depending on the amount and choice of food eaten, this diet can be adequate in energy, protein, and fat but may be inadequate in vitamins, minerals, and fiber. A daily multivitamin/mineral supplement or commercial nutritional supplement is recommended if the diet continues for more than 5 days. Consider the total calories, protein, and micronutrients in fortified liquids, to determine if they meet overall energy and nutrient needs.

CHAPTER 5

A. Overweight is BMI 25 to 29.9 kg/m²; obese is BMI 30 kg/m² or greater.

B. Type 2 diabetes, cardiopulmonary disease, stroke, hypertension, gallbladder disease, osteoarthritis, sleep apnea, and some forms of cancer.

C. See Table 5.1 for examples such as whole grain bread, whole grain cereal, fat-free milk, fresh fruits and vegetables, lean meat choices, and sugar-free condiments.

D. Eat three "meals" per day, adequate protein consumed first, serve liquids between meals, consume 48 to 64 ounces of low-calorie, noncarbonated, and caffeine-free beverages per day, include a chewable multivitamin for adequate micronutrients including iron, calcium, Vitamin D, Vitamin C, and Vitamin B_{12}

E. Consider current food and beverage products available to promote choices while providing nutrient density and reduced in calories for weight management such as fresh fruits and vegetables, sugar-free or reduced calorie condiments, low-calorie beverages, and high fiber foods.

CHAPTER 6

A. Type 1 diabetes is an autoimmune disease that affects the pancreas in a way that it does not make insulin.
    Type 2 diabetes is a disease that usually begins with insulin resistance. As diabetes progresses, the pancreas gradually loses its ability to make insulin.
    Gestational diabetes occurs only during pregnancy.
    Prediabetes is a condition where individuals have blood glucose levels higher than normal but not high enough to be diagnosed with diabetes.

B. Diet, exercise, and weight management.

C. To encourage healthy eating in order to: achieve personalized blood glucose, blood pressure, and lipid goals; reach and maintain body weight goals; prevent or postpone complications of diabetes.

D. There are none, this General diet can easily be used to plan a Consistent Carbohydrate diet.

E. One carbohydrate choice is equal to 15 grams of carbohydrate.

F. Feeling shaky, sweaty, tired, hungry, crabby, confused, rapid heart rate, blurred vision or headaches, numbness or tingling in the mouth and lips; in severe cases, loss of consciousness.

G. When low blood sugar is identified, give 15 grams of carbohydrate and recheck blood sugar in 15 minutes. If blood sugar remains low, provide another 15 grams of carbohydrate and recheck in 15 minutes. Repeat as necessary until optimal blood glucose levels are achieved.

H. Long-term care facility residents eat better when they are given liberalized diets. Making medication changes to control blood glucose rather than restricting food can reduce malnutrition. See Chapter 2 for liberalized diet justifications.

CHAPTER 7

A. Total fat is no longer restricted, limiting cholesterol is debated in literature but most no longer consider it a nutrient of concern, saturated fats should be limited but not be replaced with refined carbohydrates. *Trans* fats should be avoided.

B. *Trans* fat sources: cookies, crackers and snack cakes, commercially prepared fried foods, margarines made with partially hydrogenated oil, foods with partially hydrogenated oil in the ingredient list. Soluble fiber sources: See Table 7.4

C. Diseases of the gallbladder, liver, or pancreas; disturbances in digestion or fat absorption.

D. Less than 30% of total calories from fat per day.

E. Consider modifying recipes to include lean meat, low-fat dairy products, rinsing ground beef after cooking, trimming visible fat from meats prior to cooking, and removing skin from poultry. Replace fat in baked goods with fruit purees and other appropriate substitutes.

CHAPTER 8

A. Increase potassium, calcium, magnesium and fiber. Limit sodium to 2300 mgs per day.

B. Reduce blood pressure.

C. 3000-4000 mg/day; 2300 mg

D. A No Added Salt diet is more palatable for elderly clients who may be prone to undesirable weight loss and whole oral intake may already be limited.

E. Consider how low sodium and fresh spices may be used in food preparation to enhance the flavor of low sodium diets. For elderly patients, individual spices are less confusing to taste palettes than spice blends.

CHAPTER 9

A. Energy, carbohydrates, protein, potassium, sodium, phosphorus, and fluids.

B. Registered Dietitian.

C. Meat, poultry, fish, milk, yogurt, cheese, eggs, and soybeans.

D. To ensure that protein is used for tissue growth and repair rather than for energy needs.

E. ½-1 cup milk and phosphorus.

F. Gelatin, crushed ice, ice cream, sherbet, popsicles, and soup.

G. Potassium; because the sodium may have been replaced by potassium.

H. Consider a patient's unique food preferences in adding calories, typically through moderately increased carbohydrate and fat in foods while still limiting other required restrictions.

CHAPTER 10

A. Obesity, cardiovascular disease, type 2 diabetes, inflammatory diseases, constipation

B. 25–38 grams dietary fiber.

C. Whole grains (whole wheat, bulgur, oatmeal, whole cornmeal, brown rice, buckwheat, wild rice, whole rye, whole-grain barley, amaranth, millet, quinoa, sorghum, popcorn), fruits, vegetables, beans, nuts, and seeds.

D. Abdominal discomfort, bloating, cramping, and diarrhea.

E. Constipation or impaction in the colon.

F. Constipation.

G. Consider higher fiber breads, cereals, and other whole grains. Incorporate added fiber into baked goods. Encourage consumption of fruits and vegetables. Recipes for dietary fiber bars or puddings are available to promote bowel health while reducing the need for bowel medications.

CHAPTER 11

A. A food allergy is an abnormal response to a food triggered by the body's immune system. A food intolerance is when eating a certain food or foods triggers a negative physiological response, but does not involve the immune system.

B. Wheat, milk, eggs, fish, crustacean shellfish, tree nuts, soy, and peanuts are the most common allergens.

C. Corn, rice, potato, soy, tapioca, bean, sorghum, amaranth, buckwheat, quinoa, teff, millet, Montina™ and nut flours, and oats if certified as gluten-free.

D. Modified food starch, hydrolyzed or texturized vegetable proteins, soy sauce, soy sauce solids, and malt or malt flavoring.

E. Commercial breads and baked goods, instant potatoes, soup and breakfast drink mixes, margarine, cold cut meats (other than kosher), salad dressings, pudding, caramels, chocolate, mixes for pancakes, and biscuits.

F. There may be a risk for deficiencies in calcium, riboflavin, and vitamin D depending on food choices and if lactase enzyme is used to aid digestion.

G. FODMAPS are poorly absorbed carbohydrates and examples include fructose, lactose, fructans, galactans, and polyols.

H. Consider how to clearly communicate to caregivers and all members of the healthcare team the key diet components unique to that patient. Printed food lists and planned therapeutic menus, reviewed by the Registered Dietitian, are critical.

CHAPTER 12

A. High nutrient diets may be ordered for malnourished individuals, persons with elevated needs such as wound healing, and individuals unable to meet nutritional needs due to lack or appetite or cognitive impairment.

B. Common food fortifiers include non-fat dry milk, peanut butter, canola oil, and protein powder.

C. Lack of hunger, early satiety, loss of taste or smell, soreness in the mouth, pain, medications, inability to self-feed, dementia, chewing difficulty and swallowing difficulty.

D. Small Portions Diets are used for individuals who would benefit from a reduced portion size for weight maintenance or weight reduction, or for individuals who request small portions if food is too overwhelming.

E. Vegan diets which exclude all animal products may be lacking in protein, calcium, vitamin D, iron, vitamin $B_{12,}$ zinc, and omega-3 fatty acids.

F. Adherents of Islam (Muslims)

G. This diet eliminates all foods containing natural protein such as meat, fish, poultry, milk, yogurt, cheese, eggs, nuts, seeds, legumes, and peanut butter. Adequate protein intake is achieved with the use of a metabolic formula that has the phenylalanine removed. A prescribed amount of phenylalanine is allowed from natural food sources like fruits, vegetables, and grain products. Low protein foods are available to add calories and variety to the diet.

H. Stop smoking, reduce weight, avoid eating 3 hours before sleep, avoid wearing tight fitting clothing, sit upright when eating, consume small frequent meals, avoid foods that worsen symptoms.

I. To identify sources of special foods required for unique diets, options to procure items may be available from local retail grocers, medical supply companies and multiple online sources.

CHAPTER 13

A. See Table 13.1.

B. Maintain appropriate positioning for dining; offer foods that stimulate appetite; foster independence; focus on the patient and promote a positive dining experience; observe and report signs of chewing and swallowing problems; avoid syringe feeding; allow ample time to eat; and allow dining at off-hours to individualize to that patient's schedule.

C. Sip tip cups, plate guards, divided plates, scoop plates, straws, built-up utensils, curved-handled utensils, rubber place mats, and suction plates or bowls.

D. Overweight, underweight, gastrointestinal dysfunction, asthma, cardiovascular disease, diabetes, osteoporosis, and oral-hygiene issues.

E. Consider and review guidelines in question B to incorporate into the unique dining setting.

16

Appendix

Abbreviations

A1C. . . . . glycosylated hemoglobin (hemoglobin A1C)

ADA . . . . American Diabetes Association

AI. . . . . . adequate intakes

ALD . . . . alcoholic liver disease

AMDR . . . acceptable macronutrient distribution ranges

BMI. . . . . body mass index

c. . . . . . . cup

CAPD . . . continuous ambulatory peritoneal dialysis

CKD . . . . chronic kidney disease

DASH . . . dietary approaches to stop hypertension

DGA . . . . Dietary Guidelines for Americans

DHA . . . . docosahexaenoic acid

DRIs . . . . dietary reference intakes

EPA. . . . . eicosapentaenoic acid

ESRD. . . . end stage renal disease

FALCPA . . Food Allergen Labeling and Consumer Protection Act

FDA . . . . Food and Drug Administration

FODMAP . fermentable oligosaccharides, disaccharides, monosaccharides and polyols

FWP . . . . free water protocol

g . . . . . . gram

GERD . . . gastroesophageal reflux disease

GI. . . . . . gastrointestinal

GLP-1 . . . glucagon-like peptide-1

HACCP . . hazard analysis and critical control points

HE . . . . . hepatic encephalopathy

HDL . . . . high-density lipoprotein

HFCS. . . . high fructose corn syrup

IBS . . . . . irritable bowel syndrome

IBW. . . . . Ideal Body Weight

in . . . . . . inch

INR . . . . . International Normalized Ratio

IU . . . . . . International Units

LAGB . . . laparoscopic adjustable gastric band

lb . . . . . . pound

K+ . . . . . potassium

kcal . . . . . Calories

kg . . . . . . kilogram

LDL . . . . . low-density lipoprotein

m . . . . . . meter

mcg . . . . . microgram

MCT . . . . medium chain triglycerides

mEq . . . . milliequivalent

mg . . . . . milligram

mL . . . . . milliliter

mmHg . . . millimeter of mercury

Na+ . . . . . sodium

NAFLD . . nonalcoholic fatty liver disease

NAS . . . . no added salt

NASH . . . nonalcoholic steatohepatitis

NFDM . . . nonfat dry milk

NSAID . . . nonsteroidal anti-inflammatory drugs

oz . . . . . . ounce

PCM . . . . protein calorie malnutrition

PKU . . . . phenylketonuria

ppm . . . . parts per million

PT . . . . . . Prothrombin Time

qt . . . . . . quart

RDA . . . . recommended dietary allowances

RDIs . . . . recommended dietary intakes

RYBG . . . . roux-en-y gastric bypass

SG . . . . . . sleeve gastrectomy

Tbsp . . . . tablespoon

tsp . . . . . teaspoon

UGI . . . . . upper gastrointestinal

UL . . . . . . tolerable upper levels

Index

Entries followed by *f* indicate figures. Entries followed by *t* indicate tables.

Wheat allergy, 126-127, 126*t*
Wound healing, 141-142, 175

Z

Zinc
    nutrition for wound healing, 142
    vegetarian diets,147